S0-BMU-853

Nursing Student Retention
Second Edition

Dr. Marianne R. Jeffreys, EdD, RN, has conducted grant-funded research, consultations, publications, and professional presentations that encompass the topics of student retention and achievement, nontraditional students, cultural competence, self-efficacy, teaching, curriculum, and psychometrics. She is also the author of three other books including the award-winning book *Teaching Cultural Competence in Nursing and Health Care: Inquiry, Action, and Innovation* (first edition), over 30 articles, book chapters, and videos. Her conceptual models and questionnaires have been requested worldwide and in various disciplines. She is currently a professor of nursing at the City University of New York (CUNY) Graduate College and at CUNY College of Staten Island.

Dr. Jeffreys received a BS in nursing from the State University of New York College at Plattsburgh and MA, MEd, and EdD degrees in nursing education from Teachers College, Columbia University. She is a Fellow of the New York Academy of Medicine. She has been inducted into the Kappa Delta Pi International Honor Society in Education, Sigma Theta Tau International Honor Society in Nursing, Transcultural Nursing Society Scholars, and Teachers College NEAA Hall of Fame. Her awards include the international *Leininger Award* for Excellence in Transcultural Nursing, Teachers College, Columbia University's Award for Scholarship and Research, and the Mu Upsilon Chapter of Sigma Theta Tau Excellence in Professional Nursing Award. She was named Consultant of the Month (December 2007) by the National Center for Cultural Competence.

Her career includes more than 20 years teaching experience in associate, baccalaureate, masters, and/or doctoral programs and as an RN in various clinical settings for 9 years. Her expertise has been requested for grant-funded projects (HRSA, Kellogg), as well as for interdisciplinary and departmental workshops.

Nursing Student Retention

Understanding the Process and Making a Difference
Second Edition

Marianne R. Jeffreys, EdD, RN

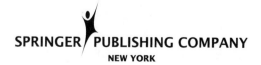

SPRINGER PUBLISHING COMPANY

NEW YORK

Copyright © 2012 Springer Publishing Company, LLC

All rights reserved.

No part of this publication may be reproduced, stored in a retrieval system, or transmitted in any form or by any means, electronic, mechanical, photocopying, recording, or otherwise, without the prior permission of Springer Publishing Company, LLC, or authorization through payment of the appropriate fees to the Copyright Clearance Center, Inc., 222 Rosewood Drive, Danvers, MA 01923, 978-750-8400, fax 978-646-8600, info@copyright.com or on the Web at www.copyright.com.

Springer Publishing Company, LLC
11 West 42nd Street
New York, NY 10036
www.springerpub.com

Acquisitions Editor: Allan Graubard
Production Editor: Lindsay Claire
Composition: Newgen Imaging

ISBN: 978-0-8261-0949-1
E-book ISBN: 978-0-8261-0950-7

13 14 15 / 5 4 3 2

The author and the publisher of this Work have made every effort to use sources believed to be reliable to provide information that is accurate and compatible with the standards generally accepted at the time of publication. The author and publisher shall not be liable for any special, consequential, or exemplary damages resulting, in whole or in part, from the readers' use of, or reliance on, the information contained in this book. The publisher has no responsibility for the persistence or accuracy of URLs for external or third-party Internet websites referred to in this publication and does not guarantee that any content on such websites is, or will remain, accurate or appropriate.

The interactive *Nursing Student Retention Toolkit* is available at www.springerpub.com/ JeffreysRetention

Library of Congress Cataloging-in-Publication Data

Jeffreys, Marianne R.
Nursing student retention : understanding the process and making a difference / Marianne R. Jeffreys.—2nd ed.
p. ; cm.
Includes bibliographical references and index.
ISBN 978-0-8261-0949-1—ISBN 978-0-8261-0950-7 (e-book)
I. Title.
[DNLM: 1. Student Dropouts. 2. Students, Nursing. 3. Education, Nursing—methods. WY 18]

610.73071'173—dc23   2012000935

Special discounts on bulk quantities of our books are available to corporations, professional associations, pharmaceutical companies, health care organizations, and other qualifying groups.

If you are interested in a custom book, including chapters from more than one of our titles, we can provide that service as well.

For details, please contact:
Special Sales Department, Springer Publishing Company, LLC
11 West 42nd Street, 15th Floor, New York, NY 10036-8002
Phone: 877-687-7476 or 212-431-4370; Fax: 212-941-7842
Email: sales@springerpub.com

Printed in the United States of America by Bang Printing.

To my son, Daniel W. Edley

Contents

Preface

Nursing and multidisciplinary college faculty, advisors, counselors, administrators, graduate students, and organizations working with academically and culturally diverse nursing student populations are called upon to

- *Enhance* student success
- *Improve* retention and graduation rates
- *Reduce* attrition rates (drop out)
- *Facilitate* academic progression and swift entry into the workforce

These goals can seem daunting and overwhelming without appropriate resources. The new edition of *Nursing Student Retention* and the *Nursing Student Retention Toolkit* offer an indispensible ensemble of hands-on, user-friendly resources. Appropriate for all undergraduate levels and settings (diploma, ADN, BS, RN-BS, and accelerated BS), the book and toolkit end the struggle to find ready-to-use materials for

- *Recognizing* factors that restrict or support retention
- *Identifying and assisting* at-risk students
- *Designing* individualized, holistic strategies for diverse learners
- *Implementing* culturally competent teaching and advisement
- *Fostering* professional development
- *Creating* an inclusive environment
- *Applying* tools and strategies to make a positive difference in student lives
- *Evaluating* strategy outcomes

Users of the book and toolkit will find the following:

- A model to guide nursing student retention and success
- A guide for identifying and assisting at-risk students
- A wide selection of educational activities
- Chapters detailing the multidimensional factors influencing retention and success
- Chapters detailing retention and success strategies

- Introductory snapshot scenarios, vignettes, case examples, illustrations, tables, and assessment tools
- Interactive retention strategy design modules
- Questionnaires for measuring and evaluating risk factors, retention strategy effectiveness, student perceptions, and satisfaction
- Techniques for diverse learners

Based on the results of doctoral and postdoctoral grant-funded studies, practical teaching experience with academically and culturally diverse learners, and multidisciplinary literature, the book and toolkit provide resources and a wealth of information for all user groups.

The book is divided into two parts: Part I: What's Happening? Exploring Student Retention and Taking Action and Part II: Making a Difference: Spotlight on Retention and Success Strategies.

Part I comprises nine chapters filled with information and action-focused resources to explore, understand, and apply essential background information about the multidimensional process of nursing student retention and success. Part II details strategies, providing case exemplars applicable across a variety of settings. The book's final chapter (Chapter 15) presents future directions, a vision for tomorrow, and proposes implications for all educators.

Readers are encouraged to pause, reflect, and question throughout the book in order to gain new insights into the multidimensional process of student retention. It is hoped that these new insights, with their holistic and multidimensional approach, will revitalize interest in nursing student retention. The ultimate goal of this book is to motivate others to further explore student retention through continued educational, theoretical, empirical, and practical endeavors. Readers are invited to contribute new insights, creative ideas, innovative strategies, empirical designs, and theoretical inquiries as they embark on their journey toward promoting nursing student retention and success. Let's make a difference!

KEY FEATURES AND HOW TO BEST USE THIS BOOK

This book and toolkit offer an ensemble of thoughtfully interconnected features in a lively, interactive, and informative fashion. Optimal benefits will be best achieved by using all the distinctive features together. A quick guide to readers on distinctive features and how to best use this book follows:

- *Opening Quotation*: Readers are asked to pause and reflect on the quotation. Later, after completing the chapter, readers are asked to reflect on the quotation again. What does it mean? How is it significant?

- *Snapshot Scenario:* A realistic scenario prompts readers to read on and discover what the multidisciplinary literature says about the issue and what solutions are available. Readers are asked to reflect on the scenario before proceeding into the chapter. What are the major points? What new information do you seek?
- *Chapter Content:* Provides a wealth of new information and evidence-based strategies reported in the nursing and higher education literature. Readers can ease into and experience the abundance of literature without feeling overwhelmed. Integrated reflection exercise boxes strategically placed throughout chapters will aid in retaining important ideas and perspectives.
- *Key Point Summary*: Highlights three to five key summary synthesis points within the chapter.
- *Easy Application Steps*: Lists quick, easy steps for immediate application in any setting.
- *Educator in Action:* This vignette synthesizes chapter information and demonstrates direct application via realistic case exemplars.
- *Toolkit Resource Box:* Suggests toolkit items for use from the book's accompanying *Nursing Student Retention Toolkit* most applicable to chapter content areas.
- *Discussion Questions:* An assemblage of questions that creatively blends chapter features and content in order to heighten awareness, deepen commitment, stimulate new ideas, and apply knowledge are found throughout all chapters. Readers are asked to answer each question individually and substantiate their answer from readings and activities in the book. Readers can then proceed to discuss questions and answers with a small group of peers, faculty, and/or administrators.
- *References*: Extensive journal and book references document relevant resources.

ABOUT THE NURSING STUDENT RETENTION TOOLKIT

This book includes access to a valuable and ready-to-use *Nursing Student Retention Toolkit* for immediate use. The toolkit consists of four sets of tools and a total of 30 distinct items. The four sets are Questionnaires, Model and Illustrated Pathways, Assessment Tools, and Faculty Interactive Retention Strategy Design Modules. Taken together, the toolkit items provide a comprehensive set of materials for planning, implementing, and evaluating retention strategies and programs. These toolkit items may be used alone or in conjunction with other items and will be of use to a broad range of readers at all levels: full-time faculty, adjunct clinical faculty, administrators, association leaders, researchers, and graduate students. The toolkit and this book will enable you to enhance nursing student retention and success.

All these toolkit items are to be found on a special website. The address of the website is www.springerpub.com/JeffreysRetention. You can download and print the toolkit items from this website, and you can also distribute them electronically.

An important note: As a purchaser of this book, you are entitled to employ these items for individual use without extra charge. Any use of the toolkit or portions of the toolkit beyond individual, personal use (such as with others in an online or institutional setting and/or in a research study) will require a license from Springer Publishing Company and payment of a modest fee for a 1-year unlimited-use license. To obtain more information regarding such an institutional license including terms and fees, please contact Springer Publishing Company at any one of the following:

Phone: 212-431-4370 or toll free at 877-687-7476
Fax: 212-941-7842
Email: customerservice@springerpub.com
Mail: Springer Publishing Company
Customer Service
11 West 42nd Street
New York, New York 10036

We thank you for your adherence to these terms of use.

Acknowledgments

Partial funding for previous research on nursing student retention, and/ or the development of an enrichment program and/or nursing student resource center was obtained from the Nursing Education Alumni Association (NEAA) of Teachers College, Columbia University Postdoctoral Research Fellowship Award; the City University of New York (CUNY) Faculty Advancement Program; PSC-CUNY Research Award Program; CUNY College of Staten Island Division of Science and Technology; and the New York State Education Department Vocational and Technical Education Act (VATEA).

PART 1

What's Happening? Exploring Student Retention and Taking Action

Part I is made up of nine chapters. Chapter 1 begins with an overview of student retention, defines key terms, and presents the Nursing Undergraduate Retention and Success (NURS) conceptual model as an organizing framework. The NURS model proposes that retention decisions will be based on the interaction of student profile characteristics, student affective factors, academic factors, environmental factors, professional integration factors, academic outcomes, psychological outcomes, and outside surrounding factors (OSF).

Chapter 2 describes student characteristics prior to beginning a nursing course and includes age, ethnicity and race, gender, language, prior educational experience, family's educational background, prior work experience, and enrollment status. The chapter elaborates upon each of these characteristics, proposing ways that they may influence retention.

Chapter 3 introduces the general concepts underlying cultural values and beliefs, self-efficacy, and motivation that can seriously influence nursing student achievement, persistence, and retention. Several tables and figures illustrate major points significant for practical application in the educational setting. Select cultural values and beliefs, especially pertinent to nursing education and student retention, are compared and contrasted.

Nurse educators are continually challenged to appraise the influence of academic factors on retention and success. Chapter 4 discusses personal study skills, study hours, attendance, class schedule, and general academic services (college library, college counseling, and computer laboratory) in relation to undergraduate nursing student retention and aims to assist nurse educators in identifying areas of student strengths and weaknesses. An in-depth exploration of each academic factor reveals several dimensions that can potentially affect students. Special issues unique to nursing education are emphasized.

Chapter 5 presents external environmental factors that may influence students' academic performance, retention, and/or success, and include financial status, family financial support, family emotional support, family responsibilities, child-care arrangements, family crisis, employment hours, employment responsibilities, encouragement by outside friends, living arrangement, and transportation. Each environmental factor is analyzed in relation to undergraduate nursing student retention and aims to assist nurse educators in identifying areas of student strengths and weaknesses.

Chapter 6 proposes professional integration factors that enhance students' interaction with the social system of the college environment within the context of professional socialization and career development. These factors include nursing faculty advisement and helpfulness, memberships in professional organizations, professional events, encouragement by friends in class, enrichment programs, and peer mentoring and tutoring. The chapter elaborates upon each of the professional integration factors, proposing ways that they can potentially and directly enhance retention through academic outcomes and psychological outcomes.

The complexity of the nursing educational experience offers unique professional, discipline-specific psychological and developmental opportunities and outcomes beyond course grades or GPA. Both academic and psychological outcomes influence persistence and retention. Chapter 7 addresses pertinent issues surrounding academic and psychological outcomes, presents proposed relationships with other variables in the NURS model, and suggests practical application strategies.

The purpose of Chapter 8 is to enhance awareness of OSF on student retention, highlight the potential significance of select factors, stimulate further inquiry, and suggest recommendations for nurse educators. OSF exist outside of the academic setting and the individual student's personal environment and can influence retention. They include world, national, and local events; politics and economics; the health care system; nursing professional issues; and job certainty.

Chapter 9 introduces select background information and main concepts involved in retention decisions and the decision-making process. Nurse educators are in a strategic position to make a difference by facilitating the process of systematic decision making and enhancing opportunities for retention and success. Steps of the decision-making process specific to nursing student retention are additionally incorporated within an illustration. Implications for nurse educators are proposed.

Overview of Student Retention

The most persistent trend in student persistence research is that student attrition persists.

SNAPSHOT SCENARIO

PROFESSOR NUMBERS: I just don't understand why we have such a high attrition rate, especially in the first nursing course. Students complete rigorous prerequisite courses prior to the nursing courses yet they still drop out or fail.

PROFESSOR PONDER: Yes, I don't understand it either. Even when some students seem to be highly motivated and possess the critical thinking skills needed for nursing, they still aren't successful.

PROFESSOR NUMBERS: It seems like our minority students drop out more frequently than our White students.

PROFESSOR ELLIS: Yes, except that some of the White students who are recent immigrants seem to have a more difficult time. Just like many of the minority students, these immigrants seem to keep to themselves inside and outside the classroom and clinical setting.

PROFESSOR PONDER: Recently, my classroom has become much more diverse. I have so many older students, men, students with full-time jobs, students caring for children, grandchildren, or aging and disabled family members, students who lived in various countries before coming to the United States, students who lost their jobs or are changing their careers because of the economy. I treat all students the same and use the same standards. So why are students dropping out, even though they have passing grades at midterm?

PROFESSOR NUMBERS: Changes in the economy have made nursing a more desirable career and many unemployed people are swarming nursing schools, desperate for admission. Once admitted, they aren't always staying. That takes seats away from other students and contributes to the nursing shortage. Something should be done about this, but I don't know where to begin.

PROFESSOR ELLIS: I was really surprised! Despite many of the obstacles and hardships that some of my students faced throughout the program, they persevered and were successful. I just can't figure out what makes a positive difference for some students [and not others]. Wouldn't it be wonderful if we could figure out why students stay, despite all their academic and personal challenges—and then help struggling students succeed—or even better—assist all students to enhance their learning and success and prevent struggles?

PROFESSOR PONDER: That would mean really understanding what's going on with our students before planning strategies. Isn't there a model that we can use to explore this? What strategies have others used that were successful? What works and what doesn't and why?

The nursing profession must be ready to embrace a new age of realism with regard to the changing student population. Currently, the dramatic shift in demographics, the restructured workforce, and a less academically prepared college applicant pool have created a more diverse nursing applicant pool (1–9). Increasingly, the "nontraditional" student is replacing the "traditional" student in nursing. The projected increases in immigration, globalization, and minority population growth have the potential to enrich the diversity of the nursing profession and to help meet the needs of an expanding culturally diverse society (3,4,7–20). Thus, the untapped potential of the nontraditional student population demands focused attention on promoting nontraditional nursing student success. Unfortunately, the retention rates of nontraditional students have been, and still remain, substantially lower than those of traditional students (3,9,10,11,21–36). Although attrition is financially costly to students, educational institutions, and society, the severest impact can be the adverse psychological costs to the students (28,37–40). The mismatch between nursing student admissions and swift entry into the workforce adversely contributes to the nursing shortage, another severe effect that impacts the nursing profession, health care, and society (Table 1.1).

Enrollment trends, retention rates, professional goals, societal needs, and ethical considerations all declare the need to prioritize the retention of nontraditional students. However, the retention of traditional students must be addressed as well. Nurse educators are in a key position to influence retention positively. As active partners in the complex process of nursing student retention, nurse educators can design theoretical and evidence-based retention strategies targeting specific student populations. Design of a diagnostic-specific strategy first requires an understanding of the dynamic phenomenon of nursing student retention, the complex interaction of influencing factors, and insight into the student's perspective (33,34,36,41).

This chapter provides an overview of undergraduate nursing student retention, defines key terms, and presents the Nursing Undergraduate Retention and Success (NURS) conceptual model as an organizing framework. The main features will be highlighted in an attempt to succinctly summarize the literature and enhance understanding of the

TABLE 1.1 Select Nursing Student Trends and Potential Future Impact on the Nursing Profession

VARIABLE	SELECT NURSING STUDENT TRENDS	POTENTIAL FUTURE IMPACT ON THE NURSING PROFESSION
Age	Consistent with global and multi-disciplinary trends, the enrollment of older students in nursing programs has increased over the last decade, with projected increases to persist in the future.	Age at entry into the nursing profession will be older, resulting in decreased number of work years until retirement.
Ethnicity and race	*Enrollment*: Recent nursing enrollment trends suggest a steady increase among some minority groups, however, no increase has been noted among Hispanic groups. *Retention*: Minority groups incur higher attrition rates than non-minority groups.	Currently, White, non-Hispanic nurses of European American heritage represent approximately 83% of all registered nurses in the United States. Mismatches between the cultural diversity in society and diversity within the nursing profession will persist into the future unless strategies for recruitment and retention are more successful.
Gender	*Men*: Although the numbers of men in nursing are increasing, they remain an underrepresented minority (6%). *Women*: Support for women entering the workforce has shifted away from encouraging traditional female professions.	Men will continue to be disproportionately underrepresented in nursing. Many academically well-qualified male and female high school students with a potential interest in nursing may never enter the nursing profession.
Language	*Enrollment*: Consistent with global and national trends in higher education, nursing programs in the United States and Canada have experienced an increase in English as second language populations over the past decade. *Retention*: English as second language student populations have unique learning needs and incur higher attrition rates.	Although individuals with personal lived experiences in other cultures and languages can potentially meet the needs of linguistically diverse and culturally diverse client populations, they will still be disproportionately represented within the nursing profession.

(continued)

TABLE 1.1 Select Nursing Student Trends and Potential Future Impact on the Nursing Profession (*continued*)

VARIABLE	SELECT NURSING STUDENT TRENDS	POTENTIAL FUTURE IMPACT ON THE NURSING PROFESSION
Prior educational experience	Consistent with trends in higher education worldwide, prior educational experiences are increasingly diverse with an academically less prepared applicant pool. Increases in the number of second-degree individuals have been noted. *Retention*: Academically underprepared students incur higher attrition rates.	Nurses with degrees in other fields can enrich the nursing profession by blending multidisciplinary approaches into nursing. Nurses with academically diverse experiences may broaden the overall perspective, especially with socioeconomic and educationally diverse client populations.
Family's educational background	Nursing programs have also seen an increase in first-generation college students, especially among student groups traditionally underrepresented in nursing. *Retention*: First-generation college students incur higher attrition rates.	First-generation college students who become nurses have the potential to enrich the diversity of the nursing profession and reach out to various socioeconomic and educationally diverse client populations.
Prior work experience	A restructured workforce, welfare-to-work initiatives, displaced homemakers, popularity of midlife career changes, and health care career ladder programs have expanded the nursing applicant pool, increasing its diversity in prior work experience. Many students work full- or part-time. *Retention*: Work-family-school conflicts may interfere with academic success and retention.	New graduate nurses may enter the nursing profession with a variety of prior work experiences that have the potential to enrich the nursing profession.
Enrollment status	Almost half of all college students attend part-time. The number of part-time nursing students, especially those with multiple-role responsibilities (work, family) has increased. *Retention*: Work-family-school conflicts may interfere with academic success and retention.	Part-time students will take longer to complete their education. Entry into practice will be delayed and total number of potential work years in nursing will be decreased.

Reprinted from Jeffreys (2010).

multidimensional phenomenon of undergraduate nursing student retention and success. Application strategies conclude the chapter.

NEED, SIGNIFICANCE, AND DEFINITIONS

What are the various trajectory pathway options for retention and attrition? How are various options defined?

Retention has been examined and discussed extensively in both higher education and nursing literature (28,42–46). Research studies, however, have been more limited and have targeted predominantly traditional students in traditional 4-year baccalaureate programs. In nursing, retention studies on new entry-into-practice programs (e.g., accelerated programs) are also limited (47). Many studies have focused on attrition through use of autopsy studies, after the student has already withdrawn. Diverse sample size, enrollment status, and methodology complicate synthesis of the literature. Although similar study variables have been examined, inconsistencies between operational definitions varied extensively, making comparison difficult (28,35,44). Additionally, voluntary attrition, due to personal reasons, and involuntary attrition, due to academic failure, are often undifferentiated (28,35,45). Tracking students via three different retention pathways (ideal, continuous, and interim/stopout), three attrition pathways (first semester failure, voluntary, and involuntary), and three licensure pathways is an important approach to document and comprehend the progress paths of nursing students today. Interestingly, the first study using this trajectory tracking pathway revealed that retention among nontraditional associate degree nursing students was almost equally distributed between ideal (26%), continuous (24%), and interim/stopout (25%). Brief stopouts for personal reasons were not predictors of failure. Rather brief stopouts could be beneficial; however, transitional interventions were recommended. Recognizing that not all students travel the same road yet still may achieve academic success and licensure is a valuable realization and a necessary first step toward understanding the multidimensional process of student retention (35). Figure 1.1 illustrates the student trajectory progression pathway. Key terms are presented in Exhibit 1.1.

What trajectory pathways have been used to track students in your course, other courses, and your program? How can clear, consistent definitions help track students within and between programs? What are the benefits of comparative retention studies?

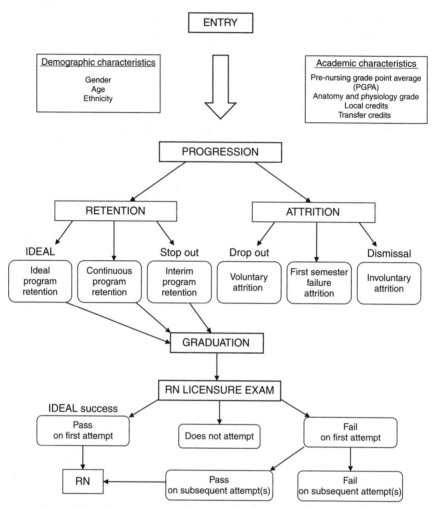

Source: Reprinted from *Nursing Education Today, 27,* M.R. Jeffreys, "Tracking students through program entry, progression, graduation, and licensure: Assessing undergraduate nursing student retention and success, pp. 406–419, 2007, with permission from Elsevier.
FIGURE 1.1 Nursing Student Progress Pathway.

MULTIDIMENSIONAL PROCESS OF STUDENT RETENTION

An extensive search in the nursing and higher education literature revealed several comprehensive conceptual models to explain undergraduate student attrition (21,26,48–51). However, only one model specifically targeted the nontraditional students (21). No models specifically targeted nursing students. What were common trends in the literature? The most persistent trend in student persistence research was that student attrition persists. Second, student attrition (or retention) was complex and multidimensional. Third, retention strategies needed to be evidence based, multidimensional, holistic, and evaluated quantitatively and qualitatively. Here,

EXHIBIT 1.1 Definitions Associated With Student Retention, Attrition, Progression, and Success

Nontraditional undergraduate nursing student refers to a nursing student who is enrolled in an entry-level undergraduate nursing program (diploma, associate degree, or generic baccalaureate) and who meets one or more of the following criteria: (1) 25 years or older, (2) commuter, (3) enrolled part-time, (4) male, (5) member of an ethnic and/or racial minority group, (6) speaks English as a second (other) language, (7) has dependent children, (8) has a general equivalency diploma, and (9) required remedial classes.

Traditional undergraduate nursing student refers to a nursing student who is enrolled in an entry-level undergraduate nursing program (diploma, associate degree, or generic baccalaureate) and who does not meet the criteria of "nontraditional undergraduate nursing student" as defined above. Specifically, such a student meets all of the following criteria: (1) 24 years or younger, (2) resides in campus housing or off-campus housing, (3) enrolled full-time, (4) female, (5) White and not a member of an ethnic and/or racial minority group, (6) speaks English as a first language, (7) has no dependent children, (8) has a U.S. high school diploma; and (9) required no remedial classes.

Course retention is the continuous enrollment in a nursing course without withdrawal.

Course success refers to passing the nursing course.

Program retention is the continuous enrollment in a nursing program (part- or full-time) by taking the required courses sequentially until meeting the program's graduation requirements, possibly including courses repeated for previous withdrawal and/or failure.

In **ideal program retention**, the student successfully completes the required courses sequentially, in the specified time period, and without evidence of withdrawal or failure.

Interim program retention is the intermittent enrollment in a nursing program (part- or full-time) by taking the required courses sequentially until meeting the program's graduation requirements, possibly including courses repeated for previous withdrawal and/or failure.

In **program success,** the student (1) successfully completes the program's graduation requirements, (2) passes the RN licensing exam, and (3) obtains a part- or full-time job as an RN and/or enrolls in a more advanced nursing program.

In **ideal program success**, the student successfully completes the program's graduation requirements within the specified time period

(continued)

and, without withdrawing or failing, passes the RN licensing exam on the first attempt, and obtains a job as a RN and/or enrolls in a more advanced nursing program.

Withdrawal is when students officially withdraw from a college course or courses due to personal and/or academic reasons.

Stopout refers to a break in continuous enrollment for one or more semesters (excluding summer sessions and intercessions).

Attrition refers to students "dropping out" of the nursing program.

Voluntary attrition is when a student drops out due to personal (nonacademic) reasons compared to **involuntary attrition** because of academic reasons (failure or dismissal). It may also be helpful to differentiate between types of involuntary attrition for the purposes of tracking students, identifying at-risk transitional periods during the academic program, and evaluating effectiveness of retention strategies initiated. For example, in some nursing programs, failure in the first nursing course necessitates a reapplication process into the program with limited seats available for reapplicants. **First semester attrition** refers to attrition from students failing the first nursing course and who either do not apply for readmission or who apply for readmission but are not readmitted. Dismissal can occur for academic reasons, misconduct, academic dishonesty, and/or failure of one or more courses as reflected in the institution's progression policy.

---

holistic means recognizing the student as a whole person with multiple roles, responsibilities, skills, knowledge, and feelings.

Subsequently, the Bean and Metzner model (21) of nontraditional undergraduate student attrition provided the underlying conceptual framework for the author's early studies on nontraditional undergraduate nursing student retention (30,32–34). Results from these studies supported that nontraditional students often juggled multiple roles such as student, parent, financial provider, and/or employee and therefore were more influenced by environmental variables than by academic variables. Additionally, students perceived family, faculty, friends, tutoring, and an enrichment program as greatly supportive (33,34). Following the preliminary studies, a series of grant-funded multidimensional retention strategies were implemented and are described later in this book.

Although many of the factors influencing nontraditional students across various disciplines are also relevant to nursing students, there are some distinguishing characteristics of the nontraditional undergraduate nursing students. As a profession, nursing also is different from liberal arts and science disciplines; therefore, applicability of these models to undergraduate nursing students in general is also limited. Retention experts recommend more focus on discipline-specific programs, nontraditional students, program completion time, student stopouts, and outcomes of education (52–54). Consequently, the Nontraditional Undergraduate Retention and Success (NURS) model was developed specifically for examining nontraditional undergraduate nursing student retention and success (55). The proposed influencing factors were clustered into variable sets and then incorporated into the original NURS model. With minor modifications, the original NURS model was easily adapted to include the traditional undergraduate nursing student population, resulting in the latest conceptualized model (Figure 1.2). Please note that in 2004, the acronym NURS was changed from "Nontraditional Undergraduate Retention and Success" to "Nursing Undergraduate Retention and Success" and encompasses components appropriate for both traditional and nontraditional students. Future reference to the NURS model in this book refers to the revised model. The latest NURS model is applicable to all entry-into-practice undergraduate nursing programs (associate degree, diploma, generic baccalaureate, accelerated second degree [baccalaureate]). It has also been effectively used to appraise retention in registered nurse-bachelor of science in nursing (RN-BSN) programs (56) and licensed practical nurse programs (57).

THE NURS MODEL: ASSUMPTIONS, PREMISES, AND OVERVIEW

The purpose of the NURS model is to present an organizing framework for examining the multidimensional factors that affect undergraduate nursing student retention and success in order to identify at-risk students, develop diagnostic-prescriptive strategies to facilitate success, guide innovations in teaching and educational research, and evaluate strategy effectiveness. Although several models have been proposed to examine college student attrition, this model specifically focuses on the aspect of retention (rather than attrition) and targets a specific student population. In other words, the emphasis is on exploring "why do nursing students stay?" as opposed to asking "why do nursing students leave?" The main goal of the model is to promote undergraduate nursing student retention and success. Educators in nursing and other college disciplines around the world have requested and used the model to first "explore the multidimensional process of student retention" and second "to take action and make a positive difference." The model is tentative and will require modification when new data become available.

Based on a review of the literature and previous studies of nontraditional undergraduate nursing student retention, several assumptions underlie the NURS model:

- Undergraduate nursing student retention is a priority concern for nurse educators.

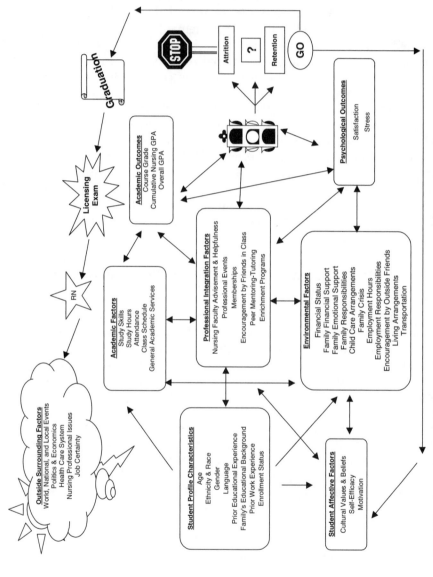

FIGURE 1.2 Jeffreys's (2004) Model of Nursing Undergraduate Retention and Success (NURS).

- Student retention is a dynamic and multidimensional phenomenon that is influenced by the interaction of multiple variables (factors).
- For undergraduate nursing students, environmental factors and professional integration factors greatly influence retention.
- All students, regardless of prior academic performance, can benefit from professional socialization and enrichment throughout preprofessional and professional education.
- Psychological outcomes and academic outcomes may interact and influence persistence.

The NURS model is presented in Figure 1.2. Briefly, the model indicates that retention decisions will be based on the interaction of student profile characteristics, student affective factors, academic factors, environmental factors, professional integration factors, academic outcomes, psychological outcomes, and outside surrounding factors. Table 1.2 defines

TABLE 1.2   Definitions Associated With Jeffreys's NURS Model

Student profile characteristics describe student characteristics prior to beginning a nursing course and include age, ethnicity and race, gender, first language, prior educational experience, the family's educational background, prior work experience, and enrollment status.

Student affective factors are students' attitudes, values, and beliefs about learning and their ability to learn and perform the necessary tasks required for course and program success, including cultural values and beliefs, self-efficacy, and motivation.

Academic factors include personal study skills, study hours, attendance, class schedule, and general academic services (e.g., college library services, college counseling services, and computer laboratory services).

Environmental factors are factors external to the academic process that may influence students' academic performance and retention and include financial status, family financial support, family emotional support, family responsibilities, childcare arrangements, family crisis, employment hours, employment responsibilities, encouragement by outside friends, living arrangements, and transportation.

Professional integration factors are factors that enhance students' interaction with the social system of the college environment within the context of professional socialization and career development. These include nursing faculty advisement and helpfulness, professional events, memberships in professional organizations, encouragement by friends in class, peer mentoring and tutoring, and enrichment programs.

Outside surrounding factors are factors existing outside of the academic setting and the student's personal environment that can influence retention such as world, national, and local events; politics and economics; the health care system; nursing professional issues; and job certainty.

Academic outcomes are represented by the student's nursing course grade, cumulative GPA for nursing courses, and overall GPA.

Psychological outcomes include satisfaction and stress.

Note: GPA, grade point average.

key model components. Outside surrounding factors have the power to affect student persistence and retention either positively or negatively despite positive academic and psychological outcomes for nursing. At the beginning of each nursing course, student profile characteristics provide information on the composition of the student group. Individual factors may interact with each other to increase or decrease persistence or risk of attrition.

Similar to the Bean and Metzner model (21), it is presumed that environmental factors are more important for nontraditional undergraduate nursing students than academic factors. Also consistent with the model, academic outcomes interact with psychological outcomes. Good academic performance only results in retention when accompanied by positive psychological outcomes for the nursing program and profession. The voluntary and/or involuntary decision to remain in a course, persist in the nursing program, graduate, take the RN licensing exam, and enter the nursing workforce and/or begin a more advanced nursing program occurs during and at the conclusion of each nursing course.

Many models explaining attrition among traditional college students have emphasized the importance of social integration in college in student adjustment, persistence, and success (48–51). For undergraduate nursing students, a different perspective of social integration is proposed. In the NURS model, professional integration factors represent variables that enhance students' interaction with the social system of the college environment within the context of professional socialization and career development. Several studies (33,34,36) consistently identified professional integration factors, such as nursing faculty advisement and helpfulness, an enrichment program, and peer mentoring-tutoring, as instrumental in assisting with nontraditional nursing student retention. Professional integration factors are at the center of the model because they are at the crossroads of the decision to persist, dropout, or stopout. It is also proposed that professional integration factors are important for traditional and nontraditional nursing student retention and for all types of nursing programs.

For example, the NURS model has applicability to undergraduates in RN-BSN programs (56); however, the manner in which factors influence student persistence is different. Basically this is true because RN-BSN students are nontraditional in the sense that they already have a professional license, do not enter baccalaureate nursing education directly after high school, most likely work full-time or part-time in the nursing profession, are older, and may have other responsibilities whereby the student role is not the main role. In addition, most students (except for diploma school graduates) have successfully completed college courses and a college degree. RN-BSN students are familiar with the college experience, may be strongly integrated and socialized within nursing (viewing nursing as an occupation or profession), and already have an established history of success in college and in nursing (having earned a college degree and passed the RN licensing exam). The professional integration and socialization is at a different point for RNs pursuing their BS degree in nursing. Professional integration and socialization occurs differently throughout one's career trajectory with advanced education and different practice roles; however, it is an irreplaceable, vital component.

In summary, within the NURS model, the proposed factors can be applied to both traditional and nontraditional undergraduate nursing student populations; however, the manner in which they impact retention may be different. Such differences will be highlighted throughout Part I of this book. Additionally, the factors interact with each other and with other variable sets in the NURS model. Such interactions will also be addressed throughout Part I.

In what ways is undergraduate nursing education different from other undergraduate majors? What are the various ways you can apply the NURS model?

KEY POINT SUMMARY

- The Nursing Undergraduate Retention and Success (NURS) model presents an organizing framework for examining the multidimensional factors that affect undergraduate nursing student retention and success in order to identify at-risk students, develop diagnostic-prescriptive strategies to facilitate success, guide innovations in teaching and educational research, and evaluate strategy effectiveness.
- The NURS model proposes that retention decisions will be based on the interaction of student profile characteristics, student affective factors, academic factors, environmental factors, professional integration factors, academic outcomes, psychological outcomes, and outside surrounding factors.
- Academic outcomes interact with psychological outcomes whereby good academic performance only results in retention when accompanied by positive psychological outcomes for the nursing program and profession.
- The voluntary and/or involuntary decision to remain in a course, persist in the nursing program, graduate, take the RN licensing exam, and enter the nursing workforce and/or begin a more advanced nursing program occurs during and at the conclusion of each nursing course.
- Professional integration factors are at the center of the model because they are at the crossroads of the decision to persist, dropout, or stopout.

APPLICATION STRATEGIES ████████████████

EASY APPLICATION ACTION STEPS

Determining Retention, Attrition, and Licensure Rate

1. Obtain data for each trajectory pathway in Figure 1.1.
2. Develop a composite of your program's trajectory pathway.
3. Propose percentages of increase or decrease for each pathway option.

Touring the Multidimensional Process of Nursing
Student Retention and Success

1. Contemplate the big picture of the NURS model (panoramic view).
2. Beginning with student profile characteristics, consider the interaction between all model components and possible outcomes, noting that professional integration factors are at the center of the model.
3. Plan to explore each area more in depth by reading each book chapter.

EDUCATOR-IN-ACTION VIGNETTE

PROFESSOR LIGHT: As a follow-up to our discussion about nursing student retention, attrition, and success, and Professor Ponder's query about finding a conceptual model to help us, I conducted a literature search and discovered the NURS model. Let me share with you the major parts and definitions.

PROFESSOR PONDER: What's the best way to use the model? How should we begin?

PROFESSOR LIGHT: It's really not any different than looking at a roadmap. Often, educators and institutions look at entry, progression, and graduation as a straight-line or a clear-cut pathway. Just like going from point A destination to point B destination may seem clear cut, there are many anticipated and unanticipated factors that can affect reaching a destination; by stopping the journey or by making it longer, shorter, more pleasant, and so on. The NURS model presents the big picture, or multidimensional nature of nursing student retention and success while also condensing the many variables (factors) influencing retention and success within variable sets (or boxes). The arrows really show movement and a method of connecting the dots (or boxes) with each other along the journey.

PROFESSOR NUMBERS: I like that the NURS model has corresponding quantitative questionnaires that we can administer to our students. We could use the Student Perception Appraisal-Revised (SPA-R) pretest and posttest to document what's supporting their retention and what's restricting their retention. For students who dropout or stopout, we can use the withdrawal questionnaire. The questionnaire items correspond with concepts in the NURS model. We can aggregate data and explain it within the context of the NURS model.

PROFESSOR GRANT: I noticed that there are several large grants available to nursing programs that aim to enhance student retention and success, especially among underrepresented groups in nursing. We could use the NURS model and quantitative data to guide our grant proposal project by providing baseline data and then planning to evaluate changes from baseline data once our retention strategies are formulated. Several past grant recipients have developed retention strategies incorporating the professional integration and socialization factors depicted in the NURS model. For example, one school developed an enrichment program with peer mentor-tutoring, enhanced faculty advisement strategies, test prep workshops, an orientation program, development of a nursing student club affiliated with the National Student Nurses Association, and opportunities for participation in professional conferences. Another school developed a Nursing Neighborhood by converting space in the nursing building to incorporate various formal and informal group and individual peer mentor-tutoring and computer-based virtual learning activities exclusively for nursing students. Satisfaction is also a component within the NURS model, so satisfaction for retention strategies implemented can be measured by using or adapting a satisfaction questionnaire (Toolkit Items 6 and 7).

PROFESSOR NOVICE: All this is very interesting to me. I'm a new adjunct faculty member and I had no idea that so many factors could influence student success. The NURS model condenses everything into one picture. I realize that being a nurse practitioner with clinical expertise will not help me fully assist my students to be successful until I learn more about the teaching-learning process and how to help students succeed. I'm enrolled in a doctoral program and want to become a tenured professor someday. Now that Professor Grant mentioned funding available for nursing student retention research, I realize that educational research has been undervalued by many nurses involved in clinical research. We can't improve quality of patient care unless we resolve the nursing shortage and we can't do that if potentially good future nurses are dropping out. Perhaps I should focus my doctoral research on nursing student retention? I really want to make a positive difference in student retention.

PROFESSOR LIGHT: Several presenters at a national conference last year presented retention strategies implemented at their programs, documenting improved student retention rates, increased National Council Licensure Examination (NCLEX) pass rates, increased student satisfaction and confidence, and reduced stress. Some of the presenters used the NURS model and the accompanying questionnaires. It was helpful to have a familiar model that linked concepts and variables within and between schools.

TOOLKIT RESOURCE BOX

Item 12—NURS Model
Item 13—Nursing Student Progress Pathway
Item 21—Who Are At-Risk Students?
Items 1–4—Student Perception Appraisal Questionnaires—Pretests and Posttests

---

DISCUSSION QUESTIONS

1. In what ways can nontraditional nursing students enhance the nursing profession and help meet the needs of diverse patient populations?
2. A nursing faculty colleague states, "I treat all my students the same and I have the same expectations for each of them. I don't know why I should change my approach just because our student population has changed. Our RN pass rate still exceeds the state average of 87%, even though our attrition rate has increased from 8% to 22% in the last 2 years." (a) How does this statement make you feel? (b) How would you respond?
3. What are the benefits of using consistent definitions, evaluation measures, and conceptual model(s) in retention research and education?
4. Professor Green says, "What's the difference between attrition research and retention research? Isn't it asking the same question and getting the same answers?"
5. What aspect of the NURS model intrigued you the most? Why?

REFERENCES

1. Kelly, E. (1997). Development of strategies to identify the learning needs of baccalaureate nursing students. *Journal of Nursing Education, 36*, 156–162.
2. Tayebi, K., Moore-Jazayeri, M., & Maynard, T. (1998). From the borders: Reforming the curriculum for the at-risk student. *Journal of Cultural Diversity, 5*, 101–109.
3. Bosher, S. D., & Pharris, M. D. (2009). *Transforming nursing education: The culturally inclusive environment.* New York, NY: Springer Publishing.
4. Grossman, D., & Jorda, M. L. (2008). Transitioning foreign-educated physicians to nurses: The new Americans in nursing. *Journal of Nursing Education, 47*(12), 544–551.
5. Harvath, T. A. (2008). A culture of learning. *Journal of Nursing Education, 47*(12), 535–536.

6. Hegge, M. J., & Hallman, P. A. (2008). Changing nursing culture to welcome second-degree students: Herding and corralling sacred cows. *Journal of Nursing Education, 47*(12), 552–556.

7. Tagliareni, M. E. (2008). Quoted in Sapers, J. Shaping the future of nursing, *TC Today, 33*(1), 13–17.

8. Schumacher, G., Risco, K., & Conway, A. (2008). The Schumacher model: Fostering scholarship and excellence in nursing and for recruiting and grooming new faculty. *Journal of Nursing Education, 47*(12), 571–575.

9. Jeffreys, M. R. (2010). *Teaching cultural competence in nursing and health care: Inquiry, action, and innovation* (2nd ed.). New York, NY: Springer Publishing.

10. Barbee, E. L., & Gibson, S. E. (2001). Our dismal progress: The recruitment of non-whites into nursing. *Journal of Nursing Education, 40*(6), 243–245.

11. Bessent, H. (Ed.). (1997). *Strategies for recruitment, retention, and graduation of minority nurses in colleges of nursing*. Washington, DC: American Nurses Publishing.

12. Department of Health and Human Services. (2000). *Healthy people 2010: Understanding and improving health* (2nd ed.). Washington, DC: U.S. Government Printing Office.

13. Department of Health and Human Services. (2009). *Healthy people 2020:* Washington, DC, Retrieved January 24, 2010, from http://www.healthpeople.gov/hp2020.

14. National League for Nursing (2009). *A commitment to diversity in nursing and nursing education*. [Reflection and Dialogue]. Available at www.nln.org/about-nln/reflection_dialogue/refl_dial_3.htm

15. American Association of Colleges of Nursing. (2008). *Cultural competency in baccalaureate nursing education*. Washington, DC: Author.

16. American Association of Colleges of Nursing (2010). *Fact sheet: Enhancing diversity in the nursing workforce*. Washington, DC: Author.

17. Wilson, D. W. (2007). From their own voices: The lived experience of African American registered nurses. *Journal of Transcultural Nursing, 18*(2), 142–149.

18. Tucker-Allen, S., & Long, E. (1999). *Recruitment and retention of minority nursing students: Stories of success*. Lisle, IL: Tucker Publications.

19. Villaruel, A. M., Canales, M., & Torres, S. (2001). Bridges and barriers: Educational mobility of Hispanic nurses. *Journal of Nursing Education, 40*(6), 245–251.

20. Yoder, M. K. (2001). The bridging approach: Effective strategies for teaching ethnically diverse nursing students. *Journal of Transcultural Nursing, 12*, 319–325.

21. Bean, J. P., & Metzner, B. (1985). A conceptual model of nontraditional undergraduate student attrition. *Review of Educational Research, 55*, 485–540.

22. Braxton, J. M. (ed.) (2000). *Reworking the student departure puzzle*. Nashville, TN: Vanderbilt University Press.

23. Dowell, M. A. (1996). Issues in recruitment and retention of minority nursing students. *Journal of Nursing Education, 35*(7), 293–297.

24. Levin, M. E., & Levin, J. R. (1991). A critical examination of academic retention programs for at-risk minority college students. *Journal of College Student Development, 32*, 322–334.

25. Manifold, C., & Rambur, B. (2001). Predictors of attrition in American Indian nursing students. *Journal of Nursing Education, 40*(6), 279–281.

26. Metzner, B., & Bean, J. P. (1987). The estimation of a conceptual model of non-traditional undergraduate student attrition. *Research in Higher Education, 27,* 15–38.

27. Yurkovich, E. E. (2001). Working with American Indians toward educational success. *Journal of Nursing Education, 40*(6), 259–269.

28. Seidman, A. (2005). *College student retention: Formula for student success.* Westport, CT: Praeger.

29. Seidman, A. (2007). *Minority student retention: The best of the Journal of College Student Retention: Research, Theory, and Practice.* Amityville, NY: Baywood.

30. Jeffreys, M. R. (1993). *The relationship of self-efficacy and select academic and environmental variables on academic achievement and retention.* Unpublished doctoral dissertation, Teachers College, Columbia University, New York.

31. Jeffreys, M. R. (1995). Joining together family, faculty, and friends: New ideas for enhancing nontraditional student success. *Nurse Educator, 20*(3), 11.

32. Jeffreys, M. R. (1998). Predicting nontraditional student retention and academic achievement. *Nurse Educator, 23*(1), 42–48.

33. Jeffreys, M. R. (2001). Evaluating enrichment program study groups: Academic outcomes, psychological outcomes, and variables influencing retention. *Nurse Educator, 26*(3), 142–149.

34. Jeffreys, M. R. (2002). Students' perceptions of variables influencing retention: A pretest and post-test approach. *Nurse Educator, 27*(1), 16–19 [Erratum, 2002, 27(2), 64].

35. Jeffreys, M. R. (2007). Tracking students through program entry, progression, graduation, and licensure: Assessing undergraduate nursing student retention and success. *Nurse Education Today, 27,* 406–419.

36. Jeffreys, M. R. (2007). Nontraditional students' perceptions of variables influencing retention: A multisite study. *Nurse Educator, 32*(4), 161–167.

37. Nora, A., Cabrera, A., Hagedorn, L., & Pascarella, E. (1996). Differential impacts of academic and social experiences on college-related behavioral outcomes across different ethnic and gender groups at four-year institutions. *Research in Higher Education, 37,* 427–451.

38. Rowser, J. (1997). Do African American students' perceptions of their needs have implications for retention? *Journal of Black Studies, 27,* 718–726.

39. Tinto, V. (1993). *Leaving college: Rethinking the causes and cures of student attrition.* Chicago, IL: University of Chicago Press.

40. Schneider, M. (Ed.) (2010). *Finishing the first lap: The cost of first-year student attrition in America's four-year colleges and universities.* Washington, DC: American Institutes of Research.

41. Harvey, V., & McMurray, N. (1994). Self-efficacy: A means of identifying problems in nursing education and career progress. *International Journal of Nursing Studies, 31,* 471–485.

42. Braxton, J. M. (2001). Introduction to special issue: Using theory and research to improve college student retention. *Journal of College Student Retention: Research, Theory, & Practice, 3*(1), 1–2.

43. Courage, M. M., & Godbey, K. L. (1992). Student retention: Policies and services to enhance persistence to graduation. *Nurse Educator, 17*(2), 29–32.

44. Garcia, M. (1987). *Community college persistence: A field application of the Tinto model.* Unpublished doctoral dissertation, Teachers College, Columbia University, New York.

45. Tucker-Allen, S. (1989). Losses incurred through minority student nurse attrition. *Nursing & Health Care, 10*, 395–397.
46. Tinto, V. (1998). College as communities: Taking research on student persistence seriously. *Review of Higher Education, 21*, 167–177.
47. Rouse, S. M., & Rooda, L. A. (2010). Factors for attrition in an accelerated baccalaureate nursing program. *Journal of Nursing Education, 49*(6), 359–362.
48. Nora, A. (1987). Determinants of retention among Chicano college students: A structural model. *Research in Higher Education, 26*, 31–60.
49. Pascarella, E. T., & Chapman, D. W. (1983). Validation of a theoretical model of college withdrawal: Interaction effects in a multi-institutional sample. *Research in Higher Education, 19*, 25–47.
50. Spady, W. (1970). Dropouts from higher education: Toward an empirical model. *Interchange, 2*, 38–62.
51. Tinto, V. (1975). Dropout from higher education: A theoretical synthesis of recent research. *Review of Educational Research, 10*, 259–271.
52. Astin, A. W. (2005). Making sense out of degree completion rates. *Journal of College Student Retention: Research, Theory, & Practice, 7*, 5–17.
53. DesJardins, S. L., Ashburg, D. A., & McCall, B. P. (1999). An event history model of student departure. *Economics of Education, 18*, 375–381.
54. DesJardins, S. L., Kim, D. O., &Rzonca, C. S. (2003). A nested analysis of factors affecting bachelor's degree completion. *Journal of College Student Retention: Research, Theory, & Practice, 4*(4), 407–436.
55. Jeffreys, M. R. (2003). Strategies for promoting nontraditional student retention and success. In M. Oermann & K. Heinrich (Eds.), *Annual review of nursing education: Volume I* (pp. 61–90). New York, NY: Springer Publishing.
56. Robertson, S., Canary, C. W., Orr, M., Herberg, P., & Rutledge, D. N. (2010). Factors related to progression and graduation rates for RN-to-bachelor of science in nursing programs: Searching for realistic benchmarks. *Journal of Professional Nursing, 26*(2), 99–107.
57. Castaldi, P. A. (2009). *Development of an evidence-based student retention model for practical nursing programs.* Unpublished doctoral dissertation, Rush University, Chicago, IL.

Student Profile Characteristics

Diversity exists in many forms and can impact upon student retention.

What diversity exists within your nursing program?

SNAPSHOT SCENARIO

At a conference coffee break:

PROFESSOR CAVE: Our nursing program really doesn't have any diversity. The students are all the same—same race, same age. They grew up in the area, enter our program right after high school, and commute.

PROFESSOR LIGHT: Well, my clinical group last semester represented much diversity. Five students were first-generation college students, one became interested in nursing while caring for a same-sex partner who died of AIDS, one was the primary caregiver of a terminally ill aunt, one was adopted by a multiracial family during infancy, one didn't learn to read until age 10 because of delayed diagnosis of dyslexia, three had prior health care experience as nursing assistants, and one was totally deaf in one ear following removal of a brain tumor 2 years ago.

PROFESSOR CAVE: I never thought of diversity in that way. Now I see we do have some diversity. But we don't have much age diversity. Some schools have many second-career students, including retirees.

PROFESSOR FRANK: Over the years, I felt privileged to work with diverse ages. Retirees are really a diverse group too—in age and other ways. Some retirees that come to mind right now include a Las Vegas dancer in her twenties, police officers and firefighters in their forties, two semi-professional ball players in their late thirties, a 55-year-old prison guard, a 30-year-old fashion model, an air force captain, and a 62-year-old mail carrier.

PROFESSOR BRIDGES: Students change careers for many reasons. I ask students to share some information on an index card. Just last year, some of my career-change students included a former physician from Russia, speech pathologist from Brazil, plumber, deli owner, mortician, nun, athletic trainer, bartender at a biker bar, social worker, chemical engineer, financial analyst from Wall Street, accountant, receptionist, sanitation worker, emergency medical technician, licensed practical nurse, massage therapist, home health aide, and secretary. Also, I had several homemakers attempting to enter the workforce for the first time, including a politician's spouse and three students in the "welfare to work" program. Some of these students were full-time, others part-time.

After reading the scenarios above, what visual images popped into your head?

What race, gender, age, weight, and other physical, mental, and professional attributes did you visualize/imagine for each of the students and professors mentioned? Why?

What feelings were evoked as you read each scenario segment? Why?

What impact can these images and feelings have on your interactions with diverse student populations?

What impact could they potentially have on student satisfaction, stress, confidence (self-efficacy), persistence, attrition, and retention?

The nursing and higher education literature reports numerous background characteristics that influence retention and academic achievement. Often, retention or attrition studies have included one or more of the background variables to search for predictors of academic success and retention. This approach does not consider the multidimensional phenomenon of student retention. Conceptual models of student attrition in the higher education literature typically include background characteristics as a component in the model (1–6). Based on the higher education literature, conceptual models, and empirical research, a composite of student profile characteristics relevant for undergraduate nursing student retention is proposed (see Figure 1.2).

Student profile characteristics are described prior to beginning a nursing course and include age, ethnicity and race, gender, language, prior educational experience, family's educational background, prior work experience, and enrollment status. These variables provide information that is integral to determining special student needs and strengths, or identifying at-risk students. Individual variables may interact to increase or decrease risk of attrition. This chapter elaborates upon each of these characteristics, proposing ways that these characteristics may influence retention. Such awareness is a necessary first step in understanding the multidimensional process of undergraduate student retention. With a detailed appraisal of student profile characteristics, nurse educators can develop individual and student group composites that will help them design specific retention strategies aimed at maximizing student strengths and addressing student weaknesses. Each section explores how the specific characteristic is relevant to undergraduate nursing student retention.

PERSONAL BACKGROUND AND IDENTITY

What thoughts and feelings do you have about age diversity in nursing education?

Age

Greater numbers of older students are entering higher education worldwide, with notable increases reported in Australia, Ireland, the United Kingdom, and the United States. Almost half of all college students in the United States are over 25 years old (7). Consistent with global and multidisciplinary trends, the enrollment of older students in nursing programs has increased over the last decade, with projected increases to persist in the future. Consequently, the variable of age as a predictor in student performance, persistence, and graduation has been explored. Awareness of actual and perceived age-related barriers for retention is necessary if nurse educators are to understand the student retention process.

Several myths concerning age have served as barriers to retention. A prevalent myth that has been perpetuated by faculty, students, and society alike has been that older students are poorly equipped to meet the challenges of higher education and perform as well as traditional-age students. The older student has often been stereotyped and stigmatized from higher education (8,9). On campuses with older students greatly in the minority, feelings of differential treatment, uncertainty, powerlessness, and low confidence among older students have been reported. In contrast, perceptions of older students were more positive on campuses with higher numbers of older students (10). The overall institutional environment, climate, and culture should be examined with respect to age diversity. Age perception in relation to others in the academic environment can influence the academic experience.

Another barrier for older students has been that colleges have typically tailored their academic and support services for the traditional-age student. Special services are needed for older students. For example, in adult learner–centered institutions, there is a unique culture that caters to the adult learner through flexible scheduling of classes and support services, active learning experiences, and academic advisement geared to assist them (11–16). Nurse educators should appraise the openness and compatibility of the educational environment for diverse age groups.

For the traditional-age students, social integration and college adjustment within the academic institution are considered to be important predictors in determining retention (6). Students who adjust well and are socially integrated in activities, clubs, and/or sports are predicted to have higher retention rates than students who feel socially isolated and adjust poorly to the college environment. This is particularly applicable for the traditional-age students who live away from home at the college. For the older, part-time, commuter students, social integration has been viewed as less critical, especially on commuter campuses (1,2).

Study findings on age as a variable in determining performance, persistence, and retention have been inconsistent in both the nursing and higher education literature. For example, some studies suggested that age is a significant predictor of academic achievement and retention, with older students persisting longer than younger students (17,18), whereas other researchers reported contrasting results (12,19). Research contradicting the myth of the older students as disadvantaged and/or at greater risk for attrition has centered on documenting higher academic performance and higher degree attainment. Other reports indicated that older students demonstrated better study habits, more goal commitment, greater motivation, better time management, more self-direction, and preference for adult learning strategies. In contrast, younger students perform better on academic outcomes only when combined with strong indicators of academic aptitude (20).

Interestingly, Darkenwald and Novak (21) reported that grades of traditional-age (younger) students were higher in classes with higher numbers of older students. This finding contests the myth that older students have a negative impact on classroom environments; in contrast, the older students brought many desirable qualities to class that positively influence the younger students. This finding is important, as younger students have reported and/or demonstrated less effective study and time management strategies (22), lower self-efficacy, and less self-seeking help behaviors (23), variables that can adversely influence performance and retention. Among younger nursing students, lower self-concept was inversely correlated with greater test worry (24). Recently, researchers have begun to realize the need to explore the relationships between psychological distress, effort-reward imbalance, and the nursing work environment among different generations: baby boomers, Generation X, and Generation Y (25). The Millennial generation challenges educators to keep pace with the social and educational technologies that these learners expect (26–29). For example, the Net generation (1980–2004) expects technology, participates actively in the learning process, wants immediate response to learning, multitasks, prefers group work, and enjoys being mentored by older generations. In contrast, those in Generation X

(1960–1980) are self-directed learners who are less technology proficient, can delay gratification, and seek learning with practical application. Baby boomers (1940–1960) are generally less technology proficient since technology is viewed as a new approach rather than an expected approach, are more familiar with passive learning styles, and expect a caring and connected work environment (30). Clearly, age is a complex variable that needs to be viewed in relation not only to other variables but also to the interaction of students of diverse ages.

The older students have also been linked to additional role responsibilities that challenge persistence and retention; therefore, higher attrition rates have been reported for these students. Overall, the inconsistent findings may be due to one common misperception—that older students are homogenous and can be viewed as one discrete group. There is great diversity among older students, and so the interaction of other student profile characteristics must be considered. Nurse educators must be cautious in labeling all younger or older students as a homogeneous group. Thorough assessment of the interaction of multiple profile variables will help promote better understanding of the retention process.

What is the age distribution (range) and average age of your nursing school applicants, first-semester nursing students, and graduates?

Is your campus an adult-centered institution?

What impact could these elements potentially have on student satisfaction, stress, confidence (self-efficacy), persistence, attrition, and retention?

Ethnicity and Race

What thoughts and feelings do you have about ethnic and racial diversity in nursing education?

The term *ethnicity* has often been used interchangeably with race (31) although ethnicity really should acknowledge the sharing of common cultural values, beliefs, language, literature, food preferences, music, art, norms, and taboos. Race is a way of categorizing people into separate and distinct groups based on physical characteristics, geographical origins of one's ancestors, and/or social status. Historically, the main purpose of dividing people into groups was to create a hierarchical tier, maintain boundaries between groups, and prevent oppressed (minority) groups from pulling power away from the dominant (nonminority) group (31). Within this power imbalance, minority groups have encountered numerous obstacles and struggles for equality in education, privileges, work, housing, lifestyle, status, prestige, and other opportunities. Most minority groups continue to be underrepresented in higher education today (7). However, a proportionately higher number of Asian Americans attend college in comparison with the overall Asian American populations within the United States (7,32).

Nursing has not been immune to the struggles within and between minority and nonminority groups, or to the effects of such imbalances. For example, in the United States, the diversity within the nursing profession does not reflect the diversity within society; White nurses of European American heritage represent approximately 83% of all registered nurses (RNs) (33). Recent nursing enrollment trends suggest a steady increase among some minority groups. However, in proportion to demographic changes, practically no increase has been noted among Hispanic groups (33–36). Intensive recruitment efforts are imperative.

Even more disturbing are the disparities in minority student persistence. As a group, minority students incur higher attrition rates in college. Unfortunately, this is also true within the nursing discipline (37–45). Lack of role models, peer solidarity, and social integration can isolate students, thus presenting another barrier. The underrepresentation of minority groups within the nursing profession can present real and/or perceived added challenges for nursing students, further compounding minority student retention. Inclusion of "ethnicity and race" as a student profile characteristic in the Nursing Undergraduate Retention and Success (NURS) model recognizes that despite the immense diversity between and within ethnic and racial minority and nonminority groups, there are several common barriers that adversely influence nursing student retention, especially among ethnic and racial groups underrepresented in nursing. These barriers include stereotyping, prejudice, discrimination, and racism. "Ethnicity and race" in the NURS model also acknowledges that ethnicity and race affects all individuals in some way; anyone may be a potential victim of stereotyping, prejudice, discrimination, and racism.

Prior experiences with stereotyping, prejudice, discrimination, and racism in contemporary society can create fear of stereotyping, prejudice, discrimination, and racism within the academic and professional arena, thus interfering with motivation, achievement, and retention. If nurse educators are to understand the numerous ways in which ethnicity and race impact retention, they must openly acknowledge that stereotyping, prejudice, discrimination, and racism exist within nursing education and the nursing profession. The myth that these problems do not exist serves as a major barrier to understanding. University environments are microcosms of the larger society and may therefore portray and perpetuate ethnically or racially insensitive practices that create feelings of cultural incongruence and isolation among underrepresented groups (46–49).

As a subculture of the university environment, nursing may also overtly or covertly reflect and perpetuate insensitive practices.

It has been well documented that stereotyping, prejudice, discrimination, and racism exist in varying levels in nursing and nursing education (39,40,49–54). Nurse educators need to move beyond passively tolerating diversity to actively embracing it. More important, nurse educators need to anticipate student fears and actively dismantle stereotyping, prejudice, discrimination, and racism within academia, nursing, health care, and society. Individual and group self-awareness may reveal that the educational environment has been "unconsciously incompetent" in cultural sensitivity, cultural competency, and active antiracist practices. According to Purnell (55), the road to cultural competency passes various stages of being "unconsciously incompetent," "consciously incompetent," "consciously competent," and "unconsciously competent." Cultural values and beliefs are discussed in greater detail in Chapter 3.

Awareness that covert or subtle racism consciously or unconsciously create feelings of isolation, stress, and cultural pain is extremely important. Nurse educators must also acknowledge that these unwanted feelings can adversely influence retention. One example of subtle racism in nursing and health care is the prevalence of physical examination "norms" that are based on the assessment of a "White" individual (51). Stereotyping subgroups of Asian Americans as one group discounts the diversity within this group; prejudicial views that Asian American students are the "model minority" and high achiever group not only negate the academic diversity within this group but create additional pressure to reach high levels of achievement with minimal instructor assistance. Such biases can adversely affect retention (32). Assuming that all African American students are academically underprepared is another common stereotype and prejudice among many nursing faculty (51). Believing that nonminority students are less confident in caring for culturally different clients than minority students is also stereotypical and inaccurate; the danger here is that minority student's special needs concerning care of culturally different clients may never be adequately addressed (56–58). Nurse educators' expectations that are more, less, or different based solely on the student's ethnic or racial background are discriminatory and racist. Individual student strengths and needs should be objectively appraised.

Ethnicity and race have been used to identify special needs of minority students and have been examined as both sample descriptors and independent variables. The literature abounds with descriptions of minority special needs that has centered on defining characteristics of the at-risk minority students through the use of precollege and/or at-college predictors. Examples of precollege predictors included measures of academic preparedness (grade point average [GPA]), adaptability, commitment to educational goals, perceptions of progress to goals, willingness to seek academic assistance, self-confidence, reasons for pursuing a degree, and family characteristics (59). Living environment, classroom experience, advisement, extracurricular activities, financial support, and perceived faculty involvement were described as at-college predictors (59). This means that ethnicity and race should not be used exclusively to identify at-risk students or to design retention strategies. Ethnicity and race must be examined in relation to the other student profile characteristics and other components of the NURS model. A holistic appraisal will enhance the design of a diagnostic-prescriptive approach to support retention.

What ethnic and racial diversity exists within your program among your student applicants, first-semester nursing students, and graduates?

What are the predominant groups represented? How does the ethnic and racial distribution compare with ethnic and racial groups in the geographic region serviced by the educational institution and health care agencies?

What ethnic and racial diversity exists among your nursing faculty, college-wide faculty, and staff?

What ethnic and racial diversity exists among RNs, unlicensed personnel, physicians, other professionals, and patients in nursing students' clinical placement sites?

What impact could these elements potentially have on student satisfaction, stress, confidence (self-efficacy), persistence, attrition, and retention?

Gender

What thoughts and feelings do you have about gender diversity in nursing education?

Bean and Metzner (1) reported gender as a background and defining variable that influenced nontraditional student attrition. Higher attrition rates were reported for nontraditional male students than for nontraditional female students among multidisciplinary college populations (1). Other studies have found no real gender effect (20). Although the numbers of men in nursing are increasing, they remain an underrepresented minority within the traditionally female profession (60). Due to the disproportionate number of men, gender has generally been examined as a sample descriptor within studies of nursing student attrition. In recent years, because the nursing literature reports the unique experience of the male nursing student, a different examination of gender has been proposed.

Understanding that the experience of the male nursing student is unique is an important first step toward enhancing retention (60–64). High school counselors' misperceptions and lack of adequate knowledge about the rigors of nursing as a profession have steered many men away from nursing as a viable career option (65–67). Societal misperceptions labeling nursing as a "feminine" profession have been a hindrance in recruiting and retaining men in nursing. In comparison with the recent support for women entering nontraditional work roles, there has been little support for men breaking gender barriers (60,62–64,68). Additionally, the support for women entering the workforce has shifted away from encouraging traditional female professions. In fact, Constantine and Watt (47) reported that gender role perception and womanist identity attitudes may actually create high levels of anger toward women who pursue traditional gender roles.

Gender-related barriers to retention within the nursing profession must be addressed if retention is to be enhanced. Such barriers include overt and covert bias and discrimination. For example, equal opportunities in clinical education and clinical work settings are often lacking, sometimes resulting in legal action (61). Among men, prevalent perceptions of being treated differently from female nurses and/or female students contribute to feelings of loneliness, isolation, and self-doubt (61,63,64,67,69–71). Fear of being perceived as unmanly and questions by others concerning sexual orientation serves to further isolate men (61,62,65,67,72). Social isolation has frequently been reported as adversely influencing retention. Lack of role modeling and professional socialization for male nursing students has been problematic as well (60,62,70).

Boughn (72) cautions against stereotyping the experiences and needs of male students, noting two distinct groups of men reported in the nursing literature. One group has been described as the older, second-career individuals who are often members of a lower socioeconomic class. The second group consists of men in their late teens or early twenties who enter nursing immediately after high school. Yet, within these two groups, much diversity exists. Like other student profile characteristics, gender must be viewed in context, recognizing the powerful interaction among factors.

What gender diversity exists within your program among your student applicants, first-semester nursing students, and graduates?

What gender diversity exists within various ethnic, racial, and age groups?

What gender diversity exists among your nursing faculty, college-wide faculty, and staff?

What gender diversity exists among RNs, unlicensed personnel, physicians, other professionals, and patients in nursing students' clinical placement sites?

What impact could these elements potentially have on student satisfaction, stress, confidence (self-efficacy), persistence, attrition, and retention?

Language

What are your thoughts and feelings about language diversity in nursing education?

Global trends and increased immigration around the world have resulted in increased numbers of students whose first language is different from that used in the educational institution. The term *first language* is defined here as the primary, native home language used for listening, speaking, reading, writing, and thinking. Some students who relocate to different countries several times over the course of their primary, secondary, and postsecondary educational process may understand, speak, read, write, and think in several languages on varying levels of fluency and comprehension. Students whose first language is not the same as the one used in school will have special academic and nonacademic needs (73–85).

For the purposes of this book, the focus will be on English as the language used in the nursing school. Students whose first language is English (EFL) will be differentiated from students whose first language is not English. Although the literal meaning of the term *English as second language* or ESL may not truly describe student populations who encountered English as a third, fourth, or fifth language, in this book the term ESL will conceptually mean anyone whose first language is other than standard English. Standard English refers to English that is commonly expected on a college level.

Consistent with global and national trends in higher education, nursing programs in the United States, Canada, the United Kingdom, and Australia have also experienced an increase in ESL populations over the past decade. ESL student populations have been identified as at-risk students, yielding higher rates of attrition and demonstrating unique educational needs. With the emphasis on student retention, the NURS model focuses on identifying the student's first language to help identify subgroups within the ESL group so that appropriate interventions can be designed to enhance retention. Categorizing all ESL students together really oversimplifies the complexity of the ESL experience.

It is important to recognize that the ESL experience is not solely focused on language but involves a multidimensional approach to understanding the ESL student holistically. Students who speak the same first language may be quite diverse in their cultural values and beliefs, ethnic and racial identities, socioeconomic level, and immigration status. Prior educational, lifestyle, and acculturation experiences of an international student are different from those of an immigrant or refugee. Each group may have different first- and second-language skills that are further complicated by the interaction of diverse factors, all of which put ESL students at greater risk for attrition.

Awareness of the complexities of the ESL experience is a necessary first step toward promoting retention. Clearly, although language considerations need to be addressed, nonacademic factors can outweigh language barriers and adversely affect learning, achievement, and retention. Acculturation stress, adaptation, assimilation, cultural values, beliefs toward education, experiences with second language, and expectations can impact greatly upon learning, achievement, and retention. These factors are discussed in greater detail in Chapters 3 and 10. Efforts at professional socialization and retention must assess the unique needs of various ESL students on a subgroup and individual basis, integrating language development skills, socialization, and acculturation measures within a culturally congruent framework (74,78,79,81–84,86,87).

What language diversity exists within your program among your student applicants, first-semester nursing students, and graduates?

What are the predominant groups represented? How does the language distribution compare with languages spoken in the geographic region serviced by the educational institution and health care agencies?

What language diversity exists among your nursing faculty, college-wide faculty, and staff?

What language diversity exists among RNs, unlicensed personnel, physicians, other professionals, and patients in nursing students' clinical placement sites?

What impact could these elements potentially have on student satisfaction, stress, confidence (self-efficacy), persistence, attrition, and retention?

EDUCATIONAL AND WORK BACKGROUND

Prior Educational Experience

What are your thoughts and feelings about students' prior educational experience, academic preparedness, educational diversity within the classroom, and predictors of academic success?

Prior educational experience includes precollege variables (high school performance or general equivalency diploma [GED]), prenursing program variables such as prenursing college course performance, and postsecondary education and degrees. For the older students who have never been to college, precollege variables may not be accurate predictors of academic aptitude, achievement, or attrition (20). They may be more appropriate for traditional students who enter college immediately after high school. Majority students with a high secondary school GPA (grade point average) and excellent attendance records are predicted to have greater success in college. High school performance, however, has been less predictive for minority (18,32,88–90), disadvantaged (91–93), and/or first-generation college students (94–96).

Use of high school performance or SAT scores as the sole predictor for college success should be avoided (97). Higher education in general is flooded with more academically diverse and less prepared students worldwide (98,99). Nursing programs are similarly challenged (78,100–103). Nurse educators will need to develop new measures to assist academically diverse student populations.

Routine assessment of other variables such as the type of secondary school program, gaps in educational experience, place of education, and language used for education will help analyze strengths and weaknesses within today's academically diverse population. Type of secondary school program (college preparatory, honors, advanced placement, vocational, technical, or general) should also be viewed in relation to GPA. Additionally, students from at-risk school districts may have other educational disadvantages that will impact college achievement and retention. For example, lack of supplies and materials in impoverished areas may have provided limited educational opportunities, thus creating an educationally disadvantaged environment and increasing risk for poor college performance. Racism, discrimination, lowered teacher expectations, and negative support from peers in at-risk school districts can further intensify an educationally disadvantaged environment and limit student success (42,90,93,94,104–106).

Gaps between the last educational experience and the current enrollment in a nursing program indicate the need for transitional (nonacademic) support, any refresher knowledge and skill updates, or remedial courses. More remedial courses are needed in proportion to older students and with the length of time elapsed between enrollments (107). Among educators, there is much disagreement about what constitutes remediation (107). Remedial courses have been defined as reading, writing, and math for college students lacking the necessary skills for performing work at the level stipulated by the educational institution (106). In nursing and the health sciences, remediation can be extended to include courses in biology, chemistry, and/or physics that would give students the necessary skills and background for performing college-level work in science courses. Test scores usually determine whether a student is able to enter required college-level courses for the nursing major. Unfortunately, scores on an exam may not differentiate between the need for remedial, refresher, or update courses.

For the purposes of this book, differentiation between terms is important. Remedial coursework is for students who never had an adequate level of skill or knowledge in an area. Refresher courses are for students who previously attained knowledge; however, gaps in education have resulted in "forgetting" information or skills. Update courses are courses for students who previously attained knowledge and skills in a particular area and have retained the knowledge and skills as presented at their last educational experience, yet are missing essential new knowledge and skills. For example, an older, second-career student with a baccalaureate degree in biology earned 20 years ago may really need an update in knowledge rather than a remedial course. In contrast, a recent immigrant who earned a GED after leaving secondary school 2 years ago may need intensive immersion in remedial work to develop skills and knowledge necessary for beginning college-level biology. Failing grades on a college placement exam may place these two students in the same remedial class despite the unique and different needs of each. This type of mismatch can be discouraging to students and interfere with persistence behaviors.

For students educated in other countries, it may be difficult to evaluate learning experiences, grades, standards, degrees, and certifications. The primary language of prior educational experience(s) may also impact retention. What can be generalized, however, is that students educated in foreign countries had different educational experiences that may create actual or perceived advantages and disadvantages for them. The learning needs and expectations of foreign-educated students may be very different from what faculty perceive, thus creating another obstacle for learning, achievement, satisfaction, and retention (85).

Prior educational experience in college includes the learning process, persistence behaviors, and outcomes (grades and degree attainment). Students with prior college degrees are believed to have higher retention rates due to prior knowledge of what to expect in college, less credits needed to complete current degree sought, and a better financial status (108). Students with and without college degrees may underestimate the academic rigor and time demands of a nursing program. Prior college transcripts should be reviewed for the number of course withdrawals, repeats, and failures, as well as overall GPA, grades achieved in science courses, and transfer history. Some research supports that science course grades serve as strong predictors of success in nursing programs and on passing the NCLEX exam (109–112). Yet other studies over the last 30 years suggest that these variables are not sufficient in explaining student retention and success (113–115). Benda (116) found that the most important predictor of success was whether prerequisite courses were taken at a junior or senior college. Science courses were less predictive if course grades were transferred from another college or if the course was taken over 2 years ago (111). Additionally, transfer history can reveal whether the student had short-term and/or long-term commitments to the previously selected institution(s) and major(s). Strong goal commitment has been identified as a positive predictor of retention (2).

Lagtime, or the number of years between a student's last enrollment at another college and the student's entry into college currently, has been explored as a predictor for retention (117). Among older students, longer lagtime has been correlated with higher GPA; however, among younger students, longer lagtime seems to be a disadvantage. Short-term interruptions, or stopouts, appear to be more prevalent among older students, and it is believed that among older students, stopouts are viewed as more acceptable than among traditional-age students (117). This phenomenon is not surprising, considering that older students often have more responsibilities external to the academic institution. The influence of environmental variables on retention are discussed in greater detail in Chapter 5.

Assessment of prior college experience can identify educationally disadvantaged students at risk for attrition and provide essential information for designing strategies to address educational weaknesses and to maximize strengths. Academically well-prepared students may be put at risk for attrition if emphasis is put on the academically weak students. A myopic view of seeing only the academically weak students as at risk for attrition will ignore and isolate the strengths and needs of academically well-prepared students. Remembering that even strong students need support is crucial. For example, Olenchak and Hebert (94) found that gifted students who are first-generation college students often underachieve in college and have high rates of attrition. Capitalizing on student strengths and assessing academically well-prepared students for other risk factors for attrition is a necessary step in promoting overall retention.

What educational diversity exists among your nursing student applicants, first-semester nursing students, and graduates?

What impact could educational diversity potentially have on student satisfaction, stress, confidence (self-efficacy), persistence, attrition, and retention?

Family Educational Background

What are your thoughts and feelings about first-generation college students? About the influence of family educational background on your nursing students' retention and success?

With greater numbers of first-generation college students entering higher education, exploring the family's educational background deserves attention. Many studies have indicated that parents' level of formal education is a powerful predictor of traditional-student persistence, placing first-generation college students at greater risk for attrition (95,96,118–123). Nursing programs have also seen an increase in first-generation college students, especially among student groups traditionally underrepresented in nursing (39,40,45,93,124,125). In the NURS model, family's educational background includes the level of formal education for the students, parents, siblings, spouse, significant other(s), children, and grandchildren.

In two studies of nontraditional nursing student retention, students who selected and actively participated in enrichment program peer mentor-tutor study groups were predominantly the first individuals in their family to attend college (126,127). Several explanations may be proposed for this phenomenon of self-selection. These first-generation college students may have perceived themselves at a disadvantage and therefore perceived a greater need for peer mentoring-tutoring than other students. Another explanation may be that these first-generation college students were more motivated, self-directed, and seeking self-help interventions. Perhaps the opportunity for socialization within college and the nursing profession was quite desirable for first-generation college students. This phenomenon warrants further exploration.

Why Is the Experience Different?

The higher education literature examining traditional-age first-generation college student persistence has identified three major areas resulting in disadvantages that increase attrition risk: precollege, transitional, and college experience (128). First, differences in planning for college, college selection, and expectations for college put students at an initial disadvantage. Students and families may not have realistic plans, choices, or expectations. Second, the transition between high school or work and college is often a cultural, as well as a social and academic, one for the first-generation college students. As the first person in a family to enter college, the student experiences losses and gains, creating sources of potential conflict and feelings of isolation. Third, first-generation college students have more difficulty integrating academically and socially within the college environment, thus increasing the risk for a stressful, unsatisfied, or unhappy college experience (94–96,121–123,128,129). Awareness of the family's educational background, and of the issues surrounding the overall experience of the first-generation college student, can help nurse educators proactively design strategies to assist students during all three phases and enhance retention through positive experiences and realistic expectations.

Several researchers suggest the need to further explore the role parental socialization has in college choice and expectations, especially among

Latinos where college enrollment is lowest (35,130,131). Family expectations for college, despite family's educational background, were highest among Asian Americans (32,131). Although emotional support may be high for the first person in the family to attend college, the student may feel much pressure to succeed, achieve high grades, and fulfill family expectations. As mentioned previously, even gifted first-generation college students often have high rates of attrition (94). Conversely, in families with multigenerational college degrees, it may also be expected that achieving a college degree is the norm. As a female-dominated profession, nursing may be particularly influenced by the degree attainments of women family members. Family expectations that conflict with student expectations and goals can adversely affect student performance. Nurse educators' sensitivity to student-perceived stress and expectations relative to family expectations is important. Additionally, recognizing the potential obstacles faced by first-generation college students is a critical step.

Among nontraditional populations, women with partners who had earned college degrees perceived less pressure to leave college (132). This finding was compounded by the influence of income as persons with college degrees generally earn higher salaries; people without college degrees usually earn lower salaries and have less realistic expectations and insight about college. It is not surprising that low-income groups apply less frequently to college (131) and have lower retention rates. Financial status as an environmental factor is addressed in Chapter 5.

What is the percentage of first-generation college students among your nursing student applicants, first-semester nursing students, and graduates?

What impact could this element potentially have on student satisfaction, stress, confidence (self-efficacy), persistence, attrition, and retention?

Prior Work Experience

What are your thoughts and feelings about prior work experience among college students? About the influence of prior work experience on your nursing students' retention and success?

Examining prior work experience in light of a restructured workforce, economic crisis, unemployment, welfare-to-work initiatives, displaced homemakers, and second-career options can be beneficial. During economic changes, increases in public university enrollment, particularly associate degree programs, have occurred due to the swift entry into the workforce, open admissions, and lower tuition investment with high earning return potential. Prior work experience suggests that the student had a commitment to a task, needed to meet certain responsibilities within a particular time frame, and is familiar with the workplace environment. Men may enter a nursing program with considerable work experience, whereas women may have little or none (133). Displaced homemakers without any prior work experience may feel insecure next to classmates who do have prior work experience. Housewives, female professionals, or paraprofessionals whose work experience was dissatisfying, low paying, and with little chance for career advancement were more motivated to persist in college and less likely to withdraw (132).

National initiatives aimed at alleviating the nursing shortage emphasize career mobility within the health care field. Although students who work in the health care field as unlicensed personnel, licensed practical nurses (LPNs), or other health care paraprofessionals have prior work experience, they may have difficulty adjusting to a new role, new worldview, more critical thinking, and decision making within a perspective guided by the professional scope of nursing practice (134). Linking students with peer mentors who are further along in the career ladder may be beneficial (134,135). Reluctance or inability to change existing views, practices, and work habits may lead to unsafe practices and poor learning outcomes. Overconfidence in self-performance and learning can lead to lack of adequate preparation, failure, and attrition (see Chapter 3).

In nursing programs where high numbers of students have prior health care experience, nurse educators should recognize that those without this experience might perceive themselves as at a disadvantage. Low self-efficacy (confidence) may lead to low goal commitment, more stress, and decreased persistence, therefore potentially challenging retention. Focusing on the unique talents and life experiences of all students may help clarify any misperceptions of deficits, particularly in the clinical area. Students with prior experience may feel pressured to never make a mistake; the need to excel may interfere with learning, performance, and retention. Nurse educators must remember that although prior health care experience may present the student with some advantages, the special transitional and socialization needs of these students must be routinely appraised and addressed if all student potentials are to be maximized. Attitudes of faculty toward LPNs and their special needs may also need modification (135).

What type of prior work experience exists among your nursing student applicants, first-semester nursing students, and graduates?

What impact could prior work experience potentially have on student satisfaction, stress, confidence (self-efficacy), persistence, attrition, and retention?

Enrollment Status

What are your thoughts and feelings about students' full-time and part-time enrollment in an undergraduate nursing program?

What are your thoughts and feelings about student enrollment at a commuter campus, a residential campus, and a commuter at a predominantly residential 4-year college? What do you feel, think, and know about the influence of enrollment status on your nursing students' retention and success?

Enrollment status refers to whether a student is enrolled full-time (12 or more credits), part-time (less than 12 credits), matriculated, non-matriculated, commuter, or campus resident. Almost half of all college students attend part-time. Consistent with trends in higher education, the number of part-time nursing students has increased. Retention rates are highest among traditional-age full-time college students who reside in campus housing (92,120,136). Nonmatriculated students and part-time students tend to withdraw more than matriculated and full-time students (120,137,138). Purely commuter campuses tend to have the lowest retention rates with more nonmatriculated students attending part-time (120,139). Part-time commuter students tend to interact less with the academic environment than do traditional full-time students (1,2,120,140). Students' enrollment status needs to be viewed in context with the type of institution (commuter versus residential and community college, 4-year college, accelerated program, or hospital school of nursing). Matriculated students have a stronger evidence of goal commitment through their already invested time, money, and credits toward the nursing major.

In combination with other environmental variables, enrollment may create multiple role conflicts for part-time but especially full-time students who have other responsibilities. Work-family-student conflict is defined as incompatible pressures arising simultaneously from the work, family, and student roles (141). The influence of environmental variables on retention is discussed in Chapter 5; the influence of stress is discussed in Chapter 7.

What is the percentage of full-time and part-time enrollment among your nursing student applicants, first-semester nursing students, and graduates?

What is the percentage of students who commute to campus among your nursing student applicants, first-semester nursing students, and graduates?

What impact could this element potentially have on student satisfaction, stress, confidence (self-efficacy), persistence, attrition, and retention?

INTERACTION WITH OTHER MODEL DIMENSIONS

Student profile characteristics have a direct influence on academic factors, cultural values and beliefs, self-efficacy, motivation, and environmental factors. A bidirectional relationship is proposed between professional integration and professional socialization. This proposition recognizes that individual and combined efforts at professional integration and socialization may positively or negatively influence how student profile characteristics are viewed. For example, a male student who perceives himself to be integrated and positively socialized within the nursing profession may not perceive gender as an obstacle to success. Similarly, an African American student at a predominantly White university who attends a conference sponsored by the National Black Nurses Association (NBNA) and who is paired with an NBNA mentor may change his or her views about race as an obstacle or as a strength within the nursing profession. Pairing ESL students at varying levels of the educational process can minimize language as a perceived obstacle. Although family educational background at the start of the nursing educational process will remain unchanged, professional socialization and integration efforts can minimize the students' concern with not belonging in college.

KEY POINT SUMMARY

- Student profile characteristics are described prior to beginning a nursing course and include age, ethnicity and race, gender, language, prior educational experience, family's educational background, prior work experience, and enrollment status.
- Nurse educators' expectations that are more, less, or different based on a single student profile characteristic are detrimental since individual student strengths and needs are not objectively appraised.
- Student profile characteristics have a direct influence on academic factors, cultural values and beliefs, self-efficacy, motivation, and environmental factors.
- A bidirectional relationship is proposed between professional integration and professional socialization. This proposition recognizes that individual and combined efforts at professional integration and socialization may positively or negatively influence how student profile characteristics are viewed.

APPLICATION STRATEGIES

EASY APPLICATION ACTION STEPS

Determining Student Profile Composites for Retention, Attrition, and Licensure Rates

1. Obtain student profile data for each trajectory in Figure 1.1.

2. Identify student profile trends within your program's trajectory pathway options.
3. Propose percentages of increase and decrease for student profile categories within each pathway option.

EDUCATOR-IN-ACTION VIGNETTE

Without appropriate background knowledge, individual appraisal, and sensitivity, educator actions may adversely impact students' academic and psychological outcomes, persistence, and retention. Consider the possible adverse effects of the following educator actions:

After the first preconference prior to the first clinical day, Professor Hurdles individually tells Marsha, a 25-year-old African American student, that she should go to the college's math and English tutoring center before administering medications and writing nursing progress notes. Marsha earned a baccalaureate degree with honors from a private university and majored in mathematics. For 3 years, she taught high school algebra, geometry, and AP calculus. After caring for a terminally ill family member, Marsha decided to return to college to become an RN.

Cindy is a 20-year-old White student who lived in many foster homes throughout much of her childhood, resulting in frequent elementary and secondary school transfers. She ran away from her last foster home at age 16 and dropped out of high school; however, she completed her GED 1 year ago. She feels insecure and has low confidence about her academic ability. She is just about to ask Professor Hurdles where she can get some extra help when Professor Hurdles says, "It's nice to see a young student have all her priorities straight and enter nursing right after high school. I expect you to excel without difficulty."

After several weeks, one male student (Juan) mentions to other students and another clinical instructor, "I wish that I would get the same clinical opportunities as the female students in my clinical group. I have not been assigned to any female patients. How will I learn to feel comfortable interviewing female patients if I never have the opportunity? Doesn't Professor Hurdles trust me?" Another student, Harry adds, "I feel the same way. It seems that I always have the assignment with male patients who require heavy lifting and physical care. I thought the nursing profession for men involved more than lifting, moving, and bed baths."

Kim is a foreign student from Korea who has only been in the United States for 2 years. She currently has a 3.7 GPA in prenursing courses. Her mastery of the English language in such a short time is remarkable, although she speaks with a heavy (but understandable) accent. Professor Hurdles assigns Kim to a Japanese patient (who only speaks Japanese) and says, "I am sure you will have no trouble communicating with your patient now."

In contrast to these examples, educator actions that embrace diverse student profile characteristics, are knowledgeable, appreciate students as individuals, maximize strengths, and improve weaknesses have the most potential for promoting positive academic and psychological outcomes, persistence, and retention. For example, during the first clinical preconference, Professor Bridges welcomes all the students stating, "I look forward to a wonderful semester. We are fortunate to have such a diverse group because each of you undoubtedly has individual strengths, experiences, insights, and talents that can be shared with others, enriching the overall group and ultimately benefiting patient care. On your index card, please write down your personal strengths. We will discuss them in a few minutes."

After ten minutes, Professor Bridges says, "Everyone may have areas that you may be concerned about or areas that you would like additional help, guidance, or experience with. On the other side of the index card, please write these areas." During the group discussion, Professor Bridges asks each student to share a perceived strength and an area for professional development, personal growth, or concern. Select student responses follow:

LUCIENNE: Many people think I am African American, but I came to the United States 3 years ago after residing in four other countries. Since I speak French and Spanish fluently, I would be happy to help anyone with translations but I don't really know about all the cultural customs among the different groups who speak these languages. Multiple-choice questions are difficult for me. This is not the type of testing I am accustomed to, especially on the computer.

ROSEANNE: I don't really have anything important to share. I am 36, and my family questions why I am going to college to become a nurse. No one in my family ever went to college. I am just a housewife and mom who attends school part-time. I always wanted to be a nurse. I love talking with people and want to work in pediatrics.

DOUGLAS: You both could be a big help to me. I worked for 10 years in the computer field until the company went bankrupt. I'm really more comfortable with computers than talking with people. Since I lived in a small town my whole life and only moved to this big city recently, I am not sure of how to interact with people of different cultures. Everything seems so fast paced. I wish I had your lifetime motivation about nursing.

After each presentation, Professor Bridges thanks each student individually for his or her contribution, offers constructive suggestions, and asks for other student input. Individual, paired, and group learning experiences are then developed throughout the semester with students building on each other's strengths. Although the sharing of student perceptions permits Professor Bridges to gain insight into the individual student experience, she also identifies potential areas of strengths and weaknesses associated with each student profile characteristic (such as acculturation stress and multiple role conflict), appraises students individually, and offers appropriate resources and support accordingly.

TOOLKIT RESOURCE BOX

Item 13—Nursing Student Progress Pathway

Item 15—Learner and Program Characteristics

Item 9—Demographic Data Sheet—Prelicensure (DDS-P)

Item 10—Demographic Data Sheet—RN-BSN (DDS-RN)

Items 1–4—Student Perception Appraisal Questionnaires—Pretests and Posttests

Item 21—Who Are At-Risk Students?

Item 23—Promoting Positive Help-Seeking Behaviors

Item 24—Appraising Teaching Strategies: Potential Effect on Diverse Populations

Item 26—Strategy Mapping Across the Curriculum

Item 29—Culturally Congruent Approach to Faculty Advisement and Helpfulness

---

DISCUSSION QUESTIONS

1. When you read the Educator-in-Action Vignette, what visual images popped into your head? What race, gender, age, weight, and other physical, mental, and professional attributes did you visualize/imagine for each student, Professor Hurdles, and Professor Bridges? Why? What feelings were evoked as you read each scenario? Why? What impact can these images and feelings have on your interactions with diverse student populations? What impact could they potentially have on student persistence, satisfaction, stress, self-efficacy (confidence), attrition, and retention?

2. Professor Hurdles's students share the information highlighted in the Educator-in-Action Vignette with you because you are the course coordinator. How would you respond?

3. Review the student profile characteristics presented in the chapter. Which one provided you with the most new information and insights? Why? How will this change your teaching, advisement, and interaction with students?

4. Complete the following demographic questions about yourself. Mark one response.

Age: ___18–21   ___22–25   ___Over 85   ___Other
Ethnicity: ___Khmer   ___Moroccan   ___Sudanese ___Hmong ___Other
Race: ___Green   ___Blue   ___Purple   ___Other
Primary
language: ___Cherokee ___Hawaiian   ___Gaelic   ___Other
Health care
profession: ___Physician ___Chiropractor ___Dentist   ___Other

How would your profile characteristics be described based on your responses? Will you be visible or invisible in relation to the groups/category choices presented? Are you in the "in" group or the "other" group? How did you feel completing the questionnaire? What concerns do you have concerning validity of data? How are student profile data collected in your program and college? What modifications would you suggest? Why?

5. What are the student profile characteristics of the students in your class, the first-semester nursing students, and graduating students? How are data collected? What changes to data collection would you suggest? Why?

REFERENCES

1. Bean, J. P., & Metzner, B. (1985). A conceptual model of nontraditional undergraduate student attrition. *Review of Educational Research, 55*, 485–540.
2. Metzner, B., & Bean, J. P. (1987). The estimation of a conceptual model of nontraditional undergraduate student attrition. *Research in Higher Education, 27*, 15–38.
3. Nora, A. (1987). Determinants of retention among Chicano college students: A structural model. *Research in Higher Education, 26*, 31–60.
4. Pascarella, E. T., & Chapman, D. W. (1983). Validation of a theoretical model of college withdrawal: Interaction effects in a multi-institutional sample. *Research in Higher Education, 19*, 25–47.
5. Spady, W. (1970). Dropouts from higher education: Toward an empirical model. *Interchange, 2*, 38–62.
6. Tinto, V. (1997). Classrooms as communities. *Journal of Higher Education, 68*(6), 599–623.
7. U.S. Department of Education, National Center for Education Statistics. (2011). *The condition of education, 2011.* Washington, DC: Author.
8. Richardson, J. T. E. (1995). Mature students in higher education: II. An investigation of approaches to studying and academic performance. *Studies in Higher Education, 20*, 5–17.
9. Richardson, J. T. E. (1994). Mature students in higher education: I. A literature survey on approaches to studying. *Studies in Higher Education, 19*, 309–325.

10. Lynch, J. M., & Bishop-Clark, C. (1998). A comparison of the nontraditional students' experience on traditional versus nontraditional college campuses. *Innovative Higher Education, 22*(3), 217–229.
11. Mancuso, S. (2001). Adult-centered practices: Benchmarking study in higher education. *Innovative Higher Education, 25*(3), 165–181.
12. Murtaugh, P. A., Burns, L. D., & Schuster, J. (1999). Predicting the retention of university students. *Research in Higher Education, 40*(3), 355–371.
13. Chaves, C. (2006). Involvement, development, and retention: Theoretical foundations and potential extensions for adult community college students. *Community College Review, 34*(2), 139–152.
14. O'Brien, F., Keogh, B., & Neenan, K. (2009). Mature students' experiences of undergraduate nurse education programmes: The Irish experience. *Nurse Education Today, 29*, 635–640.
15. Steele, R., Lauder, W., & Caperchione, C. (2005). An exploratory study of the concerns of mature access to nursing students and the coping strategies used to manage these adverse experiences. *Nurse Education Today, 25*, 573–581.
16. Fleming, S., & McKee, G. (2005). The mature student question. *Nurse Education Today, 25*, 230–237.
17. DeFelice, C. E. (1989). *The relationship between self-efficacy and academic achievement in associate degree nursing programs.* Unpublished doctoral dissertation, Teachers College, Columbia University, New York.
18. Manifold, C., & Rambur, B. (2001). Predictors of attrition in American Indian nursing students. *Journal of Nursing Education, 40*(6), 279–281.
19. Allen, C. B., Higgs, Z. R., & Holloway, J. R. (1988). Identifying students at risk for academic difficulty. *Journal of Professional Nursing, 4*(2), 113–118.
20. Hoskins, S. L., Newstead, S. E., & Dennis, I. (1997). Degree performance as a function of age, gender, prior qualifications and discipline studied. *Assessment and Evaluation in Higher Education, 22*(3), 317–328.
21. Darkenwald, G. G., & Novak, R. J. (1997). Classroom age composition and academic achievement in college. *Adult Education Quarterly, 47*(2), 108–116.
22. Devlin, M. (1996). Older and wiser? A comparison of the learning and study strategies of mature age and younger teacher education students. *Higher Education Research and Development, 15*(1), 51–60.
23. Gianakos, I. (1996). Career development differences between adult and traditional-aged learners. *Journal of Career Development, 22*(3), 211–223.
24. Waltman, P. A. (1997). Comparison of traditional and non-traditional baccalaureate nursing students on selected components of Meichenbaum and Butler's model of test anxiety. *Journal of Nursing Education, 36*(4), 171–179.
25. Lavoie-Tremblay, M., Wright, D., Desforges, N., Gelinas, C., Marchionni, C., & Drevniok, U. (2008). Creating a healthy workplace for new-generation nurses. *Journal of Nursing Scholarship, 40*(3), 290–297.
26. Bellack, J. P. (2009). Integrating diversity. *Journal of Nursing Education, 48*(9), 475–476.
27. Zalon, M. L. (2008). Using technology to build community in professional associations. *The Journal of Continuing Education in Nursing, 39*(5), 235–240.
28. Johnson, S. A., & Romanello, M. L. (2005). Generational diversity: Teaching and learning approaches. *Nurse Educator, 30*(5), 212–216.
29. Mangold, K. (2007). Educating a new generation: Teaching baby boomer faculty about millennial students. *Nurse Educator, 32*(1), 21–23.

30. Billings, D. M., & Kowalski, K. (2009). Nurses working with librarians. *Journal of Continuing Education in Nursing, 40*(1), 16–17.

31. Root, M. P. P. (1992). Within, between, and beyond race. In M. P. P. Root (Ed.), *Racially mixed people in America* (pp. 3–11). Newbury Park, CA: Sage.

32. Ting, S.-M. R. (2000). Predicting Asian Americans' academic performance in the first year of college: An approach combining SAT scores and noncognitive variables. *Journal of College Student Development, 41*(4), 442–449.

33. U.S. Department of Health and Human Services. (2010). *The registered nurse population: Findings from the March 2008 National Sample Survey of Registered Nurses.* Retrieved from http://bhpr.hrsa.gov/healthworkforce/rnsurveys/rnsurveyfinal.pdf

34. Heller, B. R., Oros, M. T., & Durney-Crowley, J. (2000). The future of nursing education: 10 trends to watch. *Nursing and Health Care Perspectives, 21*(1), 9–13.

35. Villaruel, A. M., Canales, M., & Torres, S. (2001). Bridges and barriers: Educational mobility of Hispanic nurses. *Journal of Nursing Education, 40*(6), 245–251.

36. Bond, M. L., Gray, J. R., Baxley, S., Cason, C. L., & Denke, L. (2008). Voices of Hispanic students in baccalaureate nursing programs: Are we listening? *Nursing Education Perspectives, 29*(3), 136–142.

37. Bessent, H. (1997). *Strategies for recruitment, retention, and graduation of minority nurses in colleges of nursing.* Washington, DC: American Nurses Publishing.

38. Mills-Wisneski, S. M. (2003). African-American baccalaureate nursing students' perceptions of nursing programs and factors that support or restrict academic success (Doctoral dissertation, Widener University, 2003). (UMI No. 3083001).

39. Tucker-Allen, S., & Long, E. (1999). *Recruitment and retention of minority students: Stories of success.* Lisle, IL: Tucker Publications.

40. Bosher, S. D., & Pharris, M. D. (2009). *Transforming nursing education: The culturally inclusive environment.* New York: Springer.

41. Gardner, J. (2005). Barriers influencing the success of racial and ethnic minority students in nursing programs. *Journal of Transcultural Nursing, 16*(2), 155–162.

42. Gilchrist, K. L., & Rector, C. (2007). Can you keep them? Strategies to attract and retain nursing students from diverse populations: Best practices in nursing education. *Journal of Transcultural Nursing, 18*(3), 277–285.

43. DeLapp, T., Hautman, M. A., & Anderson, M. S. (2008). Recruitment and retention of Alaska natives into nursing (RRANN). *Journal of Nursing Education, 47*(7), 293–297.

44. Evans, B. C. (2008). "Attached at the umbilicus": Barriers to educational success for Hispanic/Latino and American Indian nursing students. *Journal of Professional Nursing, 24,* 205–217.

45. Ackerman-Barger, P. W. (2010). Embracing multiculturalism in nursing learning environments. *Journal of Nursing Education, 49*(12), 677–682.

46. Brown, L. L., & Kurpius, S. E. R. (1997). Psychosocial factors influencing academic persistence of American Indian college students. *Journal of College Student Development, 38*(1), 3–12.

47. Constantine, M. G., & Watt, S. K. (2002). Cultural congruity, womanist identity attitudes, and life satisfaction among African American college women

attending historically black and predominantly white institutions. *Journal of College Student Development, 43*(2), 184–193.

48. Constantine, M. G., Robinson, J. S., Wilton, L., & Caldwell, L. D. (2002). Collective self-esteem and perceived social support as predictors of cultural congruity among black and Latino college students. *Journal of College Student Development, 43*(3), 307–316.
49. Love, K. L. (2010). The lived experience of socialization among African American nursing students in a predominantly white university. *Journal of Transcultural Nursing, 21*(4), 342–350.
50. Abrums, M. E., & Leppa, C. (2001). Beyond cultural competence: Teaching about race, gender, class, and sexual orientation. *Journal of Nursing Education, 40*(6), 270–275.
51. Barbee, E. L., & Gibson, S. E. (2001). Our dismal progress: The recruitment of non-whites into nursing. *Journal of Nursing Education, 40*(6), 243–244.
52. Farella, C. (2002). School of hard knocks: Is racism a fixture of nursing academia? *Nursing Spectrum, 14*(12), 34–35.
53. Yearwood, E., Brown, D. L., & Karlik, E. C. (2002). Cultural diversity: Students' perspectives. *Journal of Transcultural Nursing, 13*(3), 237–240.
54. Martin, D. E., & Kipling, A. (2006). Factors shaping Aboriginal nursing students' experiences. *Nurse Education Today, 26*, 688–696.
55. Purnell, L. D. (2008). Purnell's model for cultural competence. In L. D. Purnell & B. J. Paulanka (Eds.), *Transcultural health care: A culturally competent approach* (3rd ed., pp 19–55). Philadelphia, PA: FA Davis.
56. Jeffreys, M. R., & Smodlaka, I. (1999). Changes in students' transcultural self-efficacy perceptions following an integrated approach to culture care. *Journal of Multicultural Nursing and Health, 5*(2), 6–12 [Erratum, 2000, 6(2)].
57. Jeffreys, M. R., & Smodlaka, I. (1999). Construct validation of the Transcultural Self-Efficacy Tool. *Journal of Nursing Education, 38*, 222–227.
58. Jeffreys, M. R. (2010). *Teaching cultural competence in nursing and health care: Inquiry, action, and innovation* (2nd ed.). New York: Springer.
59. Levin, M. E., & Levin, J. R. (1991). A critical examination of academic retention programs for at-risk minority college students. *Journal of College Student Development, 32*, 323–334.
60. Brady, M. S., & Sherrod, D. R. (2003). Retaining men in nursing programs designed for women. *Journal of Nursing Education, 42*(4), 159–162.
61. Burtt, K. (1998). Male nurses still face bias. *American Journal of Nursing, 98*(9), 64–65.
62. Dyck, J. M., Oliffe, J., Phinney, A., & Garrett, B. (2009). Nursing instructors' and male nursing students' perceptions of undergraduate, classroom nursing education. *Nurse Education Today, 29*, 649–653.
63. Keogh, B., & O'Lynn, C. (2007). Male nurses' experiences of gender barriers: Irish and American perspectives. *Nurse Educator, 32*(6), 256–259.
64. McLaughlin, K., Muldoon, O. T., & Moutray, M. (2010). Gender, gender roles and completion of nursing education: A longitudinal study. *Nurse Education Today, 30*, 303–307.
65. Kelly, N. R., Shoemaker, M., & Steele, T. (1996). The experience of being a male student nurse. *Journal of Nursing Education, 35*(4), 170–174.
66. Sullivan, E. (2002). In a woman's world. *Reflections on Nursing Leadership, 28*(3), 10–17.

67. Anthony, A. S. (2004). Gender bias and discrimination in nursing education: Can we change it? *Nurse Educator, 29*(3), 121–125.
68. Baker, C. R. (2001). Role strain in male diploma nursing students: A descriptive quantitative study. *Journal of Nursing Education, 40*(8), 378–380.
69. Patterson, B. J., & Morin, K. H. (2002). Perceptions of the maternal-child clinical rotation: The male student nurse experience. *Journal of Nursing Education, 41*(6), 266–272.
70. Stott, A. (2004). Issues in the socialization process of the male student nurse: Implications for retention in undergraduate nursing courses. *Nurse Education Today, 24*, 91–97.
71. Wang, H., Li, X., Hu, X., Chen, H., Gao, Y., Zhao, H., et al. (2011). Perceptions of nursing profession and learning experiences of male students in baccalaureate nursing program in Changsha, China. *Nurse Education Today, 31*, 36–42.
72. Boughn, S. (1994). Why do men choose nursing? *Nursing and Health Care, 15*(8), 406–411.
73. Flege, J. E., & Liu, S. (2001). The effects of experience on adults' acquisition of a second language. *Studies in Second Language Acquisition, 23*(4), 527–552.
74. Upton, T. A., & Lee-Thompson, L.-C. (2001). The role of the first language in second language reading. *Studies in Second Language Acquisition, 23*(4), 469–495.
75. Andrade, M. S. (2009). The value of a first-year seminar: International students' insights in retrospect. *Journal of College Student Retention: Research, Theory, and Practice, 10* (4), 483–506.
76. Andrade, M. S. (2006). International students in English-speaking universities: Adjustment factors. *Journal of Research in International Education, 5*(2), 131–154.
77. Smith, R. A. (2010). Feeling supported: Curricular learning communities for basic skills courses and students who speak English as a second language. *Community College Review, 37*(3), 261–284.
78. Jeong, S. Y.-S., Hickey, N., Levett-Jones, T., Pitt, V., Hoffman, K., Norton, C. A., et al. (2011). Understanding and enhancing the learning experiences of culturally and linguistically diverse nursing students in an Australian bachelor of nursing program. *Nurse Education Today, 31*, 238–244.
79. Caputi, L., Engelmann, L., & Stasinopoulos, J. (2006). An interdisciplinary approach to the needs of non-native-speaking nursing students: Conversation circles. *Nurse Educator, 31*(3), 107–111.
80. Suliman, W. A., & Tadros, A. (2011). Nursing students coping with English as a foreign language medium of instruction. *Nurse Education Today, 31*, 402–407.
81. Cunningham, H., Stacciarini, J.-M. R., & Towle, S. (2004). Strategies to promote success on the NCLEX-RN for students with English as a second language. *Nurse Educator, 29*(1), 15–19.
82. Brown, J. F. (2008). Developing an English-as-a-second-language program for foreign-born nursing students at an historically black university in the United States. *Journal of Transcultural Nursing, 19*(2), 184–191.
83. Sanner, S., & Wilson, A. (2008). The experiences of students with English as a second language in a baccalaureate nursing program. *Nurse Education Today, 28*, 807–813.

84. Colosimo, R., & Xu, Y. (2006). Research on shame: Implications for English as a second language nursing students. *Home Health Care Management and Practice, 19*(1), 72–75.

85. Jalili-Grenier, F., & Chase, M. M. (1997). Retention of nursing students with English as a second language. *Journal of Advanced Nursing, 25,* 199–203.

86. Abriam-Yago, K., Yoder, M., & Kataoka-Yahiro, M. (1999). The Cummins model: A framework for teaching nursing students for whom English is a second language. *Journal of Transcultural Nursing, 10*(2), 143–149.

87. Kataoka-Yahiro, M. R., & Abriam-Yago, K. (1997). Culturally competent teaching strategies for Asian nursing students for whom English is a second language. *Journal of Cultural Diversity, 4*(3), 83–87.

88. Ting, S.-M. R. (1997). Estimating academic success in the first year of college for specially admitted white students: A model combining cognitive and psychosocial predictors. *Journal of College Student Development, 38*(4), 401–409.

89. Young, J. W., & Koplow, S. L. (1997). The validity of two questionnaires for predicting minority students' college grades. *Journal of General Education, 46*(1), 45–55.

90. Cerna, O. S., Perez, P. A., & Saenz, V. (2009). Examining the precollege attributes and values of Latina/o bachelor's degree attainers. *Journal of Hispanic Higher Education, 8*(2), 130–157.

91. Chaney, B., Muraskin, L. D., Cahalan, M. W., & Goodwin, D. (1998). Helping the progress of disadvantaged students in higher education: The federal student support services program. *Educational Evaluation and Policy Analysis, 20*(3), 197–215.

92. Seidman, A. (2005). *College student retention: Formula for student success.* Westport, CT: Praeger.

93. Zuzelo, P. R. (2005). Affirming the disadvantaged student. *Nurse Educator, 30*(1), 27–31.

94. Olenchak, F. R., & Hebert, T. P. (2002). Endangered academic talent: Lessons learned from gifted first-generation college males. *Journal of College Student Development, 43*(2), 195–212.

95. Vuong, M., Brown-Welty, S., & Tracz, S. (2010). The effects of self-efficacy on academic success of first-generation college sophomore students. *Journal of College Student Development, 51*(1), 50–64.

96. D'Allegro, M. L., & Kerns, S. (2011). Is there such a thing as too much of a good thing when it comes to education? Reexamining first generation student success. *Journal of College Student Retention: Research, Theory, and Practice, 12* (3), 293–317.

97. Fleming, J. (2002). Who will succeed in college? When the SAT predicts black students' performance. *Review of Higher Education, 25*(3), 281–296.

98. Ransdell, S. (2001). Predicting college success: The importance of ability and non-cognitive variables. *International Journal of Educational Research, 35,* 357–364.

99. Strage, A., Baba, Y., Millner, S., Scharberg, M., Walker, E., Williamson, R., et al. (2002). What every student affairs professional should know: Student study activities and beliefs associated with academic success. *Journal of College Student Development, 43*(2), 246–266.

100. Gallagher, P. A., Bomba, C., & Crane, L. R. (2001). Using an admissions exam to predict student success in an AND program. *Nurse Educator, 26*(3), 132–135.
101. Urwin, S., Stanley, R., Jones, M., Gallagher, A., Wainwright, P., & Perkins, A. (2010). Understanding student nurse attrition: Learning from the literature. *Nurse Education Today, 30*, 202–207.
102. Williams, M. G. (2010). Attrition and retention in the nursing major: Understanding persistence in beginning nursing students. *Nursing Education Perspectives, 31*(6), 362–367.
103. Storr, H., Wray, J., & Draper, P. (2011). Supporting disabled student nurses from registration to qualification: A review of the United Kingdom (UK) literature. *Nurse Education Today, 31*(8), e29–e33.
104. Vaquera, G., & Maestas, R. (2009). Pre-college factors impacting persistence at a diverse university. *Journal of College Student Retention: Research, Theory, and Practice, 10*(4), 425–445.
105. Palmer, R. T., & Young, E. M. (2009). Determined to succeed: Salient factors that foster academic success for academically unprepared black males at a black college. *Journal of College Student Retention: Research, Theory, and Practice, 10*(4), 465–482.
106. Nnedu, C. C. (2009). Recruiting and retaining minorities in nursing education. *Association of Black Nursing Faculty Journal, 20*(4), 93–96.
107. Merisotis, J. P., & Phipps, R. A. (2000). Remedial education in colleges and universities: What's really going on? *Review of Higher Education, 24*(1), 67–85.
108. Scott, C., Burns, A., & Cooney, G. (1998). Motivation for return to study as a predictor of completion of degree amongst female mature students with children. *Higher Education, 35*, 221–239.
109. Brennan, A. L., Best, D. G., & Small, S. P. (1996). Tracking student progress in a baccalaureate nursing program: Academic indicators. *Canadian Journal of Nursing Research, 28*(2), 85–97.
110. Campbell, A. R., & Dickson, C. J. (1996). Predicting student success: A 10-year review using integrative review and meta-analysis. *Journal of Professional Nursing, 12*(1), 47–59.
111. Griffiths, M. J., Bevil, C. A., O'Connor, P. C., & Wieland, D. M. (1995). Anatomy and physiology as a predictor of success in baccalaureate nursing students. *Journal of Nursing Education, 34*(2), 61–66.
112. Wold, J. E., & Worth, C. (1990). Baccalaureate student nurse success prediction: A replication. *Journal of Nursing Education, 29*(2), 84–89.
113. Aber, C. S., & Arathuzik, D. (1996). Factors associated with student success in a baccalaureate nursing program within an urban public university. *Journal of Nursing Education, 35*(6), 285–288.
114. Hutcheson, J. D., Garland, L. M., & Lowe, L. S. (1979). Antecedents of nursing school attrition: Attitudinal dimensions. *Nursing Research, 28*(1), 57–62.
115. Jeffreys, M. R. (2007). Tracking students through program entry, progression, graduation, and licensure: Assessing undergraduate nursing student retention and success. *Nurse Education Today, 27*, 406–419.
116. Benda, E. J. (1991). The relationship among variables in Tinto's conceptual model and attrition of bachelor's degree nursing students. *Journal of Professional Nursing, 7*(1), 16–24.

117. Malloch, D. C., & Montgomery, D. C. (1996). Variation in characteristics among adult students. *Continuing Higher Education Review, 60*(1), 42–53.

118. Berger, J. B. (2001). Understanding the organizational nature of student persistence: Empirically-based recommendations for practice. *Journal of College Student Retention: Research, Theory, & Practice, 3*(1), 3–22.

119. Eaton, S. B., & Bean, J. P. (1995). An approach/avoidance behavioral model of college student attrition. *Research in Higher Education, 36*(6), 617–645.

120. Kuh, G. D. (2001). Organizational culture and student persistence: Prospects and puzzles. *Journal of College Student Retention: Research, Theory, & Practice, 3*(1), 23–40.

121. Bryan, E., & Simmons, L. A. (2009). Family involvement: Impacts on postsecondary educational success for first-generation Appalachian college students. *Journal of College Student Development, 50*(4), 391–406.

122. Hilberg, S., Joshi, A., & House, A. (2009). Washington state achievers program: Influence of the scholarship program on low-income college students' achievement and aspirations. *Journal of College Student Retention: Research, Theory, and Practice, 10*(4), 447–464.

123. Martinez, J. A., Sher, J., Krull, J. L., & Wood, P. K. (2009). Blue-collar scholars? Mediators and moderators of university attrition in first-generation college students. *Journal of College Student Development, 50*(1), 87–103.

124. Campbell, A. R., & Davis, S. M. (1996). Faculty commitment: Retaining minority nursing students in majority institutions. *Journal of Nursing Education, 35*(7), 298–303.

125. Tayebi, K., Moore-Jazayeri, M., & Maynard, T. (1998). From the borders: Reforming the curriculum for the at-risk student. *Journal of Cultural Diversity, 5*(3), 101–109.

126. Jeffreys, M. R. (2001). Evaluating enrichment program study groups: Academic outcomes, psychological outcomes, and variables influencing retention. *Nurse Educator, 26*(3), 142–149.

127. Jeffreys, M. R. (2002). Students' perceptions of variables influencing retention: A pretest and post-test approach. *Nurse Educator, 27*(1), 16–19 [Erratum, 2002, 27(2), 64].

128. Terenzini, P. T., Springer, L., Yaeger, P. M., Pascarella, E. T., & Nora, A. (1996). First generation college students: Characteristics, experiences, and cognitive development. *Research in Higher Education, 37*(1), 1–23.

129. Padilla, R. V., Trevino, J., Gonzalez, K., & Trevino, J. (1997). Developing local models of minority student success in college. *Journal of College Student Development, 38*(2), 125–135.

130. Hernandez, J. C. (2000). Understanding the retention of Latino college students. *Journal of College Student Development, 41*(6), 575–588.

131. Hurtado, S., Inkelas, K. K., Briggs, C., & Rhee, B.-S. (1997). Differences in college access and choice among racial/ethnic groups: Identifying continuing barriers. *Research in Higher Education, 38*(1), 43–75.

132. Scott, C., Burns, A., & Cooney, G. (1996). Reasons for discontinuing study: The case of mature age female students with children. *Higher Education, 31*, 233–253.

133. Seidl, A. H., & Sauter, D. (1990). The new non-traditional student in nursing. *Journal of Nursing Education, 29*(1), 13–19.

134. Hammond, P. V., Davis, B. L., Marlin, B. W., & Montgomery, A. J. (1995). Student upward mobility: Utilization of an educational support model. *Association of Black Nursing Faculty Journal, March/April*, 51–53.
135. Sweet, S., & Fusner, S. (2008). Social integration of the advanced placement LPN: A peer mentoring program. *Nurse Educator, 33*(3), 202–205.
136. Skahill, M. P. (2002). The role of social support network in college persistence among freshman students. *Journal of College Student Retention: Research, Theory, & Practice, 4*(1), 39–52.
137. Johnson, G. M. (1996). Faculty differences in university attrition: A comparison of the characteristics of arts, education and science students who withdrew from undergraduate programs. *Journal of Higher Education Policy and Management, 18*(1), 75–91.
138. St. John, E. P., Hu, S., Simmons, A. B., & Musoba, G. D. (2001). Aptitude vs. merit: What matters in persistence. *Review of Higher Education, 24*(2), 131–152.
139. Astin, A. W. (1997). How "good" is your institution's retention rate? *Research in Higher Education, 38*(6), 647–658.
140. Napoli, A. R., & Wortman, P. M. (1998). Psychosocial factors related to retention and early departure of two-year community college students. *Research in Higher Education, 39*(4), 419–455.
141. Jeffreys, M. R. (1993). *The relationship of self-efficacy and select academic and environmental variables on academic achievement and retention.* Unpublished doctoral dissertation, Teachers College, Columbia University, New York.

Cultural Values and Beliefs, Self-Efficacy, and Motivation: Important Considerations

All students belong to one or more cultural groups before entering nursing education and therefore bring their patterns of learned values, beliefs, and behaviors into the academic and professional setting.

Despite the numerous adversities faced by many undergraduate nursing students today, some students persist while others do not; self-efficacy and motivation can influence persistence and academic performance.

SNAPSHOT SCENARIO

PROFESSOR PONDER: Several of the students in my clinical group failed the midterm exam in your lecture class. Some are thinking of withdrawing, stopping out, or even dropping out completely. What do you think happened? What can be done?

PROFESSOR CAVE: I keep my office door open so students can stop by and ask for help. If students don't ask for help, they deserve the grade they get. If it means they fail out or drop out of the nursing program, so be it. I even make it a point to look each of my students straight in the eye when I announce my office help sessions. Many of the weak students just look away quickly because they haven't kept up with the reading.

The next day, Professor Ponder asks the students to anonymously write down whether the students had sought help from professors, and why or why not. Here are some of the responses:

A: In my culture, it is considered disrespectful to ask a teacher for help. The teacher is an authority figure. It would cause the teacher great dishonor for me to ask for help.

B: When my professor announced her help session and looked me straight in the eye, I felt so embarrassed and I immediately dropped my gaze. In my culture, direct eye contact with an authority figure is extremely disrespectful. I respect my teachers and always complete a critical reading of the assigned chapters prior to class. I did not have any questions.

c: Every week last year before I was in this class, whenever I walked by my professor's office, I would glance inside. I never saw any students who looked like me. The few students I ever saw talking with her were the same background as her. I did not have any confidence about asking this professor for help.

d: In the past, I was always able to memorize and cram for my tests and still get excellent grades. So, I didn't see any reason to study that hard or to ask for help.

e: Ask for help? For what? I understand everything and don't need any help. What can be hard about nursing?

f: I am such a hopeless case. I don't think anything can help me now.

g: Of course I asked for help to improve my grade. That's what the professor gets paid for. I'm very competitive and I must get an A grade in this course.

After reading the scenarios above, what visual images popped into your head?

What race, gender, age, weight, and other physical, mental, and professional attributes did you visualize/imagine for each of the students and professors mentioned? Why?

What feelings were evoked as you read each scenario segment? Why?

What impact can these images and feelings have on your interactions with diverse student populations?

What impact could they potentially have on student satisfaction, stress, confidence (self-efficacy), persistence, attrition, and retention?

Nurse educators must seriously consider the impact of student affective factors on nursing student achievement, persistence, and retention. Student affective factors are attitudes, values, and beliefs about education, nursing, and one's ability to learn and perform the necessary tasks required for course and nursing program success. In the Nursing Undergraduate Retention and Success (NURS) model, these factors include cultural values and beliefs (CVB), self-efficacy, and motivation. Student affective factors are different from student profile characteristics in that they deal with variables that may change. Student affective factors may change over time and may be positively or negatively influenced by all other variable sets. This chapter introduces the general concepts underlying CVB, self-efficacy, and motivation that demand sincere consideration in nursing education today.

CULTURAL VALUES AND BELIEFS

What are your own CVB? What are the CVB of your students, faculty colleagues, administrators, nurses, and staff in clinical agencies?

Culture refers to patterns of learned values, beliefs, and behaviors that are shared from generation to generation within a group (1,2). All students belong to one or more cultural groups before entering nursing education and therefore bring their patterns of learned values, beliefs, and behaviors into the academic and professional setting. Values are standards that have eminent worth, meaning, and importance in one's life; values guide behavior. They are the "powerful directive forces that give order and meaning to people's thinking, decisions, and actions" (3). Cultural values influence thinking, decisions, and actions within the student role and other aspects of people's lives.

The inclusion of CVB in the NURS model recognizes that student's CVB unconsciously and consciously guide thinking, decisions, and actions that ultimately affect nursing student retention. Cultural congruence refers to the degree of fit between the student's values and beliefs and the values and beliefs of their surrounding environment (4–6). Here, the surrounding environment refers to the environment of nursing education within the educational institution and the nursing profession. The NURS model proposes that high levels of cultural congruence will serve as a bridge to promoting positive academic and psychological outcomes, thus enhancing persistence behaviors and retention. High levels of cultural incongruence are proposed as inversely related to positive academic and psychological outcomes; thus, cultural incongruence presents a barrier to retention.

Cultural styles are the "recurring elements, expressions, and qualities that characterize a designated cultural group through their [sic] series of action-patterns, beliefs, and values" (2, p. 155). The dominant values and norms of a cultural group guide the development of cultural styles (2). Nursing is a unique culture that reflects its own cultural style. Currently (within the United States), the culture of nursing reflects many of the dominant societal values and beliefs held in this country. Similarly, nursing education reflects the Western European value system dominant in U.S. universities. Although increases in culturally diverse students have been noted in higher education and in nursing, the values and beliefs underlying nursing education have been slow to change in accordance with changing student population needs. Furthermore, pedagogical changes in curriculum and teaching-learning strategies have been slow to change from the dominantly used Tylerian model despite empirical support for active learning strategies (7–13).

Ethnocentrism and cultural blindness have been major obstacles to the needed changes in nursing education. Ethnocentrism is the idea that the values and beliefs traditionally held within nursing education are supreme. Consequently, traditional teaching-learning practices are upheld. Within the context of nursing education, cultural blindness is the inability to recognize the different CVB that exist among diverse student populations. Because cultural blindness does not acknowledge that differences exist, imposition of dominant nursing education values and beliefs occurs. This imposition can cause cultural shock, cultural clashes, and cultural pain among students whose CVB are incongruent with the dominant nursing CVB.

Unfortunately, some nurse educators who acknowledge that differences exist may nevertheless expect students to instantly abandon long-held CVB and to easily adopt new values and beliefs. A nursing student does not simply "take off" old CVB and "put on" new nursing CVB as easily as changing clothes. Lack of cultural fit (cultural incongruence) can result in acculturation stress. Acculturation stress has been well documented among immigrant populations; however, it can occur whenever differences in CVB exist (4,5,14). Stress resulting from cultural incongruence adversely affects retention directly through negative psychological outcomes and indirectly through poor academic performance (see Chapter 7). Poor academic performance can occur as a result of poor psychological outcomes and/or incongruent views concerning education, learning styles, and nursing. Views of nursing and motivation for nursing education can also vary greatly among cultures; policy, learning styles, and values about education differ across cultures (15,16).

It is, however, critical to preserve certain values and beliefs within the nursing profession such as the code of ethics or standards of practice. Enculturation into nursing is a learning process that must be undertaken by all nursing students. It means that students learn to take on or live by the values, norms, and expectations of the nursing profession (17). Sufficient assistance can minimize stress and enhance enculturation (18). Enculturation is more difficult if the student's own CVB are not congruent with those of nursing. For example, a traditional Vietnamese American student who views the physician as an authority figure may find it difficult to confront one who prescribes a questionable treatment. Over time, it may become easier for that student to become assertive within the professional nursing role while still maintaining traditional CVB in other contexts. Nurse educators are challenged to explore various CVB within nursing, nursing education, and student cultures and to make culturally sensitive and appropriate decisions and actions.

Table 3.1 selectively compares and contrasts CVB of nursing education, higher education generally, and four other cultural groups. Based on a review of the literature, traditional views within the identified cultures were included but are in no ways meant to stereotype individuals within

TABLE 3.1 Comparison of Select Cultural Values and Beliefs

	NURSING EDUCATION	HIGHER EDUCATION	CHINESE AMERICAN	AFRICAN AMERICAN	MEXICAN AMERICAN	IRISH AMERICAN
Orientation	Individual	Individual	Group	Group	Group	Individual
Time perception	Present and future oriented; punctuality valued	Present and future oriented; punctuality valued	History of past important; traditionally lateness for appointments is expected; more recently, lateness is considered rude.	Present oriented; punctuality less important	Present oriented; relaxed punctuality	Past, present, future; flexible sense of time
Verbal communication	Direct, specific, and quick communication preferred; expects individuals to indicate when something is not understood	Depending on discipline, may have more or less elaboration and speed may not be as much of a priority as in the fast-paced healthcare setting common to nursing	Moderate to low tones preferred; loud tone associated with anger; answers "yes" when asked if something is understood; reluctant to talk about feelings and views	Loud tones (in comparison to other cultures) are preferred; views and feelings are shared openly with family and trusted friends	Personal topics may be taboo; feelings and views only shared with trusted family and friends; "small talk" expected to begin communication encounter	Low contextual language where meaning is explicit rather than implicit; personal topics are private; thoughts and feelings shared only with close family and friends
Nonverbal communication	Most often consistent with dominant societal values, such as direct eye contact, handshaking, and spatial distances	Same as nursing education	Avoid direct eye contact, especially with persons of authority and highly respected individuals	Direct eye contact is sometimes perceived as aggressive	Avoid direct eye contact, especially with persons of authority and highly respected individuals; handshaking demonstrates respect	Direct eye contact is maintained, indicating respect and trust

(continued)

59

TABLE 3.1 Comparison of Select Cultural Values and Beliefs *(continued)*

	NURSING EDUCATION	HIGHER EDUCATION	CHINESE AMERICAN	AFRICAN AMERICAN	MEXICAN AMERICAN	IRISH AMERICAN
Household responsibilities	The "traditional" student did not have household or outside responsibilities; student role is primary	Same as nursing education; community colleges have expanded services available to accommodate adult learner with multiple role responsibilities; examples: weekend or evening college, day care center	Household responsibilities shared; however, specific roles expected based on gender; male is head of family	Household responsibilities may be divided between men and women and children; woman is often head of family	Household responsibilities mainly part of female role; male dominance, with male as head of family; modesty.	Traditionally household responsibilities part of female role; however, in recent years, responsibilities shared between men and women
Health	Professes "holistic" view of health but still strongly based on medical model with focus on symptom alleviation, use of technology, and Western medicine	Health is not the major focus of institutions of higher education; in recent years, many colleges have eliminated or relaxed graduation requirements for courses in health, fitness, and/or physical education	Balance between "yin and yang"	Health is viewed as a harmony with nature	Balance between "hot and cold"	Determined by external forces
Nurse	Professional; seeking more respect from other health professionals and society	In comparison to other disciplines, nursing had a late start in higher education; May be viewed as a vocation rather than profession	Respected as authority figures after physicians; nurses with advanced education are more highly respected than are nurses with less education	Respected member of the healthcare team but less important than physicians	Respected member of the healthcare team; however, often viewed as an outsider	Nurses are respected as members of a service-oriented field or "occupation"

Education	Within the nursing culture, disputes surrounding minimal educational requirements still persist	Minimal education for tenure and promotion is the doctorate, although masters degree may be minimal at the community colleges	Highly valued, especially a college education	Highly valued, especially a college education	Education is valued; however, access to college education has been limited historically; families often expect females to put family first	Education is highly valued.
Teacher	Traditional pedagogy viewed teacher as "authority" who "transmits" learning to student; newer proponents of androgogy view teacher as partner or facilitator of learning who implements learner-centered approaches	Same; teaching role and load have greater emphasis at community colleges; teaching role may be secondary to scholarly activity, publication, and research at senior colleges and research institutions	Authority figure; true equality does not exist; therefore, concept of "partner" in learning may be difficult to comprehend; high expectation within group to excel academically	Respected authority figure; historically, unequal opportunities for advancing education; disproportionate numbers receive primary and secondary education in at-risk school districts (educational disadvantaged)	Teacher is viewed as a highly respected superior; rote learning and memorization predominates education in Mexico, with little emphasis on practical application, analysis, and synthesis	Respected professional
Work habits	Speed, accuracy, quality, and cost-effectiveness are valued; completion of tasks and "keeping busy" traditionally valued	"Keeping busy" is less valued than high quality, scholarly productivity, especially at senior colleges and research institutions	Speed in working is not a priority; hard work is valued	Hard work is valued	Work is secondary to family and other life activities; may be uncomfortable with authority persons checking work	Hard work highly valued

61

(continued)

TABLE 3.1 Comparison of Select Cultural Values and Beliefs *(continued)*

	NURSING EDUCATION	HIGHER EDUCATION	CHINESE AMERICAN	AFRICAN AMERICAN	MEXICAN AMERICAN	IRISH AMERICAN
Autonomy	Competition with authority; assertive; autonomous decision-making within the scope of nursing practice expected	Competitive, assertive; academic freedom highly valued; democratic governance, faculty-developed curricula, and professional unions/organizations valued	Defers to person in authority, often seeking approval before making decisions; avoids conflict and values harmony	Self-reliance and autonomy encouraged within group; past discrimination experiences may discourage autonomy; females are often head of household and decision-makers	Defers to person in authority, with males as dominant decision-makers; input of others is considered in decision-making; autonomy for females is more difficult than for males; avoids competition and conflict	Autonomy and independence outside the family is encouraged while family loyalty is still maintained
Help-seeking behaviors	Individual is expected to initiate help-seeking behaviors	Same	Stigma for seeking help for emotional disorders and stress; may be reluctant to approach for help by attempting to "save face"	Varied; may seek help within own social network before seeking outside help	Varied; may seek help within own social network before seeking outside help	May delay seeking help; denial of problems is a way of coping with physical and emotional problems
Persistence	Nursing is "hard work"; withdrawal from a nursing course is acceptable for academic and/or personal circumstances and should be decided by the individual	Among disciplines outside of nursing, nursing may not be perceived as "hard work" or academically rigorous/ challenging work for academically strong students; views on withdrawal similar to nursing education	Hard work is highly respected; withdrawal decisions may be difficult and may include the family	Withdrawal decisions may be difficult, especially if families have sacrificed greatly to assist student with educational endeavors	Withdrawal decisions may be difficult, especially if families have sacrificed greatly to assist student with educational endeavors; decisions may include the family; withdrawal would be acceptable if interfering with family responsibilities	Withdrawal decisions may be difficult since academic or personal problem must first be acknowledged

Information obtained from Andrews and Boyle (1999), Campinha-Bacote (1998), Leininger and McFarland (2002), and Purnell and Paulanka (2003), (58–61) Adapted from Jeffreys (2004).

the cultures. Nurse educators are cautioned about making stereotypes and are reminded to explore CVB of individual students. For the purposes of this chapter, the following categories were selected and deemed most relevant to nursing student retention: individual-group orientation, time perception, verbal communication, nonverbal communication, household responsibilities, health, nurse, education, teacher, work habits, help-seeking behaviors, and persistence. It is beyond the scope of this book to provide in-depth explanations about each category, yet the importance of an in-depth understanding must be recognized. The selective approach is meant to spark interest, stimulate awareness, and encourage further exploration among nurse educators before attempting the design of culturally relevant and congruent nursing educational strategies. This is critical; the need to understand, respect, maintain, and support the different CVB of culturally diverse students is a precursor to culturally relevant and competent education. Part II of this book will present strategies that incorporate an understanding of how CVB influence retention. Additionally, Chapter 10 specifically addresses cultural congruent faculty advisement and helpfulness.

> How can various CVB influence teaching, learning, satisfaction, stress, self-efficacy, motivation, retention, and success?

SELF-EFFICACY AND MOTIVATION

> What do you know about the ways self-efficacy and motivation may influence academic achievement, student retention, and persistence behaviors?

Despite the numerous adversities faced by many undergraduate nursing students today, some students persist while others do not. Self-efficacy and motivation can influence persistence and academic performance. Self-efficacy is the student's perceived confidence for learning or performing specific tasks or skills necessary to achieve a particular goal. It is the belief that one can perform or succeed at learning a specific task, despite obstacles and hardships, and that one will expend whatever energy is necessary to accomplish the task (19). Self-efficacy has been strongly linked to persistence behaviors and motivation. Empirical evidence supports it as a significant variable influencing an individual's action, performance, and persistence (20–36). Motivation has been described as the "power within the student to generate actions that will result in his or her success" (37).

What does self-efficacy have to do with persistence?

In nursing, the less frequent study of self-efficacy (confidence) on academic performance and retention of nursing students has demonstrated significant findings (38–41). In the NURS model, self-efficacy is proposed as an important factor influencing retention. Figure 3.1 traces the proposed influences of self-efficacy on student's actions, performance, and persistence for learning tasks. Details will be discussed in the sections that follow.

Background

A key concept in Bandura's (19) social cognitive theory is that learning and motivation for learning are directly influenced by self-efficacy perceptions, which are domain specific and task specific. Individuals with strong self-efficacy perceptions think, feel, and act differently from those who are either inefficacious or overly confident. Strong (resilient) self-efficacy enhances sociocognitive functioning in several ways: (1) new or difficult tasks are viewed as challenges that are accepted willingly, (2) great preparatory efforts are exhibited, (3) strong goal commitment and persistence behaviors are enhanced, (4) failures and setbacks are attributed to insufficient effort, and (5) more energy is expended to overcome failures, hardships, setbacks, and potential stressors in an effort to achieve goals (19). A strong self-efficacy to withstand failures combined with some uncertainty (task perceived as a challenge rather than self-doubts about capability) will encourage preparatory efforts and thus enhance performance outcomes (42). Students with this kind of self-efficacy are highly motivated and actively seek help to maximize their abilities.

In contrast, the inefficacious student (one with low confidence levels) is at risk for lowered persistence, poor motivation, and insufficient goal commitment, and may give up when obstacles or hardships are encountered. Such students may easily become discouraged if they do not quickly grasp new concepts, skills, or knowledge. They view academic challenges as overwhelming and insurmountable obstacles, threats, and hardships to be avoided. Consequently, they may decrease their study hours and lower persistence with study tasks and assignments. Low self-efficacy can affect retention directly if students give up without even trying and then withdraw from school or indirectly through poor academic outcomes and/or psychological outcomes. Poor academic outcomes (low grades and/or failure) may be caused by decreased class attendance, inadequate studying, and/or incomplete assignments. Such students become increasingly overwhelmed, focused on failure, dissatisfied, and stressed.

Students with low self-efficacy benefit the most with diagnostic-specific interventions designed to enhance self-efficacy and other academic and psychological outcomes (21,43–45). Early identification of inefficacious

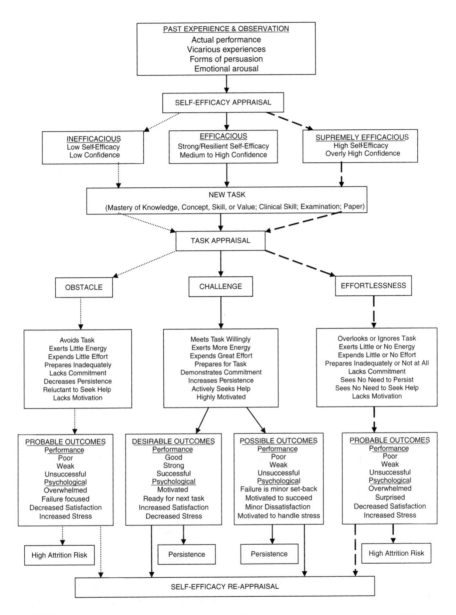

FIGURE 3.1 Proposed influences of self-efficacy on students' actions, performance, and persistence.

students followed by diagnostic-prescriptive interventions can help students maximize strengths, minimize weakness, and facilitate success. For example, students inefficacious about multiple choice test–taking skills will benefit most from intensive test-taking preparation workshops. Because inefficacious students often lose motivation and are reluctant to actively seek assistance, the nurse educator plays a key role in initiating actions with these students. Although self-efficacy appraisal is task specific, repeated failures and negative psychological outcomes decrease self-efficacy for learning and performing the necessary tasks for becoming a registered nurse, thereby lowering persistence behaviors overall.

Other at-risk students are those who are supremely efficacious (overly confident). Supremely efficacious students may be totally unaware of their weaknesses, underestimate the task or its importance, overlook the task, and overestimate their abilities and strengths (42). These students may not see the need for adequate academic preparation, restructuring of priorities, or time management to accommodate academic tasks. Therefore, they may not be adequately prepared. Retention is affected through poor academic outcomes and negative psychological outcomes. Poor, weak, or unsuccessful performances can lead to feeling overwhelmed, surprised or shocked, and dissatisfied, and to stress.

Supremely efficacious students often lack motivation for the task and see no need to seek assistance; the nurse educator can play a key role in initiating actions with them. For example, statistically significant findings in one study indicated that the at-risk students were supremely efficacious; students who perceived academic factors as highly supportive had significantly lower course grades. The results suggested that some students in the study sample did not have accurate perceptions of their academic skills required for professional nursing education (46,47). Early identification of supremely efficacious students can help students realistically appraise their strengths and weaknesses and recognize the need for adequate preparation for the achievement of successful outcomes. Because students (especially beginning students) may not know what to expect in nursing, they may need much guidance in ongoing self-appraisal. Realistic self-efficacy appraisal allows one to seek help to enhance strengths and remedy weaknesses.

Self-Efficacy Appraisal

According to Bandura (19), past experiences and observation influence self-efficacy appraisal via four information sources: actual performances, vicarious experiences, forms of persuasion, and emotional arousal (physiological indices). Actual performances are the strongest source of efficacy information. Successful performances can raise efficacy, while unsuccessful performances lower it. Lowered self-efficacy can be psychologically stressful and dissatisfying to students, further negatively impacting motivation, persistence, and retention. Individuals with low self-efficacy can initially feel devastated by failure or poor performance and further lowered self-efficacy can cause avoidance behaviors (19,42). Avoidance behaviors in nursing can be dangerous. For example, a student with low self-efficacy for assessing blood pressure reluctantly attempts the assessment, misinterprets findings, and fails to recognize severe hypertension in a client who later strokes. This student may be fearful of attempting other assessments, lack motivation, avoid help-seeking behaviors, and become increasingly dissatisfied and anxious.

Students with strong (realistic) levels of self-efficacy will not be adversely affected by an occasional failure and will view it as a temporary setback or challenge to be overcome with more effort expenditure (19,42,48). In the above case example, the realistically strong efficacious student would be motivated to seek extra assistance in the skills lab or request additional supervised opportunities in the clinical setting to take blood pressures. Most likely, such a student would initially take the task seriously, view it with some uncertainty, and exert preparatory efforts before attempting to apply blood pressure assessment in the clinical setting. In contrast, the supremely efficacious student (unrealistic and overconfident in self-appraisal) would view the task without uncertainty, prepare inadequately, and potentially jeopardize patient safety. Unsuccessful performances and/or adverse consequences will lower self-efficacy. The supremely efficacious student's new goal should be to view the task seriously and as a challenge that requires adequate preparatory efforts.

Vicarious experience, or modeling, is less influential than actual performance. Models that display effort and perform tasks successfully will be more influential than models that complete the task effortlessly. Self-efficacy perceptions will be further enhanced if models are similar to the individual in background and ability (19,49). It would be expected that beginning (novice) students have less astute skills for observing models. With little or no experience in the domain of nursing, such students will be at risk for selective observations that are myopic, slightly skewed, severely distorted, or limited, thereby increasing the risk for unrealistic self-appraisals. Through the use of various structured mentoring strategies, nurse educators can enhance the power of modeling on self-efficacy appraisal and development (refer to Part II of this book for strategies). Furthermore, by assisting students to develop keen observation skills, nurse educators can have a powerful influence on efficacy appraisal.

Forms of persuasion include positive verbal feedback from peers, teachers, and family. Positive persuasion will enhance efficacy only if students' subsequent efforts turn out positively (49). Therefore, positive verbal feedback should be given judiciously and honestly. In the NURS model, encouragement by family, faculty, or friends must be realistic, thus incorporating this important dimension of self-efficacy appraisal.

Physiological indices such as elevated pulse rate and sweating may indicate the emotional arousal such as anxiety and/or fear. Conscious awareness of anxiety symptoms over a particular task may lower efficacy beliefs (19,42,49). For example, if a student repeatedly experiences elevated pulse rate and sweating at the beginning of each clinical day's experience, despite the cognitive and psychomotor ability to perform tasks, the student's efficacy beliefs may be lowered and adversely affect learning, performance, persistence, motivation, and retention. Mild anxiety associated with some uncertainty has some benefits in that students are more attentive to detail, recognize the need for preparatory actions, and actively seek assistance. Lack of physiological changes would accompany the expected profile of supremely efficacious students and adversely affect task performance.

Self-efficacy changes over time in response to new experiences and observations (42,50,51). Several studies have supported that culturally diverse nursing students' self-efficacy perceptions were significantly influenced by the educational and health care experiences. For example, in one longitudinal study, self-efficacy perceptions for inefficacious students were raised to medium (strong) levels and self-efficacy perceptions for supremely efficacious students were lowered to medium levels following the educational experience that integrated specific skills (44). Students' course level was statistically significant in influencing perceptions in studies examining changes in transcultural self-efficacy perceptions (44,45,52–57). Novice students had overall lower self-efficacy perceptions, and more experienced students had overall higher self-efficacy perceptions. Ethnic/racial group identity was statistically insignificant, suggesting that self-efficacy measures can be designed to capture the effect of educational experiences across culturally diverse groups; however, further empirical investigation is recommended (44,45,52–56).

Carefully designed self-efficacy measures (survey tools) can be used to appraise students' initial self-efficacy levels for particular tasks and skills. Situation-specific or task-specific tools must be designed to measure self-efficacy (42). Consequently, nurse educators should selectively choose a reliable and valid self-efficacy tool specifically designed for their investigation. Often this means that a new tool must be developed. The instrument design process is complex and time-consuming; however, specific steps should be followed to enhance the validity and reliability of findings. Review of survey data to identify inefficacious and supremely efficacious individuals will allow for early intervention and assistance in enhancing realistic self-efficacy appraisal. Empirical support for self-efficacy as a predictor of retention is more difficult to evaluate than conceptually acknowledging that self-efficacy plays an important role in student achievement and retention.

What strategies are implemented to help beginning students and more advanced students engage in initial and ongoing realistic self-efficacy appraisal? What else should be implemented?

KEY POINT SUMMARY

- Student affective factors describe students' attitudes, values, and beliefs about education, nursing, and one's ability to learn and perform the necessary tasks required for course and nursing program success. In the NURS model, these factors include CVB, self-efficacy, and motivation.
- The NURS model proposes that high levels of cultural congruence will serve as a bridge to promoting positive academic and psychological outcomes, thus enhancing persistence behaviors and retention.
- Students with resilient (strong) self-efficacy beliefs perceive tasks as challenges, exert great effort in overcoming obstacles, are highly motivated, and actively seek help to maximize their abilities.
- Inefficacious students are at risk for lowered persistence, motivation, and goal commitment and may give up when obstacles or hardships are encountered.
- Supremely efficacious (overly confident) students may be totally unaware of their weaknesses, underestimate the task or its importance, overlook the task, overestimate their abilities, and overrate their strengths, thereby increasing the risk for inadequate preparation.

APPLICATION STRATEGIES

EASY APPLICATION ACTION STEPS

Appraising Your CVB

1. Compare and contrast your CVB with the traditional ones listed for higher education, the nursing profession, and the select cultural groups listed in Table 3.1.
2. What do you think and feel when your CVB are the same?
3. What do you think and feel when your CVB are different?

Appraising Your Students' CVB

1. After giving some examples (such as in Table 3.1 or other literature resources), explain to students that to best meet their needs, you would like to learn more about them (and that enhanced cultural self-awareness will assist in their own development of cultural competence with culturally diverse patients).
2. Using the CVB appraisal template, invite your students to jot down their CVB in each category (may want to do anonymously).
3. Review students' responses for common themes, noting similarities and differences between your CVB and student responses.

Touring the Proposed Influences of Self-Efficacy on Students' Action, Performance, and Persistence

1. Select a required task or skill from your course (e.g., injection, interviewing a patient, oral presentation, written paper, final exam).
2. Trace the path of each student pathway (inefficacious, efficacious, and supremely efficacious) (Figure 3.1).
3. List strategies to enhance realistic self-efficacy appraisal for the selected skill or task.

EDUCATOR-IN-ACTION VIGNETTE

As part of the Writing Across the Curriculum initiative, Professor Glass has integrated a low-stakes written "reflection" component in the first introductory nursing fundamentals and medical-surgical nursing course. Students are asked to reflect and then briefly write about a specific topic in class for which they receive class participation credit. During the second week, Professor Glass presents the students with the writing prompt "Nursing is...." Responses are diverse, and Professor Glass identifies several students with varying levels of self-efficacy. She sees this as an important opportunity to intervene and promote positive behaviors. Professor Glass returns the written assignment the next week, with constructive comments written for each student. Common themes will be addressed generally in class. Select written excerpts and instructor-written responses and actions follow:

MORTON: ...what I should be doing now. I have been a nursing assistant for five years. I really do all the nursing care for the patients in the nursing home except give medications and fill out paperwork. I know what to expect in the nursing program so it will be a lot easier for me.

ANALYSIS: Morton is supremely efficacious, appraises the task of nursing effortlessly, and is at risk for inadequate preparation and undesirable academic and psychological outcomes.

Professor Glass writes, "Thank you for sharing your views. Your work as a nursing assistant has provided you with some valuable experiences with clients and other health care personnel. Some questions to think about may be: "What patient assessments must registered professional nurses make before, during, and after medication administration? What background scientific knowledge is pertinent to decision making and planning patient care safely?" Professor Glass then asks to speak with Morton privately after class for further discussion. To help Morton gain a broader perspective, Professor Glass arranges for Joe, a third-semester student who is also a nursing assistant, to speak with him concerning the nursing profession, benefits of maximizing opportunities and efforts within the nursing program, and strategies for success. Unfortunately, it is not until Morton has the "actual experience" of failing the first exam that he reappraises his situation, seeks to learn vicariously from positive role models, appreciates Professor Glass's constructive feedback and guidance, and exerts greater preparatory efforts.

NATALIE: . . . a very important profession in the health care field. I didn't realize that nurses had so much responsibility and critical decision making. I thought that nurses just carried out the doctor's orders. I realize that nursing is very complex and that I will have to make more time to complete my reading and assignments if I am to be a good nurse.

ANALYSIS: Natalie has strong/resilient self-efficacy.

Professor Glass writes, "You have already gained much insight about the nursing profession. Nursing is complex but can be quite rewarding. Keep up your positive attitude, motivation, and hard work." Intermittently, Professor Glass asks Natalie about her perceived progress in clinical and continues to encourage her diligent efforts.

RITA: " . . . hard work. It is harder than I expected. The nurses on the unit last week were so knowledgeable and professional. I don't know if I will ever be able to be like them or if I have what it takes to become a nurse. Patients really depend on nurses for their lives. There is so much to know in such a little time."

ANALYSIS: Rita is inefficacious, perceives the task of becoming a nurse as an obstacle, and is at risk for inadequate preparation and undesirable academic and psychological outcomes.

Professor Glass writes, "Thank you for sharing your reflection. I am glad that the nurses last week were such positive role models. Some of those nurses were students here not too long ago and expressed some of the same concerns you have. Nursing is hard work; however, it can be a quite rewarding profession. Please see me for help concerning time management and effective study techniques for maximizing time spent for skill/knowledge mastery and learning." Professor Glass meets with Rita and links her with a culturally diverse study group led by a peer mentor-tutor of similar age and cultural background.

TOOLKIT RESOURCE BOX

Item 16—Cultural Values and Beliefs: Faculty Self-Assessment
Item 17—Cultural Values and Beliefs: Student Self-Assessment

Item 14—Self-Efficacy Pathway
Item 23—Promoting Positive Help-Seeking Behaviors
Item 24—Appraising Teaching Strategies: Potential Effect on Diverse Populations
Item 26—Strategy Mapping Across the Curriculum
Item 29—Culturally Congruent Approach to Nursing Faculty Advisement and Helpfulness
Items 1–4—Student Perception Appraisal Questionnaires—Pretests and Posttests

---

DISCUSSION QUESTIONS

1. Professor Green states, "The same students always ask questions in class. The others just sit there quietly, never challenging me, offering an opinion, or seeking clarification. Although I have an "open-door policy" whereby students can stop by during my office hours to ask questions and get assistance on assignments, many never do. Although I have students of different ages and backgrounds in my class, I don't discriminate against any of them. I treat all students the same; they all have the same opportunity to seek assistance. It is their fault if they get a low grade because they didn't ask for help. It's not that complicated to ask me a question."
   How would you respond to Professor Green?

2. Professor Clock says, "Trying to consider students' CVB, their self-efficacy, and motivation levels will take too much time. There is too much content to cover in the classroom. Clinical days are very hectic; often there's no time for a decent clinical postconference discussion. Some of the students are so slow in their patient care, yet others are always motivated and finding something to keep them busy."
   How would you respond to Professor Clock?

3. At the end of the course, three students who are recent immigrants from the same foreign country individually go to your office sharing similar sentiments. Here is one student's excerpt: "I feel so ashamed that I failed your course. You are an excellent teacher and offered us so much help inside and outside the classroom. In my culture, it is very disrespectful and shameful to have failed a course because a teacher is so well respected. I wanted to assure you that it is not your fault that I failed. I failed because I could not meet the requirements. You have been very fair. I thank you for the opportunity to have been in your course. Please do not feel as though it is your fault. I hope you can forgive me."
   How would you respond to this student? What proactive actions can you implement with future students?

4. What part of the chapter intrigued you the most? Why? How will this influence your future teaching, advisement, and interaction with nursing students and faculty?

5. Professor Tech says, "My course is entirely online. Most of the courses in this accelerated program are mainly online. Students' CVB aren't an issue because they don't actually converse or see each other. All communication is done through the online discussion board. Students are expected to participate in ongoing weekly discussions. Students' CVB are not an issue because all students are the same in the online learning environment."

How would you respond to Professor Tech's comments?

REFERENCES

1. Leininger, M. M. (1978). *Transcultural nursing: Theories, concepts, and practices.* New York, NY: John Wiley & Sons.

2. Leininger, M. M. (1994). *Transcultural nursing: Concepts, theories, and practices.* Columbus, OH: Greyden Press.

3. Leininger, M. M. (1995). *Transcultural nursing: Concepts, theories, research, and practice.* Blacklick, OH: McGraw-Hill College Custom Services.

4. Constantine, M. G., & Watt, S. K. (2002). Cultural congruity, womanist identity attitudes, and life satisfaction among African American college women attending historically black and predominantly white institutions. *Journal of College Student Development, 43*(2), 184–193.

5. Constantine, M. G., Robinson, J. S., Wilton, L., & Caldwell, L. D. (2002). Collective self-esteem and perceived social support as predictors of cultural congruity among black and Latino college students. *Journal of College Student Development, 43*(3), 307–316.

6. Gloria, A. M., & Kurpius, S. E. R. (1996). The validation of the cultural congruity scale and the university environment scale with Chicano/a students. *Hispanic Journal of Behavioral Sciences, 18*(4), 533–549.

7. Andrews, M. (1995). Transcultural nursing: Transforming the curriculum. *Journal of Transcultural Nursing, 6*(2), 4–9.

8. Crow, K. (1993). Multiculturalism and pluralistic thought in nursing education: Native American world view and the nursing academic world view. *Journal of Nursing Education, 32*(5), 198–204.

9. Ironside, P. (2004). "Covering content" and teaching thinking: Deconstructing the additive curriculum. *Journal of Nursing Education, 43*(1), 5–12.

10. Iwasiw, C., Goldenberg, D., & Andrusyszyn, M.-A. (2005). *Curriculum development in nursing education.* Boston: Jones & Bartlett.

11. Ulrich, D. L., & Glendon, K. J. (1999). *Interactive group learning: Strategies for nurse educators.* New York, NY: Springer Publishing.

12. Bastable, S. B. (2003). *Nurse as educator: Principles of teaching and learning for nursing practice* (3rd ed.). Boston, MA: Jones & Bartlett.

13. Lowenstein, A. J., & Bradshaw, M. J. (2004). *Fuszard's innovative teaching strategies in nursing* (2nd ed.). Boston, MA: Jones & Bartlett.

14. Fuertes, J. N., & Westbrook, F. D. (1996). Using the social, attitudinal, familial, and environmental (S.A.F.E.) acculturation stress scale to assess the adjustment

needs of Hispanic college students. *Measurement and Evaluation in Counseling and Development, 29,* 67–76.

15. Rognstad, M.-K. (2002). Recruitment to and motivation for nursing education and the nursing profession. *Journal of Nursing Education, 41*(7), 321–325.

16. Purnell, L. D. (2008). Purnell's model for cultural competence. In L. D. Purnell & B. J. Paulanka (Eds.), *Transcultural health care: A culturally competent approach* (3rd ed, pp. 19–55). Philadelphia, PA: FA Davis.

17. Leininger, M. M. (2002). Essential transcultural nursing care concepts, principles, examples, and policy statements. In M. M. Leininger & M. R. McFarland (Eds.), *Transcultural nursing: Concepts, theories, research, and practice* (3rd ed., pp. 45–69). New York, NY: McGraw-Hill.

18. Vance, C. (2011). *Fast facts for career success in nursing: Making the most of mentoring in a nutshell.* New York: Springer.

19. Bandura, A. (1986). *Social foundations of thought and action: A social cognitive theory.* Englewood Cliffs, NJ: Prentice-Hall.

20. Bean, J. P., & Eaton, S. B. (2001). The psychology underlying successful retention practices. *Journal of College Student Retention: Research, Theory, & Practice, 3*(1), 73–90.

21. Zimmerman, B. J. (1995). Self-efficacy and educational development. In A. Bandura (Ed.), *Self-efficacy in changing societies* (pp. 202–231). New York, NY: Cambridge University Press.

22. Crede, M., & Kuncel, N. R. (2008). Study habits, skills, and attitudes: The third pillar supporting collegiate academic performance. *Perspectives on Psychological Science, 3,* 425–453.

23. Feldt, R. C., Graham, M., & Dew, D. (2011). Measuring adjustment to college: Construct validity of the student adaptation to college questionnaire. *Measurement and Evaluation in Counseling and Development, 44*(2), 92–104.

24. Reason, R. D. (2009). An examination of persistence research through the lens of a comprehensive conceptual framework. *Journal of College Student Development, 50*(6), 659–682.

25. Le, H., Casillas, A., Robbins, S. B., & Langley, R. (2005). Motivational and skills, social, and self-management predictors of college outcomes: Constructing the student readiness inventory. *Educational and Psychological Measurement, 65*(3), 482–508.

26. Cox, R. D. (2009). "It was just that I was afraid": Promoting success by addressing students' fear of failure. *Community College Review, 37*(1), 52–80.

27. Vuong, M., Brown-Welty, S., & Tracz, S. (2010). The effects of self-efficacy on academic success of first-generation college sophomore students. *Journal of College Student Development, 51*(1), 50–64.

28. Zell, M. C. (2010). Achieving a college education: The psychological experiences of Latina/o community college students. *Journal of Hispanic Higher Education, 9*(2), 167–186.

29. Turner, E. A., Chandler, M., & Heffer, R. W. (2009). The influence of parenting styles, achievement motivation, and self-efficacy on academic performance in college students. *Journal of College Student Development, 50*(3), 337–346.

30. DeWitz, S. J., Woolsey, M. L., & Walsh, W. B. (2009). College student retention: An exploration of the relationship between self-efficacy beliefs and purpose in life among college students. *Journal of College Student Development, 50*(1), 19–34.

31. Gore, P. A. (2006). Academic self-efficacy as a predictor of college outcomes: Two incremental validity studies. *Journal of Career Assessment, 14*(1), 92–115.

32. Betz, N. E. (2007). Career self-efficacy: Exemplary recent research and emerging directions. *Journal of Career Assessment, 15*(4), 403–422.
33. Barry, C. L., & Finney, S. J. (2009). Can we feel confident in how we measure college confidence?: A psychometric investigation of the college self-efficacy inventory. *Measurement and Evaluation in Counseling and Development, 42*(3), 197–222.
34. Martin, A. J., & Dowson, M. (2009). Interpersonal relationships, motivation, engagement, and achievement: Yields for theory, current issues, and educational practice. *Review of Educational Research, 79*(1), 327–365.
35. Lundberg, K. M. (2008). Promoting self-confidence in clinical nursing students. *Nurse Educator, 33*(2), 86–89.
36. Friedman, B. A., & Mandel, R. G. (2010). The prediction of college student academic performance and retention: Application of expectancy and goal setting theories. *Journal of College Student Retention: Research, Theory, and Practice, 11* (2), 227–246.
37. Stage, F. K., & Hossler, D. (2000). Where is the student? Linking student behaviors, college choice, and college persistence. In J. Braxton (Ed.), *Reworking the student departure puzzle* (pp. 170–195). Nashville, TN: Vanderbilt University.
38. Ford-Gilboe, M., Laschinger, H. S., Laforet-Fliesser, Y., Ward-Griffin, C., & Foran, S. (1997). The effect of a clinical practicum on undergraduate nursing students' self-efficacy for community-based family nursing practice. *Journal of Nursing Education, 36*(5), 212–219.
39. Goldenberg, D., Iwasiw, C., & MacMaster, E. (1997). Self-efficacy of senior baccalaureate nursing students and preceptors. *Nurse Education Today, 17*, 303–310.
40. Harvey, V., & McMurray, N. (1994). Self-efficacy: A means of identifying problems in nursing education and career progress. *International Journal of Nursing Studies, 31*, 471–485.
41. Madorin, S., & Iwasiw, C. (1999). The effects of computer-assisted instruction on the self-efficacy of baccalaureate nursing students. *Journal of Nursing Education, 38*(6), 282–285.
42. Bandura, A. (1989). Regulation of cognitive processes through perceived self-efficacy. *Developmental Psychology, 25*(5), 729–735.
43. Brown, S. D., Lent, R. W., & Larkin, K. C. (1989). Self-efficacy as a moderator of scholastic aptitude: Academic performance relationships. *Journal of Vocational Behavior, 35*(1), 64–75.
44. Jeffreys, M. R., & Smodlaka, I. (1999). Changes in students' transcultural self-efficacy perceptions following an integrated approach to culture care. *Journal of Multicultural Nursing and Health, 5*(2), 6–12. [Erratum, 2000, *6*(1), 20].
45. Jeffreys, M. R. (2010). *Teaching cultural competence in nursing and health care: Inquiry, action, and innovation* (2nd ed.). New York, NY: Springer Publishing.
46. Jeffreys, M. R. (1993). *The relationship of self-efficacy and select academic and environmental variables on academic achievement and retention.* Unpublished doctoral dissertation, Teachers College, Columbia University, New York, NY.
47. Jeffreys, M. R. (1998). Predicting nontraditional student retention and academic achievement. *Nurse Educator, 23*(1), 42–48.
48. Bandura, A. (1997). *Self-efficacy: The exercise of control.* New York, NY: W. H. Freeman.
49. Schunk, D. (1987). *Self-efficacy and cognitive achievement.* Paper presented at the Annual Meeting of the American Psychological Association, New York, NY,

August 28–September 1, 1987 (ERIC Document Reproduction Service No. ED 287 880).

50. Gist, M. E., & Mitchell, T. R. (1992). Self-efficacy: A theoretical analysis of its determinants and malleability. *Academy of Management Review, 17*, 183–211.

51. Saks, A. M. (1995). Longitudinal field investigation of the moderating and mediating effects of self-efficacy on the relationship between training and newcomer adjustment. *Journal of Applied Psychology, 80*, 211–225.

52. Jeffreys, M. R. (2000). Development and psychometric evaluation of the Transcultural Self-Efficacy Tool: A synthesis of findings. *Journal of Transcultural Nursing, 11*(2), 127–136.

53. Jeffreys, M. R., & Smodlaka, I. (1996). Steps of the instrument-design process: An illustrative approach for nurse educators. *Nurse Educator, 21*(6), 47–52. [Erratum, 1997, *22*(1), 49].

54. Jeffreys, M. R., & Smodlaka, I. (1998). Exploring the factorial composition of the Transcultural Self-Efficacy Tool. *International Journal of Nursing Studies, 35*, 217–225.

55. Jeffreys, M. R., & Smodlaka, I. (1999). Changes in students' transcultural self-efficacy perceptions following an integrated approach to culture care. *Journal of Multicultural Nursing and Health, 5*(2), 6–12. [Erratum, 2000, *6*(1), 20].

56. Jeffreys, M. R., & Smodlaka, I.(1999). Construct validation of the Transcultural Self-Efficacy Tool. *Journal of Nursing Education, 38*, 222–227.

57. Jeffreys, M. R., & Dogan, E. (2012). Evaluating the influence of cultural competence education on students' transcultural self-efficacy perceptions. *Journal of Transcultural Nursing* (in press).

58. Andrews, M., & Boyle, J. (1999). *Transcultural concepts in nursing* (3rd ed.). Philadelphia, PA: Lippincott.

59. Campinha-Bacote, J. (1998). *The process of cultural competence in the delivery of healthcare services: A culturally competent model of care* (3rd ed.). Cincinnati, OH: Transcultural C.A.R.E. Associates.

60. Leininger, M. M., & McFarland, M. R. (2002). *Transcultural nursing: Concepts, theories, research, and practice* (3rd ed.). New York, NY: McGraw-Hill.

61. Purnell, L. D., & Paulanka, B. J. (2003). *Transcultural health care: A culturally competent approach* (2nd ed.). Philadelphia, PA: F. A. Davis.

Academic Factors

All personal study hours and class attendance are not equal.

SNAPSHOT SCENARIO

Consider the following students' thoughts and attitudes, their possible impact on student retention and success, and implications for nurse educators:

SALLY SPECTATOR: I just like to sit back, watch, and listen to what's going on in class. I purposely selected Professor Lecture's class. The other professor makes people talk in class and hardly lectures; instead, students have to work in class. It's the professor's responsibility to work in class, not mine.

ROSIE DOZEY: I work the night shift right before coming to class. I sit in the back and usually find myself dozing on and off. But I've never been absent yet.

TOM TARDY: I always seem to miss the boat, and then I need to wait longer for the campus bus. When I get to class, I start to jump right in and ask questions, but my classmates get annoyed because the teacher just explained what I am asking about. Now I never talk in class.

LENA LAPTOP: I get to class 15 minutes early so I can get the seat I want—in the corner by the window—with uninterrupted wireless Internet. I plan to take detailed notes on my laptop, but then I get distracted because my friends send me IMs or e-mails. I'm afraid to miss an important message. Sometimes, I even miss a message because the men's soccer team is practicing outside.

TONY TEXT: I am very respectful of the professor and my classmates. I would never be disruptive coming late to class or leaving class to answer a cell phone call like some people do. That's why I tell my friends and family to text me while I'm in class. I can multitask and pay attention to the lecture—texting only takes a few seconds; I usually get only 10 texts during a class.

TABITHA TAPE: I don't even bother to listen in class.... or to do the assigned readings before class.... I just tape the lecture and then go back and read the sections in the chapter that Professor Lecture talked about. When things get too busy, I just listen to the tape.

DELILAH DAZE: The attendance policy says we can be absent four days this semester. I didn't, have any absences yet so I'll just miss the last four classes. It's good beach weather now. I can use my new waterproof MP3 player in the ocean and listen to the podcasted lectures as I ride the waves.

PATTI PAIR: This accelerated program is so intense. I'm glad my BFF [best friend forever] is in my class. She listens and takes notes for the first half of the class; then it's my turn for the last half. We exchange notes later. We never missed a class yet.

HEATHER HIGHLIGHT: I just can't finish all the reading before class...and I'm not sure what's important to pay attention to.... There's so much. Now I bring my e-book text to class and just highlight whatever Professor Lecture mentions. I don't have to rack my brains in class.... Just follow her and highlight the book. I'll review it again in 3 weeks before the midterm.

How many of these students are engaging in active attendance? Has this occurred in your class? Have you had a problem with attendance? How did you visualize each of these characters in terms of student profile variables (see Chapter 2)? Why?

What are academic factors? Academic factors have been included in conceptual models explaining college student attrition. The conceptual and operational definitions of these academic factors have varied, making comparison of factors between studies and between selected models difficult. Bean and Metzner (1) describe academic factors as the students' primary involvement with the academic process at the college and purport that among nontraditional students, academic factors are less important than environmental factors in influencing retention. Study hours, study skills, academic advising, absenteeism, major and job certainty, and course availability are identified as academic factors (2). Academic integration has sometimes been used to describe a cluster of academic factors that can influence retention and has been defined as "the development of a strong affiliation with the college academic environment both inside and outside of class" (3). Use of college services and interaction with college faculty, students, and personnel are included in this definition.

For undergraduate nursing students, the academic factors that are deemed most important for retention include personal study skills, study hours, attendance, class schedule, and general academic services (college library, college counseling, and computer laboratory). These factors interact with the other variable sets in the NURS model (Figure 1.2). It is essential that nurse educators go beyond a superficial skimming of academic factors toward a critical appraisal of how each academic factor can influence retention and student success. An in-depth exploration of each academic factor may reveal several aspects or dimensions that can potentially affect students differently. This chapter discusses each academic factor in relation to undergraduate nursing student retention and aims to assist nurse educators in identifying areas of student strengths and weaknesses.

STUDY SKILLS AND STUDY HOURS

Personal Study Skills

What are your students' study skills like? What do you know about your students' study skills?

Personal study skills refer to specific study skills (reading skills, writing skills, note-taking, preparing papers, studying for exams, reading notes, listening in class), attitudes about the responsibility for study activities, time management and organization, and effort expended with academic pursuits. However, an alarming one-third of college students surveyed perceived deficits in one or more specific study skills (4). Other higher education studies noted diverse academic self-beliefs, study skills, habits, and attitudes (5,6). Consistent with higher education, the increasing academically diverse nursing student population presents with quite diverse study skills (7–19). Personal study skills affect nursing student retention through academic performance and psychological outcomes.

Highly developed skills in reading, writing, note-taking, paper preparation, studying for exams, and listening are good personal study skills. However, they are not enough to assure academic success and retention. Attitudes about responsibility for study activities may range from positive, adaptive, and internal locus of control beliefs to negative, maladaptive, and external control beliefs (20). Adaptive behaviors include self-direction, detailed plans, and task-focused goals relating to study activities and academic pursuits. Maladaptive behaviors include self-handicapping, learned helplessness, task avoidance, and task-irrelevant behaviors for study activities and academic pursuits (20). Promoting positive, adaptive beliefs in nursing should be a goal for nurse educators.

Excellent time management skills, organizing, and planning are reported as better predictors of academic success than is total number of study hours (4, 21). Additionally, use of varied study skills was associated with better academic outcomes (22), which in turn positively influences retention. Effort expended on planning and study activities yields better academic outcomes (23). Effort expenditure is related to students' self-efficacy perceptions and not limited to time on task. Conclusively, quality study outweighs study hours, although sufficient study hours are needed to adequately and proficiently achieve desired academic outcomes. Several studies identified a mismatch between students' perceived study skills and study hours, whereby study hours were more restrictive in comparison to perceived study skills (24–27). Such a mismatch warrants nurse educator intervention.

Student self-appraisal of personal study skills is an advantageous precursor to maximizing personal study skill strengths, remedying weaknesses, and seeking appropriate assistance. Self-appraisals are usually based upon the student's prior academic experience and performance in terms of successes and failures; however, self-perceptions may be inaccurate and/or may fail to result in appropriate help-seeking behaviors. Researchers have substantiated that many students whose self-perceptions of skills were weak, often took limited action in seeking help (6,28–30). Routinely soliciting student self-appraisals of study skills must be partnered with actively offering appropriate assistance to weaker students. Nurse educators can take an active role in assisting students with specific study skills needed for nursing courses, developing time management and organization, promoting responsible study attitudes and behaviors, and encouraging high quality study effort expenditure.

As mentioned earlier, self-appraisals may not be accurate (31). For example, in one study, beginning associate degree nursing students overestimated the supportiveness of academic supports. Students with the highest estimates of academic supports had more nursing course failures than did students with more conservative self-appraisals. Personal study skills was only one of the eleven-variable academic cluster used for correlating academic strength (AVST) with nursing course grade (24, 25). Failing students were unable to progress in the nursing program, resulting in attrition.

Guidance with self-appraisal is strongly recommended. Beginning nursing students may need special assistance in evaluating study skills in relation to nursing program requirements. Students moving from preprofessional to professional education need much guidance and often have difficulty with transition into the profession (32). Prior successful study strategies may need to be adapted to meet the special demands of the nursing professional program. Without guidance, students may not recognize the need to adapt, resulting in poor academic, psychological, and retention outcomes.

Personal Study Hours

What do you know about the quantity and quality of your students' personal study hours?

The importance of personal study hours in relation to academic achievement and retention of college students is well documented. The nursing literature is filled with reports of student multiple roles that conflict with personal study hours and adversely affect achievement and retention (7,33–46). In the NURS model, personal study hours refer to the number of hours allocated exclusively to positive study activities in which positive study behaviors and positive study attitudes are actively used. Positive behaviors and attitudes are adaptive, self-directed, planned, realistically goal-oriented, and appropriate. Maladaptive behaviors such as procrastination, learned helplessness, unrealistic goal orientation, and defeatist attitudes are not included within personal study hours. Qualifying personal study hours differentiates between desirable and undesirable study activities, behaviors, and attitudes, attempting to measure personal study hours by desirable components rather than by using an accounting mechanism in which all hours are considered equal. All personal study hours are not equal. Students may need guidance in recognizing this difference and in accurately appraising their own personal study hours.

In the NURS model, students with more personal study hours (as operationally defined here) are expected to have more positive academic outcomes and retention than will students with inadequate personal study hours. Adequate study hours are individual-based and are defined as the least number of personal study hours needed to achieve the short-term academic outcomes (passing exam, completing accurate care plan, etc.) and long-term academic outcomes (successfully completing nursing course components). Students with inadequate personal study hours are considered to be at risk for academic failure, stress, dissatisfaction, and attrition. Because personal study skills needed for success in nursing may be unknown, undeveloped, underdeveloped, or unvalued, nurse educators are challenged to actively assist students in maximizing personal study hours as defined here.

ATTENDANCE

The Metzner and Bean (1,2) model included absenteeism as an academic variable influencing attrition; however, the NURS model focuses on attendance. Attendance was substituted for absenteeism since this was more positive and considered relevant for retention, as opposed to absenteeism being correlated with attrition. Nevertheless, the literature regarding attendance reveals several interesting phenomena that are relevant for nursing education. First, attendance (or absenteeism) should be monitored to help identify at-risk students. Second, attendance should be monitored in relation to other variables with the purpose of identifying students most at risk for attrition. For example, Bean (47) notes that among college students with high GPAs, class attendance may not be related to attrition or failure. Among college students with low GPAs, class absence may be a warning sign indicating student dissatisfaction, stress, and/or academic difficulty. Such students are at great risk for attrition and/or failure. A large meta-analysis study demonstrated that class attendance is significantly correlated with college grades (48); however, others still question the importance of attendance in academic achievement (49,50) and oppose the monitoring of attendance from a philosophical standpoint (49).

In nursing, attendance is somewhat more complex than among the general college population. As an academic factor influencing retention, it requires further discussion; thus, specific implications for nursing education will be introduced. First, national and state accreditation guidelines provide a framework for attendance policies; therefore, most nursing programs have strict attendance policies. Second, nursing program attendance policies may be stricter than the parent institution's policy. Consequently, nursing students may not comprehend, value, or expect rigid attendance policies in nursing. Additionally, students may not expect that attendance policies will be upheld, especially among beginning nursing students who have had no prior exposure to nursing courses.

Despite strict nursing program attendance policies, students are permitted a maximum number of absences (or a minimum number of attendance hours). Attendance may be further differentiated between various nursing course components such as theoretical (classroom hours), skills laboratory, and/or clinical hours. Clearly, clinical attendance is a valuable dimension to learning and assists the student in connecting theoretical information, nursing skills, and client care. Unlike most college majors, nursing deals with a humanistic, caring, and life-and-death component. Clinical absences can result in the student being minimally prepared to care for clients competently. Absences create complicated disadvantages; attendance creates valuable advantages. With limited opportunities to apply learning, students may be at more risk for failure, dissatisfaction, and stress, putting the student at greater risk for voluntary or involuntary attrition. By identifying students with minimal attendance, tardiness, and surveying other variables to develop a comprehensive student composite, nurse educators can offer appropriate interventions to enhance academic achievement, satisfaction, stress reduction, and retention.

Early identification suggests the need for an evaluative mechanism for identifying which students are at risk for "minimal" attendance. In one study of nontraditional first-semester associate degree students, most students were "highly confident" that they would attend all lecture classes, all skills laboratory classes, and all clinical laboratory classes, yet several students were not confident (24) (see Toolkit Item 5). This study did not correlate end-of-semester attendance records with student survey responses; however, surveying students' self-expectations for attendance may help identify students with lower expectations who may be at risk for lower attendance, insufficient academic achievement, and poor retention. Nurse educators could initiate prophylactic interventions to assist at-risk students.

Although attendance is commonly defined as a dichotomous variable, (either one is present or one is not present), upon closer examination, attendance is more complex. For example, a student may be physically present but mentally absent. Such a student is not benefiting educationally by being present. Another scenario may be the student spectator. Attendance as a spectator limits the potential active learning and critical thinking that occurs with attendance as an active learner. One limitation of mandatory attendance or strict attendance policies is that it may be difficult to differentiate between physical presence, mental presence, spectator attendance, and active attendance. Naturally, active learning will be obvious with group discussions, skills practice, or care of clients in the clinical setting; however, it may be more difficult to discern in large classes when lectures, videos, or PowerPoint presentations are the sole means of the passive teaching-learning activity. Attendance needs to be viewed in relation to other variables and to the other dimensions of the NURS model if at-risk students are to be identified early.

> What is the current attendance policy in your class, nursing program, college? What is the attendance rate in your class? How many students are in active attendance? What strategies can enhance students' participation as active attendees?

CLASS SCHEDULE

Availability of courses, flexibility of courses, and convenience are factors that can influence retention through academic and psychological outcomes (1,51). Consistently, across several study samples, most nursing students have identified "class schedule" as influencing retention. Responses ranged from "severely restrictive" to "greatly supportive" (24–27,39,40). Class schedule is included in the NURS model because student's perceptions of class schedule, with its physical demands and time constraints, can influence retention positively or negatively and in varying degrees. Student perception of class schedule is the most important aspect to assess.

Class schedule interacts with other academic and environmental factors, and professional integration variables in influencing retention. For example, a 2-day class schedule compatible with a nursing student's other roles and responsibilities increases the probability for greater class attendance, more study hours, participation in professional events, satisfaction, and academic achievement. In contrast, a 4-day class schedule may require a financially challenged single parent to commute 3 hours to a distant clinical site via public transportation, pay for additional child-care services, and change work hours. The incompatible class schedule increases the student's risk for attrition because of multiple-role stress, financial strain, and a probability for decreased class attendance, decreased study hours, limited participation in professional events, dissatisfaction, and lowered academic achievement. Some students may have difficulty clearly evaluating the disadvantages and advantages of various class schedules and the effect of class schedule selection on other aspects of their lives. Maintaining a rigorous class schedule is a key issue in accelerated undergraduate nursing programs (17,52–55). As faculty advisors, nurse educators have a major responsibility to effectively guide students in selecting the best class schedule most compatible with balancing other roles and responsibilities, so that students can achieve positive academic outcomes and enhance positive psychological outcomes for nursing.

> To what degree do your students perceive nursing class schedule options as supportive or restrictive to their retention and success?

GENERAL ACADEMIC SERVICES

> What do you know about the general academic services available to your students? How do students perceive general academic services at your college?

General academic services are designed to assist students with their academic goals and are available to all college students, regardless of academic major. They include the library, counseling, and computer laboratories. Although it is important that general academic services have the adequate facilities, staffing, and technology to assist college students, it is the students' perception of these services that most strongly influences retention. If students perceive the lack of adequate academic support, attrition will increase. Retention will be enhanced if academic support services follow a student-centered rather than an institutional-centered philosophy, meaning that student academic services must be accessible and convenient, especially to adult learners. General academic services that are convenient, accessible, and helpful will encourage more active use of these support services. Active involvement in the learning process is an important indicator of academic behavior, is essential for academic integration, and enhances student retention (56).

The assessment of nursing student's perceptions concerning general academic services is valuable (57). Consistent findings across three study samples revealed that most undergraduate associate degree nursing students perceived the library, counseling, and computer laboratory to influence retention, stating that these general academic services "moderately support" or "greatly support" retention (24–27,40). Students who perceive services to be valuable will expend greater effort in using them. Greater, comprehensive use of services, in conjunction with other academic factors, positively influences retention by enhancing academic and psychological outcomes. For example, maximizing use of various library services appropriate to course objectives can assist with improved study skills and academic integration, thus enhancing retention. Counseling services have been beneficial to nursing student academic and psychological outcomes (57). Higher education literature reports that counseled students have higher retention rates than noncounseled students (58–60). Kraemer (61) stated that commuter students who frequently use computer laboratory facilities on campus are more involved in cognitive development than other students; enhanced cognitive development enhances retention.

To fully comprehend the significance of general academic services on nursing student retention, nurse educators need to assess three dimensions of general academic services. First, they should assess whether students perceive the individual service to be valuable and important to academic achievement, positive psychological outcomes, and retention. Second, they should evaluate whether the services are convenient and accessible from both the student and educator perspective. Third, they should survey the frequency and duration of services used. Even if students do not use general academic services as frequently as nurse educators would recommend, students' perception that the services are available and important is a necessary precursor for strategy design. Strategies should integrate use of these general academic services to enhance nursing outcomes. Mismatches among any of the three dimensions may indicate a need for an intervention strategy aimed at the student, educator, and/or educational institution.

KEY POINT SUMMARY

- Academic factors include personal study skills, study hours, attendance, class schedule, and general academic services (college library, college counseling, and computer laboratory).
- Personal study skills refer to specific study skills (reading skills, writing skills, note-taking, preparing papers, studying for exams, reading

notes, listening in class), attitudes about the responsibility for study activities, time management and organization, and effort expended with academic pursuits.

- Personal study hours refer to the number of hours allocated exclusively to positive study activities in which positive study behaviors and positive study attitudes are actively used. Positive behaviors and attitudes are adaptive, self-directed, planned, realistically goal-oriented, and appropriate.
- Attendance is presented as a multidimensional variable that differentiates between active learning and the "mentally absent" or "spectators."
- Class schedule interacts with other academic and environmental factors, and professional integration variables in influencing retention.

APPLICATION STRATEGIES

EASY APPLICATION ACTION STEPS

Appraising Attendance Policies and Actions

1. Review the attendance policy in your course, required non-nursing courses, other nursing courses, nursing program, college, and state licensing eligibility.
2. After identifying consistent and inconsistent faculty actions taken to enforce attendance policies, consider what impact these similarities and differences have on students' perceptions about attendance.
3. Develop strategies to enhance consistent implementation of published policies.

Assisting Students to Enhance Active Attendance

1. Using the introductory scenarios at the beginning of the chapter, ask students to read aloud their randomly assigned part and invite class discussion.
2. On one half of a piece of paper, ask students to list their active attendance behaviors; on the other half, ask students to list behaviors interfering with active attendance.
3. Discuss strategies for enhancing active attendance behaviors.

EDUCATOR-IN-ACTION VIGNETTE

Several students complain that despite "studying all the time" and completing the required readings, they did not achieve the grade they expected. Sharon states, "For the amount of time I put into nursing, I should have gotten a better grade. All my free time is spent studying and reading nursing. I just don't understand it." Several other students echo the same disconcerting, unhappy sentiments. To guide students with their own personal self-appraisal, Professor Booke asked each student privately to describe details about his or her personal study hours and study skills. Questioning was directed at uncovering adaptive and maladaptive study behaviors and attitudes. Consider Professor Booke's initial questions and the diverse student responses that follow:

Questions

- What were you thinking about before you got ready to read the prerequisite reading (chapter 12) for the last class? What were you feeling?
- How did you prepare (get ready to read)?
- What were you doing while you were reading chapter 12?
- How much time was actually spent on reading chapter 12? How much of this time was uninterrupted?
- How did you read the chapter? Did you engage in active reading or passive reading strategies?
- What did you do after reading the chapter?
- What were you thinking about after you read the chapter? What were you feeling?

Student Responses

SHARON: I read the chapter from beginning to end while I was riding my exercise bike for 45 minutes. I prepared by selecting the "beginner level" on the exercise bike and positioned my book on the handles. I was thinking that I could exercise my mind and body at the same time. I guess I didn't really engage in active reading since I just read the chapter like a novel. Afterwards, I took a shower. I felt as though I got one more thing off my homework list.

ANDREW: I started the chapter while at the bus stop. The bus was crowded so I didn't get a seat for about 15 minutes. Then I finished the main parts of the chapter on the bus. I did the summary, nursing case study, and practice questions the next morning on the bus to class. I guess I had many interruptions, especially because the bus was noisy. Without interruptions, it probably would have taken 45 minutes or longer if I actually stopped to think about what I read as I went along. I felt as though no matter how much I read, I will never understand what the instructor wants me to know.

BARBARA: I read during the warm-up and halftime of my son's football game. I was thinking that I could skim over the chapter during warm-up and then go back to read the important parts during halftime. The chapter had so many details, so I highlighted the main points, and then I went back to skim it again after everyone was asleep. That day, I was too tired, so I went to bed at 11 p.m. and set my alarm clock for 3 a.m. to get up and finish. I was just thinking about how tired I was and how it took me almost 12 hours to finish chapter 12.

JANE: I went to the library and didn't leave until I had written all my notes from the chapter. I don't like to use a highlighter. I spent 4 hours at the library but most of the time was probably spent writing notes. I stop to think about whether something might be important and if it may be something that could be on the next test. I don't really trust myself, so I just write down everything.

TAMARA: Honestly, I was still trying to read from the last two classes. I thought that I would get started on my reading during the first week but I kept putting it off so I fell behind. My roommate was really homesick, so I tried to spend extra time with her. I start to read in our room but then she wants to talk. I go back and reread the part I just read before I was interrupted to make sure I remember everything. Sometimes, I reread the same part ten times and never finish a chapter.

Professor Booke's subsequent questions are directed at identifying individual student strengths and weaknesses:

- What thoughts and actions promote or support positive learning?
- What thoughts and actions interfere with or restrict learning?
- What will you do in the future?

Following a guided, realistic self-appraisal, students in the above scenarios discovered that all personal study hours are not equal. Individual appraisal permitted a mutually developed, diagnostic-prescriptive study plan for the future. To further facilitate ongoing positive study behaviors and attitudes, Professor Booke paired students with peer mentors, encouraged students to join an enrichment program reading and study group, and met with individual students bimonthly.

TOOLKIT RESOURCE BOX

Items 1–4—Student Perception Appraisal Questionnaires—Pretests and Posttests
Item 5—Educational Requirements Subscale (ERS)

DISCUSSION QUESTIONS

1. Identify two academic factors about which you learned the most. Discuss what you learned that was new and how this would impact upon your future role as a nurse educator in an undergraduate associate degree program mainly comprised of nontraditional students, an

accelerated baccalaureate program for second degree students, and/or an RN-BSN program.

2. What positive, adaptive study skill behaviors and attitudes are exhibited by students in your course? What strategies do you implement to promote positive, adaptive study skill behaviors and attitudes? What other strategies will be helpful?

3. What negative, maladaptive study skill behaviors and attitudes are exhibited by students in your course? What strategies do you implement to discourage negative, maladaptive study skill behaviors and attitudes? What other strategies will be helpful?

4. Professor Green says, "I don't think attendance really makes a difference in students' academic achievement. I wait to pass around the attendance sheet for signatures during the middle of class because so many students arrive late. It doesn't really matter because my lectures are available for download and after teaching this class the same way for 5 years, I'm sure that my lectures have been transcribed into notes. I've correlated attendance records with class grades and there is no correlation. I think we should just be more lenient about class attendance and permit students to miss up to one-third of the lecture classes." How would you respond?

5. How can the Snapshot Scenarios and the Educator-in-Action Vignette be adapted for use with students in your course?

REFERENCES

1. Bean, J. P., & Metzner, B. (1985). A conceptual model of nontraditional undergraduate student attrition. *Review of Educational Research, 55,* 485–540.

2. Metzner, B., & Bean, J. P. (1987). The estimation of a conceptual model of nontraditional undergraduate student attrition. *Research in Higher Education, 27,* 15–38.

3. Nora, A. (1993). Two-year colleges and minority students' educational aspirations: Help or hindrance?.*Higher Education: Handbook of Theory and Research, 9,* 235.

4. Strage, A., Baba, Y., Millner, S., Scharberg, M., Walker, E., Williamson, R., & Yoder, M. (2002). What every student affairs professional should know: Student study activities and beliefs associated with academic success. *Journal of College Student Development, 43*(2), 246–266.

5. Crede, M., & Kuncel, N. R. (2008). Study habits, skills, and attitudes: The third pillar supporting collegiate academic performance. *Perspectives on Psychological Science, 3,* 425–453.

6. Mattern, K. D., & Shaw, E. J. (2010). A look beyond cognitive predictors of academic success: Understanding the relationship between academic self-beliefs and outcomes. *Journal of College Student Development, 51*(6), 665–678.

7. Bosher, S. D., & Pharris, M. D. (2009). *Transforming nursing education: The culturally inclusive environment.* New York, NY: Springer Publishing.

8. Flinn, J. B. (2004). Teaching strategies used with success in the multicultural classroom. *Nurse Educator, 29*(1), 10–12.

9. Grossman, D., & Jorda, M. L. (2008). Transitioning foreign-educated physicians to nurses: The new Americans in nursing. *Journal of Nursing Education, 47*(12), 544–551.

10. Harvath, T. A. (2008). A culture of learning. *Journal of Nursing Education, 47*(12), 535–536.

11. Hegge, M. J., & Hallman, P. A. (2008). Changing nursing culture to welcome second-degree students: Herding and corralling sacred cows. *Journal of Nursing Education, 47*(12), 552–556.

12. Heller, B. R., Oros, M. T., & Durney-Crowley, J. (2000). The future of nursing education: 10 trends to watch. *Nursing and Health Care Perspectives, 21*(1), 9–13.

13. Jeffreys, M. R. (2010). *Teaching cultural competence in nursing and health care: Inquiry, action, and innovation.* (2nd ed.). New York, NY: Springer Publishing.

14. Johnson, S. A., & Romanello, M. L. (2005). Generational Diversity: Teaching and learning approaches. *Nurse Educator, 30*(5), 212–216.

15. McCleary-Jones, V. (2008). Strategies to facilitate learning among NURSING students with learning disabilities. *Nurse Educator, 33*(3), 105–106.

16. Schumacher, G., Risco, K., & Conway, A. (2008). The Schumacher model: Fostering scholarship and excellence in nursing and for recruiting and grooming new faculty. *Journal of Nursing Education, 47*(12), 571–575.

17. Seldomridge, L.A., & DiBartolo, M. C. (2007). The changing face of accelerated second bachelor's degree students. *Nurse Educator, 32*(6), 240–245.

18. Storr, H., Wray, J., & Draper, P. (2011). Supporting disabled student nurses from registration to qualification: A review of the United Kingdom (UK) literature. *Nurse Education Today, 31*(8), e29–33.

19. Tagliareni, M. E. (2008). Quoted in Sapers, J. Shaping the future of nursing. *TC Today, 33*(1), 13–17.

20. Nurmi, J-E., & Aunola, K. (2001). How does academic achievement come about: Cross-cultural and methodological notes. *International Journal of Educational Research, 35*, 403–409.

21. Ransdell, S. (2001). Predicting college success: The importance of ability and non-cognitive variables. *International Journal of Educational Research, 35*, 357–364.

22. Napoli, A. R., & Wortman, P. M. (1998). Psychosocial factors related to retention and early departure of two-year community college students. *Research in Higher Education, 39*(4), 419–455.

23. Flowers, L. A. (2002). The impact of college racial composition on African American students' academic and social gains: Additional evidence. *Journal of College Student Development, 43*(3), 403–410.

24. Jeffreys, M. R. (1993). *The relationship of self-efficacy and select academic and environmental variables on academic achievement and retention.* Unpublished doctoral dissertation, New York: Teachers College, Columbia University.

25. Jeffreys, M. R. (1998). Predicting nontraditional student retention and academic achievement. *Nurse Educator, 23*(1), 42–48.

26. Jeffreys, M. R. (2001). Evaluating enrichment program study groups: Academic outcomes, psychological outcomes, and variables influencing retention. *Nurse Educator, 26*(3), 142–149.

27. Jeffreys, M. R. (2002). Students' perceptions of variables influencing retention: A pretest and post-test approach. *Nurse Educator, 27*(1), 16–19 [Erratum, 2002, 27*(2), 64].

28. Alexitch, L. R. (2002). The role of help-seeking attitudes and tendencies in students' preferences for academic advising. *Journal of College Student Development, 43*(1), 5–19.

29. Chaney, B., Muraskin, L. D., Cahalan, M. W., & Goodwin, D. (1998). Helping the progress of disadvantaged students in higher education: The federal student support services program. *Educational Evaluation and Policy Analysis, 20*(3), 197–215.

30. Ofori, R. (2006). Measuring motivational orientations toward support-seeking: The development and predicative validity of the motives for tutorial support-seeking questionnaire. *Nurse Education Today, 26*, 228–239.

31. O'Donnell, H. (2011). Expectations and voluntary attrition in nursing students. *Nurse Education in Practice, 11*, 54–63.

32. Schon, D. (1987). *Educating the reflective practitioner.* San Franscisco, CA: Jossey-Bass.

33. Bessent, H. (1997). *Strategies for Recruitment, Retention, and Graduation of Minority Nurses in Colleges of Nursing.* Washington, DC: American Nurses Publishing.

34. Colalillo, G. (2007). Mentoring as a retention strategy in a diverse, multi-cultural, urban associate degree nursing program. *Teaching and Learning in Nursing, 2*, 28–33.

35. Dante, A., Valoppi, G., Saiani, L., & Palese, A. (2011). Factors associated with nursing students' academic success or failure: A retrospective Italian multicenter study. *Nurse Education Today, 31*, 59–64.

36. Evans, B. C. (2008). "Attached at the umbilicus": Barriers to educational success for Hispanic/Latino and American Indian nursing students. *Journal of Professional Nursing, 24*, 205–217.

37. Fleming, S., & McKee, G. (2005). The mature student question. *Nurse Education Today, 25*, 230–237.

38. Griffiths, M. J., & Tagliareni, M. E. (1999). Challenging traditional assumptions about minority students in nursing education. *Nursing and Health Care Perspectives, 20*, 290–295.

39. Jeffreys, M. R. (2007). Tracking students through program entry, progression, graduation, and licensure: Assessing undergraduate nursing student retention and success. *Nurse Education Today, 27*, 406–419.

40. Jeffreys, M. R. (2007). Nontraditional students' perceptions of variables influencing retention: A multisite study. *Nurse Educator, 32*(4), 161–167.

41. O'Brien, F., Keogh, B., & Neenan, K. (2009). Mature students' experiences of undergraduate nurse education programmes: The Irish experience. *Nurse Education Today, 29*, 635–640.

42. Presho, M. (2006). Earning and learning: Recruitment and retention in post registration nurse education. *Nurse Education Today, 26*, 511–518.

43. Schoofs, N., Bosold, S., Slot, V., & Flentje, J. (2008). Nursing student employment: Impact on academic achievement. *Nurse Educator, 33*(2), 57–58.

44. Steele, R., Lauder, W., & Caperchione, C. (2005). An exploratory study of the concerns of mature access to nursing students and the coping strategies used to manage these adverse experiences. *Nurse Education Today, 25*, 573–581.

45. Stolder, M. E., Rosemeyer, A. K., & Zorn, C. R. (2008). In the shelter of each other: Respite care for students as a partnership model. *Nursing Education Perspectives, 29*(5), 295–299.

46. Tucker-Allen, S., & Long, E. (1999). *Recruitment and retention of minority students: stories of success*. Lisle, IL: Tucker Publications.
47. Bean, J. P. (1986). Assessing and reducing attrition. In D. Hossler (Ed.), *Managing College Enrollments*. New Directions for Higher Education, 53. (pp. 47–61). San Francisco, CA: Jossey-Bass.
48. Crede, M., Roch, S. G., & Kieszcynka, U. M. (2010). Class attendance in college: A meta-analytic review of the relationship of class attendance with grades and student characteristics. *Review of Educational Research, 80*, 272–295.
49. Lipscomb, M., & Snelling, P. C. (2010). Student nurse absenteeism in higher education: An argument against enforced attendance. *Nurse Education Today, 30*, 573–578.
50. Young, P., Yates, S., Rickaby, C., Snelling, P., Lipscomb, M., & Lockyer, L. (2010). Researching student absence: Methodological challenges and ethical issues. *Nurse Education Today, 30*, 291–295.
51. Burr, P. L., Burr, R. M., & Novak, L. F. (1999). Student retention is more complicated than merely keeping the students you have today: Toward a "seamless retention theory." *Journal of College Student Retention, 1*(3), 239–253.
52. Bentley, R. (2006). Comparison of traditional and accelerated baccalaureate nursing graduates. *Nurse Educator, 31*(2), 79–83.
53. Hegge, M., & Larson, V. (2008). Stressors and coping strategies of students in accelerated baccalaureate nursing programs. *Nurse Educator, 33*(1), 26–30.
54. Raines, D. A. (2007). Accelerated second-degree program evaluation at graduation and 1 year later, *Nurse Educator, 32*(4), 183–186.
55. Stuenkel, D., Nelson, D., Malloy, S., & Cohen, J. (2011). Challenges, changes, and collaboration evaluation of an accelerated BSN program. *Nurse Educator, 36*(2), 70–75.
56. Tinto, V. (1997). Classrooms as Communities. *Journal of Higher Education, 68*(6), 599–623.
57. Lehna, C., Jackonen, S., & Wilson, L. (1996). Navigating a nursing curriculum: Bridges and barriers. *Association for Black Nursing Faculty Journal, 7(July/August)*, 98–103.
58. Lee, D., Olson, E. A., Locke, B., Michelson, S. T., & Odes, E. (2009). The effects of college counseling services on academic performance and retention. *Journal of College Student Development, 50*(3), 305–319.
59. Turner, A. L., & Berry, T. R. (2000). Counseling center contributions to student retention and graduation: A longitudinal assessment. *Journal of College Student Development, 41*(6), 627–636.
60. Wilson, S. B., Mason, T. W., & Ewing, M. J. M. (1997). Evaluating the impact of receiving university-based counseling services on student retention. *Journal of Counseling Psychology, 44*(3), 316–320.
61. Kraemer, B. A. (1997). The academic and social integration of Hispanic students into college. *Review of Higher Education, 20*(2), 163–179.

5

Environmental Factors

While some environmental factors are perceived as barriers to retention, other students perceive the same factors as supportive.

SNAPSHOT SCENARIO

During a conference coffee break, Professor Numbers says, "Last year, we admitted 100 new nursing students who had prenursing course GPAs ranging from 4.0 to 3.39. After the first semester, only 77% of them progressed to the second nursing course. Twelve students failed and 11 students withdrew by the college's withdrawal date. I just don't understand it."

Professor Frank replies, "Well, students aren't just numbers. Students are people. People have lives that constitute more than nursing school. The reality is that environmental factors can influence student retention, persistence, and success more than academic factors."

PROFESSOR CAVE: I don't really know what you mean. The students in my class all come from the same local environment and commute to school.

PROFESSOR LIGHT: Well, I had ten students in my clinical group last semester and discovered that there was much diversity concerning their environmental factors. One student lives in a seven-bedroom colonial house and drives a brand new luxury car; another student lives in a cramped two-room trailer with five family members and then carpools with a neighbor. During the semester, a destructive fire forced one student to live out of a car for 8 weeks. Another student cleans office buildings part-time and works full-time in the clothing factory to financially support and provide health insurance coverage for aging grandparents and six younger orphaned siblings. Two students are single parents of toddlers and are pleased about the campus day-care center services. Another student shares parenting of teenage twins with a same-sex partner. One student arrived at preconference and then fainted due to some domestic violence head trauma experienced that morning, afterward saying that going to school was the only thing to look forward to every day.

PROFESSOR CAVE: I guess our students' lives are more complex than I thought. I guess it's because we are a commuter school. Environmental factors probably aren't that important at a selective, residential school.

PROFESSOR LIGHT: "Well, before I started teaching at our commuter college, I taught for 5 years at a highly selective, residential college. Freshmen were required to live on campus, and most students elected to live in campus housing throughout the 4 years. Environmental factors were still influential. I'll give you some examples from my last clinical group of eight students. At the beginning of the semester, one student became pregnant and then miscarried after 7 weeks. Another student experienced a racial bias incident with two suite mates and had to receive an emergency housing change. Three students worked 10 to 20 hours on campus as part of the work–study program. Another student worked 4 nights a week from 11 p.m. until 3 a.m. at a bar to pay for college and living expenses because the parents would not provide support past age 18 despite their middle-class income. Unfortunately, this student was not eligible for financial aid or scholarships for disadvantaged students because of the parents' income. The student walked 30 minutes to and from work and appreciated getting a free cooked meal and unused leftovers every workday. Regardless of where students attend school, environmental factors are very influential."

After reading the scenarios above, what visual images popped into your head?

What race, gender, age, weight, and other physical, mental, and professional attributes did you visualize/imagine for each of the students and professors mentioned? Why?

What feelings were evoked as you read each scenario segment? Why?

What impact can these images and feelings have on your interactions with diverse student populations?

What impact could they potentially have on student satisfaction, stress, confidence (self-efficacy), persistence, attrition, and retention?

What are environmental factors? Environmental factors may broadly be defined as factors external to the academic process that may influence students' academic performance and retention (1,2). Traditionally, environmental factors have received little attention in college student attrition or retention studies. Therefore, it is not surprising that environmental factors have been absent or minimally addressed in college student retention or attrition models. The Bean and Metzner (1) model of nontraditional undergraduate student attrition proposed that environmental factors, which included finances, hours of employment, outside encouragement, family responsibilities, and opportunity to transfer, were more influential than other variable sets. Two compensatory effects or interacting variables are proposed in the model. The first is between environmental variables and academic support. Environmental support is believed to compensate for weak academic support; however, the opposite does not hold true. Academic support is not thought to compensate for weak environmental support (2).

The Bean and Metzner (1) model provided the underlying conceptual framework for several studies on nontraditional undergraduate nursing student retention (3–6). One aim of the studies was to measure student perceptions concerning the restrictiveness or supportiveness of select environmental variables and their influence on retention. Several researcher-developed instruments were used to measure student perceptions prospectively (at the beginning of the semester) and/or retrospectively (at the end of the semester) (see Toolkit Items 1–4). Overall, students perceived that environmental variables were more influential than academic variables in their impact on retention.

The environmental factors were then incorporated into the original NURS model (7) which aimed to explain nontraditional undergraduate retention and success. For the traditional student, one major factor influencing retention is college adjustment and social integration into the college residential/life environment. Because "living arrangements" can support or restrict nontraditional student retention and success as well, it seemed logical to include it in the new NURS model (Figure 1.2). Please note that in 2004, the acronym NURS was changed from "Nontraditional Undergraduate Retention and Success" to "Nursing Undergraduate Retention and Success" and it encompassed components appropriate for both traditional and nontraditional students. In the NURS model, environmental factors are defined as factors external to the academic process and include financial status, family financial support, family emotional support, family responsibilities, child care arrangements, family crisis, employment hours, employment responsibilities, encouragement by outside friends, living arrangements, and transportation.

Environmental factors may be applicable to both traditional and nontraditional undergraduate nursing student populations; however, the manner in which they impact upon retention may be different. Differences will be highlighted in this chapter. Additionally, environmental factors interact with each other and with other variable sets in the NURS model. Like the appraisal of academic factors, it is essential that nurse educators critically evaluate how each environmental factor can influence student retention and success. A detailed and holistic appraisal of student profile characteristics and student affective factors is a necessary to determine how environmental factors are perceived by individual students and specific student subgroups. This chapter discusses each environmental factor in relation to undergraduate nursing student retention and aims to assist nurse educators in identifying areas of actual and/or perceived student strengths and weaknesses.

FINANCES, FAMILY, WORK, AND FRIENDS

Financial Status

How do your students meet their expenses?

Financial status refers to the student's financial standing in meeting all expenses including tuition, college fees, books and other learning materials, living expenses, financial obligations, and commitments. Nontraditional students, especially older students, generally have greater financial obligations and commitments than do younger students, although all students can potentially be affected by financial status. Financial obligations are expenses that are clearly defined by an external source, such as car payments and car insurance. Financial commitments are expenses that are intrinsically defined and sometimes vague, such as supporting elderly family members who reside in a foreign country. Financial status, if perceived as a barrier, may adversely affect retention directly or indirectly. For example, a student who is unable to pay tuition may choose to drop out or work while attending school. The first option has a direct effect on retention through immediate attrition. The second option may have an indirect effect on retention through academic performance (failure) because of decreased study hours and/or decreased class attendance. Stress and dissatisfaction may also occur and adversely influence retention.

Financial status as a barrier to student academic success and retention has been well documented (8–10). Various terms describe this phenomenon: financial burden, financial concerns, financial difficulties, financial pressure, financial strain, and financial stress. Numerous empirical approaches have examined financial status as a variable influencing student success. One approach identified particular student profile characteristics that increase the likelihood for financial barriers. Several studies reported that financial status as a barrier is particularly prevalent among nontraditional students, especially minority students (8) older students (11), women with dependent children (12–14), and economically disadvantaged students (9,15–17).

Nurse educators should avoid stereotyping students as at risk for attrition due to financial barriers solely on meeting one of the above demographic categories. A holistic appraisal is needed. For example, assuming that a minority student is economically disadvantaged and confronted with severe financial strain based on the student's ethnic background may not only be inaccurate, but is biased and unethical. Economically disadvantaged students represent many different ethnic, racial, and religious groups.

Economically disadvantaged students perceive financial constraints as a barrier, are less likely to enroll in college, and are even less likely to earn a college degree. However, current financial aid policies and limited scholarships present financial challenges or "resource barriers" for middle-class students and for students who demonstrate small amounts of financial need (8,9,18,19). Resource barriers are real or perceived obstacles that interfere with the ability to secure adequate finances for anticipated expenses. The uncertainty of financial aid or scholarships, and/or concern about anticipated expenses is another burden that adversely affects retention, either directly or indirectly.

Among diverse samples, student perceptions of the influence of the supportiveness or restrictiveness of financial aid and scholarships on retention have been varied. Although financial problems are often cited as a reason for withdrawal, this is usually done after the student weighs the benefits, costs, and overall academic experience. Student satisfaction or dissatisfaction may tip the scale in favor of retention or attrition (20). Satisfaction with the academic experience is a desirable outcome that can influence retention; however, being able to meet financial expenses also affects persistence behavior (8,9,21–27).

Student perception of financial status is the most critical element for nurse educators to evaluate in this area. If the student perceives financial status to be a barrier, retention is adversely affected. Student appraisal of financial status and satisfaction in relation to all the other possible interacting variables is complicated. It is an individualized process that is influenced by age, gender, and culture. Perceptions are often influenced externally by political agendas concerning "underprivileged" groups and financial assistance priorities (28,29). One study indicated that White middle-class college students perceived greater difficulty in getting loans, grants, and scholarships than did minority middle-class college students. Additionally, White middle-class students who faced the loss of financial aid had greater concerns than other students about dropping out (30). Among Black students, loan attainment positively influenced degree attainment; however, loan attainment negatively influenced degree attainment among Asian, Latino, and White students (31). Among nontraditional nursing students enrolled in a public university system, financial status ranked as one of the most restrictive factors influencing retention (32). In the United States, the modest increase in federal direct student aid aimed to assist community college persistence and degree attainment is grossly insufficient to meet the demands of over 2 million new student enrollees and a 40% tuition increase (33). In other words, it has become financially more challenging for students to attain college degrees nationwide. The nursing literature worldwide also reported financial strain and economic changes adversely influencing student retention (10,34–37). (Also see Chapter 8, on politics and economics).

It is not surprising that student perceptions about the influence of financial status on retention are quite varied among diverse ethnic, racial, and socioeconomic groups. Perceived responsibility for paying for college may influence student perceptions and guide decisions on persistence. Cultural values and beliefs, as well as intergenerational differences within cultures, may be influential. For example, whether the student as an individual assumes total financial responsibility for college expenses or whether the family is expected to financially support the student can influence perceptions.

> What do you know about the financial aid and scholarship services available to your students? How do students perceive their financial status? To what degree do your students perceive their financial status as supportive or restrictive to their retention and success?

Family Financial Support

Family financial support and assurance of funds should be considered in attrition studies (9,38). Among minority nursing students, family financial support was a perceived asset and often a necessity for academic persistence (39,40). Among students enrolled in professional study programs, family financial support was also viewed as a significant factor (41). Family financial support for school is more complex than it may initially seem. Several major points will be explored here. Nurse educators are encouraged to consider each point carefully when appraising financial factors influencing retention.

First, family financial support for school should be closely viewed in relation to beliefs concerning responsibility for paying college expenses. As perceived by the student, does the family have the financial resources available to assist with college expense? Does the family intend to assist the student financially to the best of its ability? Does the family *actually* provide financial assistance to the student to the best of its ability? Finally, does the student perceive the family as financially supportive, adequate, or restrictive? Students may need guidance in evaluating financial status and planning at the beginning of the semester.

Beliefs concerning gratitude and responsibilities of the student toward family members providing financial support can also affect student perceptions and retention. For example, a student whose family is sacrificing greatly to assist with college expenses may feel extreme pressure to excel academically and persist in school. In contrast, a student whose family has available resources yet is unwilling to assist the student may feel overburdened with financial concerns and frustrated with limited financial aid resources; such perceived overwhelming barriers can adversely affect persistence behaviors and increase attrition risk.

> To what degree do your students perceive their family financial support as supportive or restrictive to their retention and success?

Family Emotional Support

Family emotional support is the active emotional involvement of family members in the student's academic endeavors and career goals. It is manifested by encouraging educational and career goals, promoting positive feelings of self-worth, believing in the student's ability to succeed, listening to problems and concerns, showing interest in academic progress, expressing optimism, offering assistance, and presence. Presence means caring about the student as a whole person and being available for emotional support. A support person does not actually need to be bodily present, but needs to be perceived as caring and encouraging. Although this is the definition used in the NURS model, surveyed students may define family emotional support differently. Nurse educators may expect a positive correlation between family emotional support for school and academic achievement and retention, but this is not always true. The sections that follow will explore the impact of family emotional support on retention. New perspectives about family emotional support aim to guide nurse educators in closely evaluating it in a variety of contexts. Being open to various worldviews or perspectives will broaden nurse educators' ability to understand the multidimensional process of student retention and assist students appropriately.

Students' perceptions of their family's emotional support are essential to evaluate. They may be realistic, clouded, or unrealistic, and yet they are what will influence decisions to persist or withdraw. They are influenced by previous educational success, struggles, and failures, and may change over time and throughout the educational process. The impact of family emotional support on the educational experience will also change. For example, in one longitudinal study, student perceptions were more optimistic at the beginning of the semester than at the end. When asked prospectively to rate the supportiveness or restrictiveness of family emotional support on their ability to remain in the nursing course that semester, students were optimistic. Initially, none perceived family emotional support as "severely restrictive," yet at the end of the semester, 11% of the sample perceived that family emotional support severely restricted their ability to remain in the nursing course. Another 18% perceived that family emotional support would "neither restrict nor support" retention prospectively; however, at the end of the semester, only 7% of the students responded this way (6). The study was limited to persisters and may have had quite different results if nonpersisters had been surveyed. Despite the small sample size, this longitudinal study offered new information for nurse educators and can provide a basis for further study. Awareness that students may be more optimistic at first or undervalue the impact of family emotional support on retention suggests that students need guidance initially in evaluating their individual situations.

The importance of environmental variables, especially family emotional support, has been thought to be most important for older, commuter students (2). End-of-semester questionnaire data from 1,156 culturally and generationally diverse undergraduate commuter nursing students indicated that family emotional support was the most frequently selected "greatly supportive" variable influencing students' ability to remain in a nursing course during the targeted semester, thereby lending validity to this assumption (32) (see Toolkit Item 4). Findings from another multi-institutional study reported that emotional support from family positively assisted second-degree students to cope with the stressors of an accelerated nursing program (42). However, other literature provides new insights into the impact of family support for different student populations, which needs to be viewed in context with student profile characteristics, cultural values and beliefs, and self-efficacy. Family conflict can adversely affect retention. In contrast, Maville and Huerta (43) indicated that perceived social support was inversely related to academic progress. Here, a strong family cohesiveness influenced the student to prioritize family first; the allegiance to family was predominant, despite support for school.

Among traditional-age minority students residing on college campuses, (especially in predominantly White institutions), strong family emotional support was significant for college adjustment and retention (44–46). Family emotional support was consistently present, despite the absence of family members within students' living environment. Other studies have suggested that strong emotional support may be perceived as an added pressure for students to succeed, especially among traditional age students (48–50). Within some cultures, group decision making among immediate and extended family members is the expected norm. Therefore, the decision to go to college, persist, withdraw, or drop out would be influenced by more than just the student's decision.

Lack of family emotional support is not always perceived as a barrier to academic success. Cultural norms, values, and beliefs related to the family role, emotional support, and decision making must be considered. Defining who the family is, from the student's perspective, is an essential step. For example, among African American traditional-age college students who did not choose to identify a paternal figure, lack of father's support was not perceived as important. Among students who perceived a paternal figure, lack of a father's support was viewed as important (44). Other researchers indicated that parental attachment significantly predicted some aspects of college adjustment differently for White, Black, and Latina/Hispanic women (51); the influence of parental expectations and attachment on adjustment and achievement varies culturally (52). Nurse educators should be aware that cultural values and beliefs concerning familial ties, expectations, and emotional support vary; individual variations within cultures frequently occur, as do variations in interfamily dynamics.

Family dynamics may influence the incidence of role conflicts and perceived emotional support. Characteristics of well-functioning families include strong, stable marital alliance, clear interpersonal boundaries, and the absence of inappropriate coalitions (53). A coalition refers to an "intrafamily alignment wherein two individuals ally against a third person" (53, p. 46). It is well documented that a dysfunctional family environment adversely affects retention and/or college adjustment among traditional-age college students; a dysfunctional family environment can also affect nontraditional students adversely.

Family emotional support is a multidimensional environmental factor that interacts with other factors and variable sets within the NURS model and should be viewed in context with the other factors and variable sets. Additionally, family emotional support may have different meanings for different students; therefore, generalizations should be avoided. When surveying student perceptions about family emotional support for school, nurse educators should be aware of the potential diversity in responses and varied significance within a cultural context. In some cases, strong family support is not always desirable, and lack of family emotional support is not always a barrier. No support is better than perceived obstacles that are viewed as deliberate and/or insurmountable. What is most desirable is a healthy family support system, especially by the students' significant other(s) (54).

> To what degree do your students perceive their family emotional support as supportive or restrictive to their retention and success?

Family Responsibilities

> What do you know about your students' family responsibilities?

Family responsibilities are the daily tasks, expectations, behaviors, attitudes, and values that are needed to adequately perform the expected role within the family setting/environment. They may or may not be compatible with academic and employment responsibilities. Mutually compatible responsibilities will enhance academic success and minimize stress; incompatible responsibilities will hinder academic success and create multiple role stress. Family responsibilities influence retention indirectly through academic and psychological outcomes and interact with other environmental factors and variable sets in the NURS model. It is presumed that family responsibilities are most applicable for commuter students, as residential students do not have daily tasks and responsibilities within the family. Residential students may be influenced adversely if their inability to participate in previously held family responsibilities is perceived negatively.

It is expected that having more family responsibilities interferes with study skills, attendance, academic performance, faculty and peer interaction, satisfaction, academic performance, and retention. Family responsibilities have been identified as a significant obstacle for nontraditional nursing student success (10,34,45,46,55–64). Both time-based pressure and strain-based pressure may result in perceived family–school role conflict. Strain-based pressure refers to strain symptoms (tension) in one role that affects performance in others (65). Family responsibilities combined with school responsibilities may compete for limited time to complete responsibilities adequately. Inability to meet family responsibilities adequately may result in decreased ability to concentrate on school responsibilities.

Nursing students may perceive family responsibilities as influencing retention in markedly different ways. For example, in a study of first-semester nontraditional associate degree nursing students, 51% perceived that family responsibilities were moderately restrictive and 6% perceived them as severely restrictive (3,4). However, samples composed of associate degree student participants in enrichment program (EP) study groups across varying course levels presented different findings. Most notable was the shift from family responsibilities as moderately restrictive (14%) to severely restrictive (25%) at the end of the semester (6). Beginning students may need additional faculty guidance to manage time, juggle roles, and effectively meet family and academic responsibilities. Approximately, 20% to 28% of the enrichment program study group participants reported family responsibilities as moderately supportive, yet many family responsibilities may have prevented other students from participating in the EP study groups, thereby skewing the results. It is reasonable to surmise that the general population of associate degree nursing students was faced with multiple family responsibilities that adversely affected retention directly or indirectly. Another study of predominantly associate degree nursing students generated results indicating that students perceived family responsibilities as mainly moderately or severely restrictive (32). These findings are consistent with the higher education and nursing literature concerning nontraditional students.

Students with dependent children frequently feel overburdened with family and domestic responsibilities. However, perceptions vary with spousal expectations, cultural expectations, number and ages of children, number and ages of other dependent family members, socioeconomic status, child-care arrangements, and other variables (13,66). Students with dependent children have family responsibilities that pertain to child-care issues. Combined with other family responsibilities, child care creates further challenges for student success and persistence. Because of its complexity, nurse educators may wish to explore child-care arrangements separately in relation to student retention.

> To what degree do your students perceive their family responsibilities as supportive or restrictive to their retention and success?

Child-Care Arrangements

> What child-care facilities and services are available at your campus? What do you know about your students' child-care needs, concerns, and issues?

Child-care arrangements are the needs, concerns, and issues surrounding child care. The increasing number of women who have dependent children and who are enrolled in nursing programs demands attention to child-care concerns. A neglected area concerns men and child-care concerns—especially with increased shared parenting responsibility, divorce, and single-parenting. Generally, dependent children and child-care arrangements have been depicted as a barrier to academic achievement and retention. Often, the presence of dependent children was seen as a predictor for attrition without fully surveying individual differences. Students with dependent children are not a homogenous group, and it behooves the nurse educator to avoid stereotypical assumptions about them.

The number and ages of children, presence of support systems, and student perceptions of child-care arrangements are necessary to assess. For example, Scott, Burns, and Cooney (12,13) indicated that younger women with younger children were more likely to leave school due to family responsibilities, financial strain, and child-care problems. Quality child care for infants and toddlers is not easily found and is more expensive, and thus creates financial strain. In general, financial aid often does not consider child-care costs, thus putting a financial burden on students (33,67). Worry over child-care issues is stressful and influences satisfaction and the overall academic experience (68). Perceived multiple-role stress for women who are mothers and students is a complex phenomenon that encompasses emotional role ambiguity, person–role conflict, and inter-role conflict (69,70). The issue goes beyond finding a safe, reliable caretaker to the emotional component of nurturance. Child-care arrangements in the NURS model take into account the emotional aspect and the physical environment and caretaker.

Insight into student perceptions of child-care arrangements as supportive or restrictive for academic achievement and retention is valuable. Consistently, across three study samples, responses were diverse for associate degree nursing students. Among respondents for whom child care was applicable, much disparity between restrictiveness and supportiveness was noted. In one study, almost 60% reported child care as supportive, although approximately 30% reported it as restrictive both at the beginning of the semester and then again at the end. Others perceived that their child-care arrangements did not influence retention in any way. Notably, all of these students remained in nursing courses throughout the semester and successfully passed the course (6). Previous studies showed that approximately two-thirds of the students with child-care arrangements felt that the arrangements restricted academic achievement and retention. Subsequently, a large multisite study also indicated disparate responses: supported (39%), restricted (30%), or did not affect (31%) (32).

> To what degree do your students perceive their child-care arrangements as supportive or restrictive to their retention and success?

Family Crisis

> What type of family crises have your students faced while enrolled in your course, other courses, and throughout the nursing program? How do family crises affect student retention and success?

Of course, family crisis adversely affects retention, doesn't it? Or does it? A family crisis is a severe, unexpected family problem that often results in increased family responsibilities, stress, and family–school conflicts. Most literature supports that family crisis adversely affects class attendance, academic performance, and retention. Depending on the type of crisis, effects may be short term or long term. For example, a student whose child is rushed to the emergency room for appendicitis may perceive this as a crisis with short-term effects. After the child's successful recovery from the appendectomy, the student can resume usual routines. Long-term effects may be psychological and/or tangible. For example, a student whose husband unexpectedly dies may experience long-term psychological effects (grievance) and tangible effects (lack of husband's income). The student will not be able to resume usual routines (including school) due to emotional distress and financial strain. Repeated crises with short-term effects may take their toll on student's persistence indirectly through stress or directly through failure due to excessive absences.

Surprisingly, some research supports that family crisis can have a positive effect on persistence behaviors. Napoli and Wortman (71) found that students with more outside negative life events were more likely to seek support from within the college environment, thereby positively affecting persistence. Strong persistence behaviors are inversely related to voluntary attrition and decrease the risk for involuntary attrition. This rather unexpected finding suggests the reconceptualization of the direction of causality between family crisis and retention. Furthermore, in several studies, it explains the diversity in nursing student responses regarding the effect of family crisis on retention. Upon superficial perusal, the diversity in student responses for this survey item may have raised questions concerning validity. However, upon further scrutiny, the responses make sense. First, most students perceived that a family crisis would not occur, would neither be restrictive or supportive, or would be restrictive. Second, posttest data demonstrated a shift from 21% to 7%, perceiving that a family crisis did not influence their ability to remain in the nursing course (6). Finally, five data sets consistently show diversity in responses (3–6,32). These studies did not explore the type of family crisis and the psychological and/or tangible impact on student academic performance and retention was not done. In the future, qualitative studies may lend insight into students' perspectives.

> To what degree do your students perceive family crisis as supportive or restrictive to their retention and success?

Employment Hours

> How many of your students are employed? How many hours do your students work daily and weekly? What is their work schedule? What is the commute time to and from work? How easy or difficult is it for students to commute to work?

With the growing number of college students who work at least part-time, employment hours becomes an environmental factor that can influence student performance and retention. In nursing, the number of nontraditional, older students who are employed is also increasing; however, the number of traditional-age college students working 30 or more hours has also increased (72,73). Work hours, in this context, refer to both the number of hours worked and the compatibility of work hours with school and family responsibilities. Long employment hours and inflexible work schedule adversely influences academic achievement and retention of nontraditional students.

Several studies correlating the number of work hours with college student outcomes provide interesting findings. One study found that the number of hours worked was only marginally associated with academic success; students who worked 1 to 5 hours weekly had statistically significant higher GPAs than students who did not work or who worked more hours (74). Other researchers reported that the number of work hours adversely affected GPA by decreasing study hours (72,75–78). The idea of work hours detracting from study hours has also been substantiated by other researchers (9,79). It is logical to acknowledge that the time spent in one role limits the time spent in another.

Although employment hours should be compared closely with work responsibilities and other environmental factors and variable sets, student perception of how work hours influence retention is important. A survey of nursing student perceptions concerning work hours supported the employment trends among college students; approximately two-thirds of the students were employed (3–6,32). Of the employed students, responses were almost equally divided between supportive and restrictive when the students were surveyed at the beginning of the semester. In a study that measured nursing student perceptions at the beginning and at the end of the semester, a shift toward employment hours as restrictive occurred (6). Again, the shift from a more conservative view to a more restrictive view retrospectively is consistent with trends in several other environmental factors. These studies did not differentiate between number of work hours and compatibility of work hours; future researchers may wish to distinguish between the two dimensions. Results of an end-of-semester multisite cross-sectional study revealed that more than half of the employed students perceived employment hours as restrictive to their ability to remain in a nursing course during the semester. Notably, in this study, the impact of employment hours was explored using the factors generated from the factor analysis of the Student Perception Appraisal-Revised (SPA-R). Statistically significant differences were noted for unemployed students and for the number of hours worked. The mean for "Environmental Factors" was highest (indicating more supportive) for unemployed students and then decreased significantly with each additional 10 hours to over 40. For personal academic factors, the same phenomenon with incrementally raised means for each additional 10 hours occurred; significant differences were noted for unemployed students as compared with those working 21 to 30 hours and 31 to 40 hours (32). This finding is consistent with educational literature suggesting that employment past 20 hours per week presents barriers to academic achievement, social and academic integration, and retention (9,72,80).

> To what degree do your students perceive their work hours as supportive or restrictive to their retention and success? How compatible are your students' work hours to successfully meeting family and school responsibilities?

Employment Responsibilities

> What do you know about your students' employment responsibilities? Does what, where, why, and how students are employed make a difference? How can work responsibilities influence student achievement, satisfaction, self-efficacy, stress, and retention?

Employment responsibilities are the tasks, expectations, behaviors, attitudes, and values that are needed to adequately perform the roles within a particular employment setting. Mutually compatible responsibilities will enhance academic success and minimize stress; incompatible responsibilities will hinder academic success and create multiple-role stress. Employment responsibilities influence retention indirectly through academic and psychological outcomes and interact with other environmental factors and variable sets in the NURS model. On-campus employment has been linked with positive effects through social integration and values congruent with the academic environment. Off-campus employment has been correlated with decreased persistence (9,30). In addition, employment responsibilities meant less time on campus and less opportunity for academic and social integration (9,72,81). For the most part, the nursing literature has not differentiated between types of employment as a study variable. However employment responsibilities as a hindrance to successful academic outcomes and retention has been discussed (10,34,43,45,46,55,80,82–86).

Student perceptions about employment responsibilities as restricting or supporting retention are often diverse. The striking change between prospective and retrospective perceptions suggests that students are more optimistic initially. For example, in one study, students initially expected employment responsibilities to be supportive (36%) but later only 14% perceived employment responsibilities as having been supportive (6). Another retrospective study revealed that more than half of employed nursing students perceived their employment responsibilities as restrictive (32). Nurse educators can proactively assist students in realistically appraising their employment hours and responsibilities and periodically guide students throughout the semester in effective time management between multiple roles.

> To what degree do your students perceive their employment responsibilities as supportive or restrictive to their retention and success? How compatible are employment responsibilities to successfully meeting family and school responsibilities?

Encouragement by Outside Friends

> What do you know about the influence of your students' outside friends on retention and success?

Outside friends are those outside of the student's classes and the college environment. They do not include family members. Encouragement by outside friends is their active emotional involvement in relation to the student's academic endeavors and career goals. Positive encouragement is manifested by supporting these goals, promoting positive feelings of self-worth, believing in the student's ability to succeed, listening to problems and concerns, showing interest in academic progress, expressing optimism, offering assistance, and presence.

The literature presents conflicting evidence about the influence of outside friends on academic performance, persistence, and retention. One study reported that students with more outside friends who attended college were more academically involved than peers with one-half the number or fewer who attended college (74). Similarly, Hernandez (47) noted more positive persistence behaviors among Latino students with outside friends who provided them with helpful and substantive information about college and who gave them ongoing encouragement. Other researchers found that outside friends significantly influence persistence in White college students, whereas minority students were often discouraged because of time spent away from family and friends and/or lack of support for college (30,54,68). What is consistently evident is that "encouragement by those most significant in a student's life is instrumental in affecting the overall college experience and persistence decisions" (54, p. 52). Cultural values and beliefs concerning friendships, views on education, and general worldview need to be considered when evaluating the impact of outside friends on retention.

Pressure by friends to participate in outside (nonacademic) activities, such as social engagements, that conflict with the student's ability to successfully complete academic and career goals is incongruent with positive encouragement behaviors. Difficulty setting limits on friends and social activities negatively influences academic performance and retention (87). Among several samples of nontraditional associate degree students, students perceived encouragement from outside friends as supportive. Most of the students were older (over 25) and were perhaps more experienced in maintaining friendships with people who provided encouragement (3–6). A subsequent multi-institutional factor analysis study indicated that friends outside of class was "greatly supportive" in influencing retention and clustered together with the variable of "friends in class," resulting in a factor labeled "Friend Support." To further explore the influence of age and other demographic variables on friend support, several other analyses were conducted, indicating that regardless of age, students whose first language was English demonstrated higher scores, suggesting that encouragement from friends was more important for EFL students (32). Among other mature access or diverse-age student groups, outside friend support was important to the students' support network in Australia (34), Ireland (88), and accelerated U.S. programs (42).

Nurse educators may wish to further explore and consider the impact of outside friends in relation to the student's age and other demographic variables. For example, several studies concerning male nursing students revealed that outside friends often made unsupportive comments, perpetuated stereotypes, questioned sexuality, and contested rationale for entry into a traditional female-dominated career that was often perceived as less desirable than other careers (89,90).Views about nursing as a desirable or undesirable profession must be considered within societal and cultural contexts. In contrast, among predominantly female ESL nursing student samples, cultural pressure and high expectations from friends encouraged students to be successful, yet the high pressure for success actually created a need for more psychosocial support and understanding from friends (91).

Another dimension to the influence of outside friends is social adjustment and institutional attachment. For example, among European American students, satisfaction with outside friendships and contacts was negatively correlated with social adjustment and institutional attachment (92). For disadvantaged students, outside friends who are not academically successful or college-focused can create conflicts and feelings of isolation within the academic environment (93).

Especially among traditional-age students, strong social adjustment and institutional attachment are expected to enhance academic performance, persistence, and retention. Students who reside at the college, especially students with outside friends who attend other colleges, have more difficulty with college adjustment than other students, thus creating a potential retention barrier (94). More recently, texting, cell phones, Internet with webcam, social networking, and virtual friends offer new opportunities for friendships, necessitating new research to explore the impact of technological advances on new and old friendships (95).

> To what degree do your students perceive encouragement by outside friends as supportive or restrictive to their retention and success?

Living Arrangements

> What do you know about your students' living arrangements?

Living arrangements include the needs, concerns, and issues concerning students' residential environment while attending college. Generally, living arrangements are quite different for commuter students than for noncommuter students. For the campus resident, one major factor influencing retention surrounds college adjustment and social integration into the college residential environment. Living at college is a new experience that requires adjustment. The NURS model takes into account the emotional aspect of living arrangements as well as the physical environment and the other individuals who share it. Consistent with the literature, it is proposed that living arrangements can support or restrict student retention and success.

The literature on college adjustment presents contrasting views. Tinto (96) proposed that successful adjustment depends on the student's ability to disassociate from past communities of friends and family and to engage in a smooth transition to a new community, developing new friends and creating a new family or community. However, other researchers stated that for minority students, positive family attachments eased transition to the college environment (41,54,97). Barriers that impede a smooth transition to a new living environment include far distance from home, friends who attend other colleges, differences in geographic area or size of town, cultural background different from the majority, and difficulty with parental separation. Nurse educators should be aware that the developmental task of parental separation is influenced by culture, gender, family dynamics, and/or interpersonal conflicts. For example, within some families and cultures, parental separation to attend college is valued, encouraged, and expected. In other families and cultures, parental separation for reasons other than marriage is discouraged. Traditional-age students from tumultuous living environments may look forward to leaving home; their perceptions may be that their college living arrangements are much improved over their previous ones.

Insight into student perceptions of living arrangements as supportive or restrictive for academic achievement and retention is valuable. Perceived satisfaction with a social support network on campus assists with college adjustment and is particularly crucial for minority students attending predominantly White universities. An environment perceived as uncaring and culturally different has caused feelings of dissatisfaction and difficult college adjustment (9,66,98–100). Positive college adjustment and the perception that living arrangements are conducive to facilitating academic outcomes, satisfaction, and career outcomes will positively influence retention. Among surveyed alumni, positive feelings about assigned living arrangements during freshman year that encouraged social interaction across racial and ethnic groups was viewed as desired and a positive factor in their college adjustment and satisfaction (101).

Living arrangements can also influence commuter student academic achievement and retention (32). Lack of a safe, nurturing living environment conducive to studying will affect retention directly or indirectly through academic outcomes. For example, a nursing student living in a homeless shelter will face many adversities in living arrangements that will interfere with academic achievement. A noisy home environment (on campus or off campus) without adequate study space will also adversely affect retention through academic outcomes and interfere with study hours. Safe, nurturing, and quiet living arrangements that are located far away from the college campus and/or clinical sites present transportation challenges.

> To what degree do your students perceive their living arrangements as supportive or restrictive to their retention and success?

Transportation

> What modes of transportation are used by your students? What transportation issues do your students face?

Transportation is more pertinent for commuter students than for noncommuter students. However, because nursing programs may require students to travel to sites outside the university setting for clinical experiences, it may also be a concern for residential nursing students. Transportation issues involve dependability, distance, parking, safety, time, energy, and money. In some areas, public transportation is not available and presents transportation challenges to nursing students who need to travel great distances for clinical work and who may not have access to a car. Real or perceived transportation difficulties serve as a barrier to attendance, punctuality, academic performance, and retention.

Transportation as a barrier may influence retention indirectly through academic and psychological outcomes. Additionally, it interacts with other environmental factors (such as family responsibilities and financial status) and academic factors (attendance and study hours). For example, long travel time will take away from family responsibilities and study hours. Unreliable and/or lengthy transportation puts an added stress on students (102). Traveling expenses may sometimes prevent students from attending classes in an effort to save money. Financial aid and scholarships usually do not cover transportation expenses, so this can be a serious impediment for economically disadvantaged students (33,63,67,103) and a cost that must be absorbed by students (104). Obviously, transportation issues need to be individually appraised. In several studies conducted at one commuter college and a large multi-institutional study, it was not surprising that nursing student perceptions about transportation were quite diverse. The surveyed students commuted various distances, traveled through different neighborhoods, and used one or more modes of transportation (subway/rail, bus, ferry, car, motorcycle, taxi, bike, foot) (3–6,32).

> To what degree do your students perceive their transportation as supportive or restrictive to their retention and success?

KEY POINT SUMMARY

- In the NURS model, environmental factors are those that are external to the academic process and include financial status, family financial support, family emotional support, family responsibilities, child-care arrangements, family crisis, employment hours, employment responsibilities, encouragement by outside friends, living arrangements, and transportation.
- Financial status refers to the student's financial standing in meeting all financial expenses including tuition, college fees, books and other learning materials, living expenses, financial obligations, and commitments.
- Family emotional support for school is the active emotional involvement of family members in the student's academic endeavors and career goals. It is manifested by encouraging educational and career goals, promoting positive feelings of self-worth, believing in the student's ability to succeed, listening to problems and concerns, showing

interest in academic progress, expressing optimism, offering assistance, and presence.

- A detailed and holistic appraisal of student perceptions concerning the influence of each environmental factor on academic success and retention reveals several dimensions that potentially affect students differently. While some environmental factors are perceived as barriers to retention, other students perceive the same factors as supportive.
- Environmental support is believed to compensate for weak academic support; however, the opposite does not hold true. Academic support is not thought to compensate for weak environmental support.

APPLICATION STRATEGIES

EDUCATOR-IN-ACTION VIGNETTE

Educators' actions concerning environmental factors can make a considerable difference in student academic and psychological outcomes, persistence, and retention. Without appropriate background knowledge, individual appraisal, and sensitivity, educators' actions may adversely impact upon these areas. Consider the possible adverse effects of the following educator actions:

Pamela's elderly mother-in-law usually cares for Pamela's infant and toddler. However, sudden diarrhea from food poisoning renders the mother-in-law incapable of providing care. Family traditions hold the mother-in-law as the most esteemed family member and head of the family, who must be cared for by the daughter-in-law when ill. Day care is not considered an appropriate option. Pamela has never been late or absent from class, and only two absences are permissible. When she calls Professor Hurdles and tells her that child care and other family responsibilities prevent her from attending class, Professor Hurdles says, "You should have called me yesterday so I wouldn't have made out the patient assignment. That is very unprofessional. If you sent your children to the day care center, you wouldn't have this problem."

Jo-Ann is a 19-year-old student who was abused by her parents until adopted at age 10 by her cousin. Her cousin recently died after a lengthy and costly illness. When registering for classes, Jo-Ann says, "If there is an opening, I would like to register for the two-day college class schedule and clinical at Children's Hospital. I live within walking distance from the hospital. Since I am an independent student, it would save me money." Professor Hurdles replies, "It sounds like you should learn to manage your money better. Why don't you ask your parents?"

In contrast, educator actions that seek to actively acknowledge the importance of environmental factors, appreciate students as individuals, objectively appraise diverse environmental situations, maximize strengths and improve weaknesses, and have the most potential for promoting positive academic and psychological outcomes, persistence, and retention. For example, Professor Bridges lists environmental factors on the course orientation agenda, adding credence to their importance. Brief sample student scenarios with various environmental factors are presented in written handouts and then read aloud. Student actions, including the effective use of family, faculty, and friend support networks are suggested by students and then further discussed.

As the group's interests about the fictitious case scenarios are stimulated, Professor Bridges seizes the opportunity to offer guidance and assist the current students. "If there are any environmental factors that you would like to talk with me about, or would like further guidance with, please write them down on your index card. If there is something you would like me to address in class further, please let me know. There is no need to write down your name. If there is something you would like to speak with me about individually, please include your name. Feel free to see me during office hours, call me, or send an e-mail. Several students write:

TRINA: After our class discussion, I realized that I may need help with balancing my work, family, and school responsibilities. Maybe applying for a student loan would allow me to work fewer hours and have more time for school and my family. Previously, I thought that student loans were only for young students. Is it too late to get a loan for this semester?

ANNA: At first, I felt overwhelmed by my family responsibilities. I thought that I was alone. The discussion and handouts made me realize that I wasn't alone and didn't have to struggle through this by myself. Thanks.

LEON: My parents didn't want me to apply for financial aid or loans. I've been working full-time to pay for school. I get passing grades, but I want to do better in school. The nurse externship program combines work and a forgivable loan without needing parental permission and financial aid forms. Thanks for telling us about it. Can you help me with the application process?

JACKIE: I don't have any questions now but it's helpful knowing that instructors think factors other than school are important in our lives. It is nice to know that faculty care.

Professor Bridges follows up with individual student requests and refers students to additional resources as appropriate. In class, she continues to remind students about the importance of ongoing self-appraisal of environmental factors and their effect on academic responsibilities, achievement, stress, satisfaction, and progress in nursing.

TOOLKIT RESOURCE BOX

Items 1–4—Student Perception Appraisal Questionnaires—Pretests and Posttests

DISCUSSION QUESTIONS

1. Identify the two environmental factors about which you learned the most. Discuss what you learned that was new and how this would impact upon your future role as a nurse educator in an undergraduate associate degree program mainly composed of nontraditional students, an undergraduate generic program, accelerated BS program for second degree students, and/or an RN-BSN program.

2. When you read the Educator-in-Action vignette at the end of the chapter, what visual images popped into your head? What race, gender, age, weight, and other physical, mental, and professional attributes did you visualize/imagine for each student, Professor Hurdles, and Professor Bridges? Why? What feelings were evoked as you read each scenario? Why? What impact can these images and feelings have on your interactions with diverse student populations? What impact could they potentially have on student persistence, satisfaction, stress, self-efficacy (confidence), attrition, and retention?

3. Professor Cave says, "It's so sad. Melissa, a 21-year-old highly motivated student in my clinical group, had no contact with her father for over 10 years and does not know his address. I was reviewing her application for a nursing scholarship for disadvantaged students and noticed that she submitted a waiver for supplying her father's contact and financial information as noncustodial parent. Her mother's information indicates that she never received any child support, yet works two jobs and contributes her modest wages to cover 40% of Melissa's college expenses. I was planning to speak with Melissa about using advanced Internet search resources so she can reestablish emotional and financial support from her father. Technology is so wonderful and it may enable her to reconnect with her father. She may not need the scholarship after all. I would rather award the scholarship to a student who has two parents at home providing emotional support." How would you respond to Professor Cave?

4. Professor Swift says, "This is an accelerated BS nursing program for students with a previous college degree. These students already were successful in college, so we don't need to allocate class time to talk about environmental or academic factors. They already know what to do to balance their time. I don't know why some accelerated nursing programs have such high attrition and failure rates. They must not select students with high GPAs." How would you respond to Professor Swift?

5. A colleague says, "I don't really understand how environmental support is believed to compensate for weak academic support; however academic support is not thought to compensate for weak environmental support." How would you explain this to your colleague?

REFERENCES

1. Bean, J. P., & Metzner, B. (1985). A conceptual model of nontraditional undergraduate student attrition. *Review of Educational Research, 55*, 485–540.
2. Metzner, B., & Bean, J. P. (1987). The estimation of a conceptual model of nontraditional undergraduate student attrition. *Research in Higher Education, 27*, 15–38.
3. Jeffreys, M. R. (1993). *The relationship of self-efficacy and select academic and environmental variables on academic achievement and retention.* Unpublished doctoral dissertation, New York, NY: Teachers College, Columbia University.
4. Jeffreys, M. R. (1998). Predicting nontraditional student retention and academic achievement. *Nurse Educator, 23*(1), 42–48.
5. Jeffreys, M. R. (2001). Evaluating enrichment program study groups: Academic outcomes, psychological outcomes, and variables influencing retention. *Nurse Educator, 26*(3), 142–149.
6. Jeffreys, M. R. (2002). Students' perceptions of variables influencing retention: A pretest and post-test approach. *Nurse Educator, 27*(1), 16–19 [Erratum, 2002, 27(2), 64].
7. Jeffreys, M. R. (2003). Strategies for promoting nontraditional student retention and success. In Oermann, M., & Heinrich, K. (eds.). *Annual review of nursing education: Volume I* (pp. 61–90). New York, NY: Springer Publishing.
8. College Board. (2008). *Fulfilling the commitment: Recommendations for reforming federal student aid.* Report from the Rethinking Student Aid Study Group. Retrieved from http://www.collegeboard.com
9. Seidman, A. (2005). *College student retention: Formula for student success.* Westport, CT: American Council on Education, Praeger.
10. Last, L., & Fulbrook, P. (2003). Why do student nurses leave? Suggestions from a Delphi study. *Nurse Education Today, 23*, 449–458.
11. Hurtado, S., Inkelas, K. K., Briggs, C., & Rhee, B-S. (1997). Differences in college access and choice among racial/ethnic groups: Identifying continuing barriers. *Research in Higher Education, 38*(1), 43–75.
12. Scott, C., Burns, A., & Cooney, G. (1998). Motivation for return to study as a predictor of completion of degree amongst female mature students with children. *Higher Education, 35*, 221–239.
13. Scott, C., Burns, A., & Cooney, G. (1996). Reasons for discontinuing study: The case of mature age female students with children. *Higher Education, 31*, 233–253.
14. Williams, E. (1997). How women experience social support as mature adult learners in a vocational setting. *Journal of Vocational Education Research, 22*(1), 39–53.
15. Chaney, B., Muraskin, L. D., Cahalan, M. W., & Goodwin, D. (1998). Helping the progress of disadvantaged students in higher education: The federal

student support services program. *Educational Evaluation and Policy Analysis,* *20*(3), 197–215.

16. Olinger, B. H. (2011). Increasing nursing workforce diversity: Strategies for success. *Nurse Educator, 36*(2), 54–55.

17. Ramsburg, L. (2007). Strive for success: A successful retention program for associate of science in nursing students. *Teaching and Learning in Nursing, 2,* 12–16.

18. Padilla, R. V., Trevino, J., Gonzalez, K., & Trevino, J. (1997). Developing local models of minority student success in college. *Journal of College Student Development, 38*(2), 125–135.

19. Braxton, J. M., & McClendon, S. A. (2001). The fostering of social integration and retention through institutional practice. *Journal of College Student Retention: Research, Theory, & Practice, 3*(1), 57–72.

20. Tinto, V. (1993). *Leaving college: Rethinking the cause and cures of student attrition.* Chicago: University of Chicago Press.

21. St. John, E. P., Hu, S., Simmons, A. B., & Musoba, G. D. (2001). Aptitude vs. merit: What matters in persistence. *Review of Higher Education, 24*(2), 131–152.

22. U. S. Department of Education, National Center for Education Statistics. (2011). The condition of education, 2011, Washington, DC: Author.

23. Nora, A., Barlow, L., & Crisp, G. (2006). Examining the tangible and psychosocial benefits of financial aid with student access, engagement, and degree attainment. *American Behavioral Psychologist, 49*(12), 1636–1651.

24. Oseguera, L., Denson, N., & Hurtado, S. (2009). Hispanic students and the Gates Millennium scholarship program: Promising results extending to the third year. *Journal of College Student Retention: Research, Theory, and Practice,* *10* (3), 307–338.

25. Joo, S-H., Durband, D. B., & Grable, J. (2009). The academic impact of financial stress on college students. *Journal of College Student Retention: Research, Theory, and Practice, 10* (3), 287–305.

26. Hornak, A. M., Farrell, P. L., & Jackson, N. J. (2010). Making it (or not) on a dime in college: Implications for practice. *Journal of College Student Development,* *51*(5), 481–495.

27. Northern, J. J., O'Brien, W. H., & Goetz, P. W. (2010). The development, evaluation, and validation of a financial stress scale for undergraduate students. *Journal of College Student Development, 51*(1), 79–92.

28. Nurmi, J-E., & Aunola, K. (2001). How does academic achievement come about: Cross-cultural and methodological notes. *International Journal of Educational Research, 35,* 403–409.

29. Dowd, A. C. (2008). Dynamic interactions and intersubjectivity: Challenges to causal modeling in studies of college student debt. *Review of Educational Research, 78*(2), 232–259.

30. Nora, A., Cabrera, A., Hagedorn, L. S., & Pascarella, E. (1996). Differential impacts of academic and social experiences on college-related behavioral outcomes across different ethnic and gender groups at four-year institutions. *Research in Higher Education, 37*(4), 427–451.

31. Museus, S. D. (2010). Understanding recial differences in the effects of loans on degree attainment: A path analysis. *Journal of College Student Retention: Research, Theory, and Practice, 11* (4), 499–527.

32. Jeffreys, M. R. (2007). Nontraditional students' perceptions of variables influencing retention: A multisite study. *Nurse Educator, 32*(4), 161–167.

33. Kennamer, M. A., Katsinas, S. G., & Schumacker, R. E. (2011). The moving target: Student financial aid and community college retention. *Journal of College Student Retention: Research, Theory, and Practice, 12* (1), 87–103.

34. Steele, R., Lauder, W., & Caperchione, C. (2005). An exploratory study of the concerns of mature access to nursing students and the coping strategies used to manage these adverse experiences. *Nurse Education Today, 25*, 573–581.

35. Urwin, S., Stanley, R., Jones, M., Gallagher, A., Wainwright, P., & Perkins, A. (2010). Understanding student nurse attrition: Learning from the literature. *Nurse Education Today, 30*, 202–207.

36. Glogowska, M., Young, P., & Lockyer, L. (2007). Should I go or should I stay? A study of factors influencing students' decisions on early leaving. *Active Learning in Higher Education, 8*(1), 63–77.

37. Ali, P. A., & Naylor, P. B. (2010). Association between academic and non-academic variables and academic success of diploma nursing students in Pakistan. *Nurse Education Today, 30*, 157–162.

38. Eaton, S. B., & Bean, J. P. (1995). An approach/avoidance behavioral model of college student attrition. *Research in Higher Education, 36*(6), 617–645.

39. Lehna, C., Jackonen, S., & Wilson, L. (1996). Navigating a nursing curriculum: Bridges and barriers. *Association of Black Nursing Faculty Journal, 7(July/ August)*, 98–103.

40. Vecchione, E. (1995). Looking at problems that hinder nontraditional students' achievements. *Nursing Leadership Forum, 1*(3), 94–98.

41. Hendricks, A. D., Smith, K., Caplow, J. H., & Donaldson, J. F. (1996). A grounded theory approach to determining the factors related to the persistence of minority students in professional programs. *Innovative Higher Education, 21*(2), 113–126.

42. Hegge, M., & Larson, V. (2008). Stressors and coping strategies of students in accelerated baccalaureate nursing programs. *Nurse Educator, 33*(1), 26–30.

43. Maville, J., & Huerta, C. G. (1997). Stress and social support among Hispanic student nurses: Implications for academic achievement. *Journal of Cultural Diversity, 4*(1), 18–25.

44. Hinderlie, H. H., & Kenny, M. (2002). Attachment, social support, and college adjustment among black students at predominantly white universities. *Journal of College Student Development, 43*(3), 327–340.

45. Tucker-Allen, S., & Long, E. (1999). *Recruitment and retention of minority students: Stories of success.* Lisle, IL: Tucker Publications.

46. Bosher, S. D., & Pharris, M. D. (2009). *Transforming nursing education: The culturally inclusive environment.* New York, NY: Springer Publishing.

47. Hernandez, J. C. (2000). Understanding the retention of Latino college students. *Journal of College Student Development, 41*(6), 575–588.

48. Olenchak, F. R., & Hebert, T. P. (2002). Endangered academic talent: Lessons learned from gifted first-generation college males. *Journal of College Student Development, 43*(2), 195–212.

49. Ting, S-M, R. (2000). Predicting Asian Americans' academic performance in the first year of college: An approach combining SAT scores and noncognitive variables. *Journal of College Student Development, 41*(4), 442–449.

50. Wilkie, C., & Redondo, B. (1996). Predictors of academic success and failure of first-year college students. *Journal of the Freshman Year Experience, 8*(2), 17–32.
51. Melendez, M. C., & Melendez, N. B. (2010). The influence of parental attachment on the college adjustment of white, black, and Latina/Hispanic women: A cross-cultural investigation. *Journal of College Student Development, 51*(4), 419–435.
52. Yazedjian, A., Toews, M. L., & Navarro, A. (2009). Exploring parental factors, adjustment, and academic achievement among white and Hispanic college students. *Journal of College Student Development, 50*(4), 458–467.
53. Lopez, F. G., Campbell, V. L., & Watkins, C. E. (1989). Effects of marital conflict and family coalition patterns on college student adjustment. *Journal of College Student Development, 30*, 46–52.
54. Nora, A. (2001). The depiction of significant others in Tinto's "Rites of Passage": A reconceptualization of the influence of family and community in the persistence process. *Journal of College Student Retention: Research, Theory, & Practice, 3*(1), 41–56.
55. Aber, C. S., & Arathuzik, D. (1996). Factors associated with student success in a baccalaureate nursing program within an urban public university. *Journal of Nursing Education, 35*(6), 285–288.
56. Burris, R. F. (2001). Teaching student parents. *Nurse Educator, 26*(2), 64–65, 98.
57. Griffiths, M. J., & Tagliareni, M. E. (1999). Challenging traditional assumptions about minority students in nursing education. *Nursing & Health Care Perspectives, 20*, 290–295.
58. Hegge, M., Melcher, P., & Williams, S. (1999). Hardiness, help-seeking behavior, and social support of baccalaureate nursing students. *Journal of Nursing Education, 38*(4), 179–182.
59. Bagnardi, M., & Perkel, L. K. (2005). The learning achievement program: Fostering student cultural diversity. *Nurse Educator, 30*(1), 17–20.
60. Henry, P. R. (2006). Making groups work in the classroom. *Nurse Educator, 31*(1), 26–30.
61. Gardner, J. (2005). Barriers influencing the success of racial and ethnic minority students in nursing programs. *Journal of Transcultural Nursing, 16*(2), 155–162.
62. Seldomridge, L. A., & DiBartolo, M. C. (2007). The changing face of accelerated second bachelor's degree students. *Nurse Educator, 32*(6), 240–245.
63. Stolder, M. E., Rosemeyer, A. K., & Zorn, C. R. (2008). In the shelter of each other: Respite care for students as a partnership model. *Nursing Education Perspectives,29*(5), 295–299.
64. O'Brien, F., Keogh, B., & Neenan, K. (2009). Mature students' experiences of undergraduate nurse education programmes: The Irish experience. *Nurse Education Today, 29*, 635–640.
65. Greenhaus, J. H., & Beutell, N. J. (1985). Sources of conflict between work and family roles. *Academy of Management Review, 10*, 76–88.
66. Wycoff, S. E. M. (1996). Academic performance of Mexican American women: Sources of support that serve as motivating variables. *Journal of Multicultural Counseling and Development, 24*, 146–155.
67. Cejda, B. D., & Hoover, R. E. (2011). Strategies for faculty-student engagement: How community college faculty engage Latino students. *Journal of College Student Retention: Theory, Research, and Practice. 12*(2), 135–153.

68. Martin, D. E., & Kipling, A. (2006). Factors shaping Aboriginal nursing students' experiences. *Nurse Education Today, 26,* 688–696.
69. Gigliotti, E. (1999). Women's multiple role stress: Testing Neuman's flexible line of defense. *Nursing Science Quarterly, 12*(1), 36–44.
70. Gigliotti, E. (2001). Development of the perceived multiple role stress scale (PMRS). *Journal of Nursing Measurement, 9*(2), 163–180.
71. Napoli, A. R., & Wortman, P. M. (1998). Psychosocial factors related to retention and early departure of two-year community college students. *Research in Higher Education, 39*(4), 419–455.
72. Torres, V., Gross, J. P. K., & Dadashova, A. (2011). *Journal of College Student Retention: Research, Theory, and Practice, 12* (1), 51–68.
73. Riggert, S. C., Boyle, M., Petrosko, J. M., Ash, D., & Rude-Parkins, C. (2006). Student employment and higher education: Empiricism and contradiction. *Review of Educational Research, 76*(1), 63–92.
74. Strage, A., Baba, Y., Millner, S., Scharberg, M., Walker, E., Williamson, R., & Yoder, M. (2002). What every student affairs professional should know: Student study activities and beliefs associated with academic success. *Journal of College Student Development, 43*(2), 246–266.
75. Ransdell, S. (2001). Predicting college success: The importance of ability and noncognitive variables. *International Journal of Educational Research, 35,* 357–364.
76. Ransdell, S. (2001). Discussion and implications. *International Journal of Educational Research, 35,* 391–395.
77. Ransdell, S., Hawkins, C., & Adams, R. (2001). Models, modeling, and the design of the study. *International Journal of Educational Research, 35,* 365–372.
78. Ransdell, S., Hawkins, C., & Adams, R. (2001). Results of the study. *International Journal of Educational Research, 35,* 373–389.
79. Toutkoushian, R. K., & Smart, J. C. (2001). Do institutional characteristics affect student gains from college? *Review of Higher Education, 25*(1), 39–61.
80. Schoofs, N., Bosold, S., Slot, V., & Flentje, J. (2008). Nursing student employment: Impact on academic achievement. *Nurse Educator, 33*(2), 57–58.
81. Kraemer, B. A. (1997). The academic and social integration of Hispanic students into college. *Review of Higher Education, 20*(2), 163–179.
82. Merrill, E. B. (1998). Culturally diverse students enrolled in nursing: Barriers influencing success. *Journal of Cultural Diversity, 5*(2), 58–67.
83. Andrew, S., Salamonson, Y., Weaver, R., Smith, A., O'Reilly, R., & Taylor, C. (2008). Hate the course or hate to go: Semester differences in first year nursing attrition. *Nurse Education Today, 28,* 865–872.
84. Watts, T. E. (2011). Supporting undergraduate nursing students through structured personal tutoring: Some reflections. *Nurse Education Today, 31,* 214–218.
85. Seago, J. A., Wong, S. T., Keane, D., & Grumbach, K. (2008). Measuring attributes of success of college students in nursing programs: A psychometric analysis. *Journal of Nursing Measurement, 16*(3), 184–200.
86. Love, K. L. (2010). The lived experience of socialization among African American nursing students in a predominantly white university. *Journal of Transcultural Nursing, 21*(4), 342–350.
87. Campbell, A. R., & Davis, S. M. (1996). Faculty commitment: Retaining minority nursing students in majority institutions. *Journal of Nursing Education, 35*(7), 298–303.

88. Fleming, S., & McKee, G. (2005). The mature student question. *Nurse Education Today, 25*, 230–237.

89. Dyck, J. M., Oliffe, J., Phinney, A., & Garrett, B. (2009). Nursing instructors' and male nursing students' perceptions of undergraduate, classroom nursing education. *Nurse Education Today, 29*, 649–653.

90. Wang, H., Li, X., Hu, X., Chen, H., Gao, Y., Zhao, H., & Huang, L. (2011). Perceptions of nursing profession and learning experiences of male students in baccalaureate nursing program in Changsha, China. *Nurse Education Today, 31*, 36–42.

91. Cunningham, H., Stacciarini, J-M. R., & Towle, S. (2004). Strategies to promote success on the NCLEX-RN for students with English as a second language. *Nurse Educator, 29*(1), 15–19.

92. Kenny, M. E., & Stryker, S. (1996). Social network characteristics and college adjustment among racially and ethnically diverse first-year students. *Journal of College Student Development, 37*(6), 649–658.

93. Zuzelo, P. R. (2005). Affirming the disadvantaged. *Nurse Educator, 30*(1), 27–31.

94. Turner, A. L., & Berry, T. R. (2000). Counseling center contributions to student retention and graduation: A longitudinal assessment. *Journal of College Student Development, 41*(6), 627–636.

95. Morris, J., Reese, J., Beck, R., & Mattis, C. (2010). Facebook usage as a predictor of retention at a private 4-year institution. *Journal of College Student Retention: Research, Theory, and Practice, 11* (3), 311–322.

96. Tinto, V. (1997). Classrooms as communities. *Journal of Higher Education, 68*(6), 599–623.

97. Cabrera, A. F., Nora, A., Terenzini, P. T., Pascarella, E. T., & Hagedorn, I. S. (1999). Campus racial climate and the adjustment of students to college: A comparison between white students and African American students. *Journal of Higher Education, 70*(2), 134–160.

98. Manifold, C., & Rambur, B. (2001). Predictors of attrition in American Indian nursing students. *Journal of Nursing Education, 40*(6), 279–281.

99. Villaruel, A. M., Canales, M., & Torres, S. (2001). Bridges and barriers: Educational mobility of Hispanic nurses. *Journal of Nursing Education, 40*(6), 245–251.

100. Yurkovich, E. E. (2001). Working with American Indians toward educational success. *Journal of Nursing Education, 40*(6), 259–269.

101. Luo, J., & Jamieson-Drake, D. (2009). A retrospective assessment of the educational benefits of interaction across racial boundaries. *Journal of College Student Development, 50*(2), 115–134.

102. Evans, B. C. (2007). Student perceptions: The influence of a nursing workforce diversity grant on retention. *Journal of Nursing Education,46*(8), 354–359.

103. Bond, M. L., Gray, J. R., Baxley,S., Cason, C. L., & Denke, L. (2008). Voices of Hispanic students in baccalaureate nursing programs: Are we listening? *Nursing Education Perspectives, 29*(3), 136–142.

104. Stuenkel, D., Nelson, D., Malloy, S., & Cohen, J. (2011). Challenges, changes, and collaboration evaluation of an accelerated BSN program. *Nurse Educator, 36*(2), 70–75.

6

Professional Integration and Socialization

Faculty can make a difference by increasing professional integration and eliminating social isolation.

SNAPSHOT SCENARIO

Several student representatives gather for lunch at the National Student Nurses Association (NSNA) conference.

Leila says, "It feels so good to meet students from other nursing programs across the country who are experiencing the same things as me. Now I really feel connected to nursing. I was thinking about dropping out last year after failing a test. My advisor saw me crying in the hallway and took me to her office. We had a long talk. Then she paired me up with a peer mentor-tutor (PMT), who was a senior. We reviewed strategies for success. Until that day, I couldn't even visualize myself inside the nursing profession. When was the first time you felt part of nursing? Did any of you ever think about dropping out?"

HELEN: During the 2-hour orientation program, when the professor had us close our eyes and visualize ourselves in a nursing uniform, wearing a name tag with our name and RN after it. Our teacher told us to practice this visualization as a prereading and prestudy strategy to get us motivated, focused, and concentrated on active reading to apply information within the context of nursing. I do this whenever thoughts of dropping out creep into my mind and it keeps me going.

JAMES: During my nursing orientation, we had just watched a 2-minute movie about nursing. It was very inspiring to quickly see all the many types of important roles RNs have. It was very action oriented with a good balance between technology and human caring. I was pleased to see men of different ages and backgrounds depicted in the film. I often wondered if I really belonged in nursing. Now I think I do because I could see myself in some of the roles.

SARENA: For me, it started when I was walking by a bulletin board outside the nursing office. I was an undeclared major but always felt like I wanted to be in a health profession. The bulletin board showed patients and nurses of many different cultural backgrounds and ages working in different settings. I saw a nurse who wore religious clothing like me and I could identify with her. The elderly patient she was caring for had such a relaxed, comforted look upon her face...and in the photo, the patient's family members were receptive to the nurse's review of patient teaching brochures. They seemed to be respectful of the nurse even though they were culturally different from her. I saw myself as the nurse in that photo, and it felt good. A nursing professor was walking by with some nursing students and saw me staring at the photo. She facilitated introductions and invited me to a nursing student club luncheon later that week, pairing me with one of the students so I wouldn't feel alone.

LORI: My teacher, the vice president of the honor society chapter, invited all the students to attend the guest presenter's presentation. It was free. Even so, I would not have gone except it was part of the requirement for a class in my accelerated nursing program. I went with some of my new friends in class. My teacher randomly assigned us to groups and I was resentful and scared at first, but now I am glad I went outside my comfort circle of friends to learn different perspectives and make new friends. My PMT was there and introduced me to some senior nursing students. During the reception afterward, my teacher introduced me to the guest speaker and to some other nurses in the community. They were very welcoming, and I felt included. Some of them invited me to attend a conference on diabetes at the local hospital. They treated me like they really wanted me to make it and join them in the ranks of nursing. I felt good.

ANABELLE: We have an enrichment program (EP) with organized peer mentoring and tutoring and study groups at my school that takes place in a resource center called the Nursing Neighborhood. It's great that there is a place for just nursing students to go to seek academic help and peer support, work together, get inspired, or just let off some steam. I always feel welcomed there and I can be myself. My classmates and the PMTs accept me for who I am, and we support each other. Even though we come from different backgrounds and neighborhoods, we all belong in the nursing neighborhood. It's comforting to have a place to call home in nursing when the nursing profession seemed so foreign and unreachable in the beginning.

Leila says, "These stories are important and can help other students. I also feel good sharing my story, and it's unfortunate that there are many students who cannot be at a national convention to share in its benefits. Let's start a blog so students around the country can share their stories of success.

Here is a blog posting:

KRYSTAL: I work full-time and have three small children. I didn't have time for the extra things like socializing on campus, so I really always felt outside the loop. But, when I got my student club membership card in the mail and my first issue of the NSNA journal, I really began to feel different. I was now an official member of something that was just about me. Looking at the card motivated me before exams and validated my purpose as part of a group that welcomed me and offered me resources for success in nursing. My family was not supportive and didn't understand why I wouldn't just stay home and collect welfare. They even accused me of thinking that I was better than them, so I was now an outsider in my own circle of friends and family. The membership made me feel like I was not alone in my journey to become a nurse.

PROFESSIONAL INTEGRATION AND SOCIALIZATION

What are your views about professional integration and socialization and their impact/influence on student persistence and retention? What professional integration and socialization strategies do you implement and evaluate in your course? In your program? What are students' perceptions about this? When did you first feel socialized in nursing? How did it feel before then?

Many models explaining attrition among traditional-age college students have emphasized the importance of social integration in college in student adjustment, persistence, and success (1–4). Social integration refers to the "degree of congruency between the student and the social system of the college" (4, p. 107). It is achieved through formal and informal faculty interactions, peer interactions, and extracurricular activities. Students with limited social integration experience greater isolation, thus adversely impacting upon academic performance and retention. Difficulty with integration may result in increased stress and anxiety (negative psychological outcomes), increasing the risk for academic difficulty and attrition (5).

In the higher education literature, the importance of social integration and academic integration in college student retention is frequently discussed (6–8). Researchers have noted the powerful influence of social integration with specific populations of students such as African American males (9,10), Dominican American males (11), male nursing students (12,13), African American female nursing students (14), Korean female nursing students (15), minority students (6,16–25), multiracial students (26), adult students (27–29), first-generation students (6,30–32), students who speak English as a second (other) language (33,34), Appalachian students (34), American Indian and Alaska native students (19,35), Aboriginal students (36), and Hispanic students (37–44). Bean and Metzner (42,43) propose that for nontraditional students (older, part-time, and/or commuter students), social integration is less influential than environmental factors on retention, although it may have indirect effects through psychological outcomes. Conclusively, social integration is a factor that should be closely considered among all populations; however, the conceptualization and the significance of social integration may vary within and between specific student subgroups.

For undergraduate nursing students, a new perspective of social integration is proposed in the NURS model (Figure 1.2). Professional integration factors are those that enhance students' interaction with the social system of the college environment within the context of professional socialization and career development. These factors include nursing faculty advisement and helpfulness, memberships in professional organizations, professional events, encouragement by friends in class, EPs, and peer mentor-tutoring. Results from recent studies have consistently identified nursing faculty advisement and helpfulness, EP, and peer mentor-tutoring as instrumental in assisting with nursing student retention (44–47). Other reports have documented the significance of EPs that incorporate nonacademic components and recognize the power of faculty mentoring, peer mentoring, and professional mentoring (20,21,35,48–59). Professional socialization is important for professional growth and development as well as retention. Additionally, professional socialization is particularly powerful in encouraging students underrepresented in the nursing profession such as men and minority students. Accelerated cohort programs have the potential to promote positive professional integration and socialization, but may be challenged to do so due to time constraints and perceived irrelevance by students and faculty, especially, if many second-career and -degree students are enrolled. Both students and faculty may perceive professional socialization as a time waster; therefore, pointing out its importance, sharing relevant articles, showcasing student and graduate supportive testimonies, and personal story-telling (narrative pedagogy) are particularly indicated with these groups to change negative attitudes and shift energy into professional integration and socialization endeavors.

Professional integration factors are at the center of the NURS model because it is believed that they are at the crossroads of the decision to persist, drop out, or stop out. Lack of professional integration increases the risk of attrition, whereas strong professional integration increases professional commitment, persistence behaviors, and retention. It is also proposed that professional integration factors are vitally important for both traditional and nontraditional nursing student retention; however, students must be actively involved in such activities throughout the educational process. Nurse educators are the key initiators and advocates of professional integration because they have the power to actively promote EPs, professional events, memberships, encouragement by friends in class, and peer mentoring and tutoring. Faculty can make a difference by increasing professional integration and eliminating social isolation.

Nurse educators must first recognize that professional integration is a multidimensional process that incorporates cognitive, affective, and practical dimensions, and that it will be best enhanced through the careful orchestration and planned coordination of activities that creatively combine these dimensions. It is also proposed that professional integration will be exponentially augmented through the initial and ongoing use of various professional integration factors that complement each other. This complementary coordination of the various professional integration factors can be emphasized through faculty interventions that aim to maximize student's experience with these factors. Although each individual factor can have a positive difference on retention, the combined effect greatly outweighs the individual effect. This is consistent with the holistic perspective that views the whole dimension of professional integration as greater than the mere total of each separate and distinct part. Affective growth and development, leading to holistic changes, will occur cumulatively after the combination of various strategies (60,61). The acronym HOLISTIC COMPETENCE can assist nurse educators in remembering several essential elements for holistic retention strategy design (see Figure 6.1).

Before designing strategies, nurse educators must understand the potential power of each professional integration factor. This chapter elaborates upon each of the professional integration factors, proposing ways that the factors can potentially enhance retention through academic and psychological outcomes. The individual benefits of each professional integration factor will be highlighted. Potential barriers to successful professional integration will conclude the chapter. Awareness of actual and perceived barriers to professional integration strategies is necessary if nurse educators are to understand the student retention process and to develop ways of preventing obstacles and removing barriers before designing strategies. Strategies for promoting retention and success will be discussed in Part II of this book.

FACULTY AND PROFESSIONAL NETWORKS

Faculty Advisement and Helpfulness

Faculty advisement and helpfulness means the active involvement of nursing faculty in the student's academic endeavors, career goals, and professional socialization. Faculty advisement involves the interaction with students in a formal, preset meeting such as in the classroom or during weekly office hours. Faculty helpfulness goes beyond the formal domain into the informal setting when, for example, a faculty member stops in the hallway to talk with a student about an upcoming professional conference congratulates a student about an excellent performance with a challenging hospitalized client.

Human-connectedness	between faculty and students makes a powerful difference in retention
Optimization	focuses on enrichment for everyone to achieve maximum potential
Learner-centered	strategies engage learners in immediate professional application and relevance
Individualized	strengths and weaknesses of diverse students must be addressed
Scientifically based	retention strategies provide a beginning repertoire of ideas and data
Teamwork	must be emphasized at all levels (faculty, staff, administration, students)
Integrated	retention efforts must be carefully woven throughout the organizational fabric
Creative	ideas and innovations must address academic and non-academic issues
Caring	sincerely about holistic needs of students is the first step in fostering success
Ongoing	and coordinated retention interventions throughout the program is essential
Multidimensional	strategies must correspond with multidimensional factors influencing retention
Proactive	strategies are initiated before problems occur and at key transitional periods
Ethics	and accountability underscore the need for full faculty involvement
Trust	is an essential component for building an open, caring learning environment
Education	for meeting the holistic needs of students includes formal & informal forums
Networks	with experts and others on best practices for student retention expands ideas
Confidence	influences student commitment, motivation, and persistence behaviors
Evaluation	of strategies implemented provide guidance for future innovations

FIGURE 6.1 HOLISTIC COMPETENCE acronym.

Faculty helpfulness is offering to meet with students outside scheduled hours for a study group or for a resume-writing workshop. Faculty advisement and helpfulness is manifested by encouraging educational and career goals, promoting positive feelings of self-worth, believing in the student's ability to succeed, listening to problems and concerns, showing interest in academic progress, presenting a realistic outlook, expressing optimism, offering assistance, and presence. Presence means caring about the student as a whole person and being available as a resource, making appropriate referrals when needed. Nurse educators should be clear about establishing boundaries for appropriate helpfulness within the faculty role, remembering that fostering over-dependence is counterproductive and that the caretaker role, while appropriate when hired for the registered nurse role is not appropriate when hired for the professorial role; referrals to the health center or counseling office should be incorporated into the nurse educator's role when the situation calls for it.

Although the faculty member needs to be present at designated (expected) times such as in class or in the faculty office, the most impor-tant factor is that the student perceives the faculty member as caring and encouraging. Student's perceptions and expectations about advisement vary and can be influenced by student profile characteristics, environ-mental factors, academic factors, and affective factors. Similarly, faculty expectations and perception of the advisor role may be quite varied. The faculty advisor role may be undervalued, and the significance of the qual-ity of faculty interactions may be underestimated among faculty. How-ever, the advisor role is pivotal in promoting socialization and retention. The faculty advisor is often the first person who the student encounters within the educational institution and perhaps the nursing profession. The faculty advisor has the potential to help students prevent problems, develop strengths, eliminate weaknesses, and feel integrated within the nursing profession. A negative first experience with a faculty advisor has the potential to turn away students who could ultimately make a signif-icant contribution to the nursing profession and health care.

Although the developmental advisement approach is strongly sup-ported in the literature as offering the most benefits to enhance student academic and psychological growth and development, not all nursing faculty may value, support, or practice developmental advisement. In a developmental approach, student–faculty relationships encourage open communication, shared responsibility and power, caring, mentoring, total student development, self-direction, active help-seeking behaviors, and decision making. Developmental advisement is more focused on the *pro-cess* of learning, whereas prescriptive advisement is grade-oriented, or focused on the attainment of a prescribed product. Prescriptive advise-ment views the faculty advisor as the authority person who dispenses information and prescribes the measures needed for students to complete their curriculum requirements (62,63).

The NURS model advocates developmental advisement, which necessitates a commitment on the part of both faculty member and stu-dent. The advisor–advisee relationship changes over the educational process. Developmental advisement and helpfulness is proactive, with faculty members often initiating contacts with students and encouraging informal contacts. Lack of preparation in effective advisement strategies appropriate for various students throughout the educational process has led to the design of faculty development workshops. Faculty advisement strategies will be discussed in Chapter 10.

Although the developmental approach is advocated in the NURS model, students may view faculty advisement and helpfulness differently. Not all students may value a developmental advisement approach. Often, student perceptions and expectations about the faculty advisement role are different from that of the faculty (64–71). Additionally, expectations about helpfulness can be different than that of faculty (21,72–73). A mismatch between student and faculty expectations and perceptions creates another barrier, whereby students become disappointed and dissatisfied and poor psychological outcomes for the nursing program increases the risk for attrition. The value of student perceptions concerning faculty advisement and helpfulness is critical in determining whether satisfaction or dissatisfaction will result. For example, in several studies, student perceptions of faculty advisement and helpfulness was consistently reported to be one of the top three "greatly supportive" factors for student retention (44–47).

The most important experiences to students are often the informal faculty–student interactions that occur outside the classroom, routine advisement, and scheduled office hours (74). In general, out-of-classroom experiences have powerful influence on retention (61,75,76), especially among minority students in predominantly White institutions (20,77) and adult students (28). The informal socialization process helps nurture professional growth, development, and integration into the nursing culture. The nursing culture refers to "the learned and transmitted lifeways, values, symbols, patterns, and normative practices of members of the nursing profession of a particular society" (78, p. 208). Students are invited into the nursing culture and are guided by expert mentors through the open sharing of nursing values, beliefs, norms, and practices.

Nurse educators must recognize students' holistic needs, expand the teaching and advisor role into a mentor role, and create innovative strategies to enhance student success. However, the nurse educator alone cannot best promote professional socialization. Capitalizing on the strengths of other professional integration factors can only help broaden the supportive collaborative network for students.

> What are your students' perceptions concerning faculty advisement and helpfulness in your course, other nursing courses, and the college?

Memberships

Membership in one's professional association is viewed as an essential activity for professional career growth, development, and mobility, as well as an activity that promotes an added opportunity for professional socialization and integration (79–83). Within the NURS model, memberships refer to affiliation or participation within nursing organizations or associations as a member prescribed by the respective bylaws. Nursing organizations/associations include the NSNA, the school's student nurse club (SNC), and specialty nursing organizations that permit student nurse membership. Memberships promote professional integration through various benefits and privileges that may include voting rights, newsletters, journals, free items, listserv announcements of professional issues, discounts at professional events, networking, referrals, mentoring services, job postings, and legal advice.

The NSNA provides an opportunity for student nurses to be actively involved in professional nursing issues, health care issues, and nursing student/education issues. Active involvement includes a variety of activities such as voting for NSNA officers, writing a letter to the editor of the NSNA journal, *Imprint*, representing the nursing program at a NSNA meeting, or running for a NSNA office. Because the NSNA is exclusively for undergraduate nursing students throughout the United States, students may feel a common bond with other nursing students beyond the limited enclaves of one nursing program. Positive solutions from student role models and the knowledge that nursing students throughout the country may be experiencing similar anxieties, concerns, obstacles, fears, and feelings may enhance professional integration, self-efficacy, motivation, persistence behaviors, and retention. Additionally, the NSNA provides unique opportunities for mentoring by nursing leaders and student leaders (82,83).

One benefit of the SNC may be that all nursing (and sometimes prenursing) students are usually considered automatic members; new students are often welcomed by more advanced students at a special event or ceremony. A second benefit is that students can develop close networks and feelings of solidarity with students throughout various stages of the nursing program's educational process, thereby enhancing professional integration. Students involved in the SNC are often aware of special nuances pertinent to that particular nursing program. Another benefit of the SNC is the opportunity to interact with peers, faculty, and/or nurses during SNC-sponsored social events. If positive psychological outcomes result, student motivation, persistence, and retention will be enhanced.

Many specialty nursing organizations, such as the international Transcultural Nursing Society, permit, and/or actively encourage student nurse membership and participation. Other specialty nursing organizations that permit student membership include the American Association of Critical Care Nurses, the Association of Child and Adolescent Psychiatric Nurses, Association of Nurses in AIDS Care, National Gerontological Nursing Organization, and International Association of Forensic

Nurses. Specialty organizations provide additional opportunities for student nurses to network with other student nurses, as well as registered nurses and noted leaders in the specialty field. Students who have a particular interest in a subfield of nursing may benefit greatly from early exposure to organizations and individuals with a common shared interest, and may become more motivated with their educational endeavors through the positive role modeling, mentoring, and active encouragement by nursing professionals with similar specialty interests and goals. Ethnic nursing organizations, such as the National Black Nurses Association, and religious nursing organizations, such as the Nurses Christian Fellowship, provide opportunities for students to network with other student nurses and registered nurses with whom students closely identify in identity, background, ideals, and/or concerns. The positive influence of role models as mentors can greatly promote professional integration, satisfaction, stress reduction, self-efficacy, motivation, persistence behaviors, and retention.

Unfortunately, many nurse educators and nursing students undervalue and underestimate the significance of student memberships. Chapter 11 will describe strategies for enhancing professional integration and socialization via memberships.

> How many students in your course and other courses hold memberships in organizations? What are your students' active membership benefits, roles, and responsibilities?

Professional Events

Professional events are nursing conferences, workshops, meetings, volunteer services, and social activities that have specific goals relevant for nursing education, practice, research, or theory. They are often sponsored by professional organizations or associations that actively encourage student participation and/or membership. Participation in professional events is valuable since it encourages interaction with other nursing students and nurses within a professional context (80,81). Such events offer unique opportunities for students to engage in socialization activities and networking and expand professional knowledge and skills. Nursing conferences and workshops exemplify a professional commitment to lifelong learning that can be motivating and uplifting to students. Professional nurses can serve as role models through their commitment to learning and the nursing profession. Positive role models can enhance self-efficacy and motivation, in turn enhancing persistence and retention.

Events that encourage active participation on the part of students either through discussion or through implementation of specific nursing roles offer students validation for their achievements so far in their professional development and their educational process. For example, students who volunteer to assist a nursing organization with blood pressure screening at a community wellness fair gain personal and professional validation by nurses and peers and from members of the community as well. Validation is especially important for nontraditional students (older, commuter, and/or minority) and has been positively linked with persistence behaviors and retention (85,86). Students who are recognized and thanked by members of the professional and lay community for their nursing knowledge, skill, and time are receiving positive feedback for their professional nursing actions.

It is proposed that within the NURS model, positive experiences in professional event participation positively affect retention by enhancing self-efficacy and motivation, promoting professional integration, and facilitating positive psychological outcomes. Individual students may view the importance of professional events differently, necessitating individual appraisal on the part of the nurse educator. For example, if a nursing student views attendance at a professional conference as unimportant or fears feeling out of place then the student may never elect to attend a conference. His or her professional integration will be limited without the extra opportunities for peer interaction, faculty interaction outside the classroom, networking with nursing professionals, and/or exposure to the other added benefits of professional nursing conferences. The use of network systems has been positively linked to enhanced persistence (87). Strategies that enhance opportunities to participate in various professional integration factors will ultimately benefit students. Chapter 11 will discuss such creative strategies.

What types of professional events did your students and those in other courses engage in this past year? How many students participated? What were their perceived benefits of event participation?

POWER OF FRIENDS AND PEER SUPPORTS

Friends in Class

What types of friendships and peer interaction exist in your course, other courses, and throughout the nursing program?

The higher education literature supports that encouragement by friends in class has the potential to positively influence students' academic and psychological outcomes, persistence behaviors, and retention (6–8,31,76,87–96). The nursing education literature similarly acknowledges the significance of class friendships, especially among groups underrepresented in nursing (20,21,50,97–101). Accordingly, encouragement by friends in class is included as a component of the NURS model. It is proposed that encouragement by friends in class will actively promote positive psychological outcomes, self-efficacy, professional socialization, persistence, and retention. Lack of class friends will adversely affect retention through social isolation, dissatisfaction, stress, low self-efficacy, and decreased motivation.

Friends in class are peers who interact positively with each other by establishing and maintaining friendships in class that are continued within the context of the college learning environment. (Required off-campus clinical placement sites are considered part of the college learning environment). Friends in class do not include family members. They are mutually bonded in career goals, expectations, and stage of educational and professional development. The main focus of in-class friends is on the common academic goal of successfully completing course requirements and becoming a registered nurse. Friends in class may also elect to participate in outside social events; however, this is secondary.

Encouragement by friends in class refers to the active emotional involvement of class friends in relation to the student's academic endeavors and career goals. Positive encouragement is manifested by supporting realistic career and educational goals, promoting positive feelings of self-worth, believing in the student's ability to succeed, listening to problems and concerns, showing interest in academic progress, expressing optimism, offering assistance, and presence. Mutual assistance or reciprocation of academic and nonacademic (emotional) supports by class friends can enhance confidence and independence. Friendships that encourage mutual reciprocation and individual independence, rather than dependence, can help with professional integration, growth, and development. Recently, Facebook usage among class friends expands the opportunities to provide a network of support that can positively influence retention (91).

Pressure by friends to participate in outside activities (such as social engagements) that conflict with the student's ability to successfully complete academic and career goals is incongruent with positive encouragement behaviors. Becoming overly dependent on another student or attempting to cause dependence by others is also incongruent. Positive encouragement behaviors recognize the unique contributions of the other class friend and facilitate mutual collaboration with valued contributions from each individual, while promoting independent behaviors. An unequal balance between class friends is counterproductive to professional development and integration. Difficulty setting limits on friends and social activities negatively influences academic performance and retention (102).

Nursing faculty and students alike may underestimate the potential influence of class friends in academic achievement, professional development, satisfaction, stress, and retention. Students' perceptions about friendships, learning, education, and peers can be influenced by students' profile characteristics, affective factors, and environmental factors. Among several samples of nontraditional associate degree students, approximately 80% of subjects perceived encouragement from friends in class as supporting retention. Most of the students were older (over 25) and were perhaps more experienced in maintaining friendships with people who provided encouragement (44–47). Nurse educators may wish to further explore and consider the impact of class friends in relation to the student's age. A subsequent multi-institutional factor analysis study indicated that friends in class were "greatly supportive" in influencing retention and clustered together with the variable of "friends outside class," resulting in a factor labeled "Friend Support." To further explore the influence of age and other demographic variables on friend support, several other analyses were conducted, indicating that regardless of age, students whose first language was English (EFL) demonstrated higher scores, suggesting that encouragement from friends was more important for EFL students. Further investigation about this phenomenon is warranted (101).

Although encouragement by in-class friends offers many unique advantages (see Chapter 12), there are some limitations. One barrier to the potential benefits achieved by positive encouragement by friends in class is that students may be reluctant to join new groups and make new friends. They may elect to band together with students of similar academic ability or background. Such banding together limits the diversity in ideas, views, and strategies that can enhance academic achievement and professional development. For example, weaker students may attempt to cluster together. Nurse educators have the unique opportunity to encourage the development of diverse, positive friendships in class through learning activities within the classroom, clinical work, online environment, and outside class assignments. Chapter 12 discusses strategies to promote positive peer interactions and maximize desired outcomes from in-class friendships.

Another limitation is that friends in class may be unable to see the whole picture, rationale for prerequisites or sequencing of courses, benefits of course assignments within the whole scope of the educational process, preparation for the RN licensing exam, the next course, employment as a RN, or continued education. Class friends are at the same point in the educational process so that their view of the interconnectedness between courses along the path to professional development is myopic, sometimes unknown, and prospective. In contrast, previous experience and retrospective appraisal can lead to a broader insight. Partnership connections with PMTs who are further advanced in the educational process can assist in minimizing this limitation.

Peer Mentoring and Tutoring

In the NURS model, peer mentoring and tutoring is a formalized, structured collaborative partnership in learning and professional development between a PMT and one or more students (protégé). A PMT is a student who is at a more advanced level of the educational process and who has demonstrated academic and professional excellence. Usually this means that the student is enrolled in a more advanced nursing course; however, an academically strong and caring peer colleague could serve as a PMT. With a peer colleague, the role of tutor would probably be more dominant than the mentor role because both students would be at the same point in the educational process; therefore, the experience of connecting pieces along the educational journey would be limited.

The NURS model proposes that peer mentoring and tutoring offers the utmost possibility in professional integration and socialization. While mentoring alone can have positive effects on professional integration and socialization, it is presumed that tutoring alone does not have this effect. Peer tutoring focuses solely on the learning of cognitive knowledge and/or psychomotor skills rather than affective learning; therefore, it may do little in the realm of professional integration and socialization. As conceptualized here, tutoring is not interchangeable with remediation, but instead focuses on enrichment and enhancement. Remediation focuses on fixing deficits in students who have not mastered basic skills and knowledge, whereas the tutoring component in the NURS model focuses on realistic self-appraisal of strengths and weaknesses, maximizing strengths, addressing weaknesses, and assisting students in achieving their optimal academic potential. Peer tutoring without mentoring, however, does not enhance professional integration and socialization to any great degree.

In mentoring, professional nursing values, beliefs, practices, expectations, and attitudes can be nurtured. The "mentor connection is a developmental, empowering, and nurturing relationship extending over time in which mutual sharing, learning, and growth occur in an atmosphere of respect, collegiality, and affirmation" (83, p. 5). Both the mentor and mentee will benefit from their interactions, thus enhancing their professional integration, socialization, and acculturation into the nursing student role and future RN role. Furthermore, the opportunity to share experiences and watch role models and peers struggle with similar academic and nonacademic challenges can help increase self-efficacy and motivation to persist (103–106).

"Mentoring is complex and elusive—difficult to define and to measure. It cannot be seen, but is a powerful, enriching phenomenon that can be described by those who experience it" (83, p. 5). For example, quantitative results from students participating in study groups led by PMTs indicated that participants were greatly satisfied with their interactions. Respondents indicated that their tutoring experience enhanced retention. Qualitative comments from student participants substantiated and added richness to the quantitative data by describing the positive emotional and academic outcomes from their experience with their PMTs. Several students who were mentored then became PMTs, further enriching their opportunities for professional growth and development. Many students reported that they now aimed for a higher level of academic and professional excellence, rather than merely settling for minimal achievement levels or passing standards. Furthermore, many students were motivated to persist in their nursing courses beyond the associate degree because of the influence of their PMTs, who were RNs enrolled in the RN-to-BSN program (46,47). Subsequently, many mentored students and PMTs have pursued masters and doctoral education and roles as adjunct faculty or clinical preceptors.

In the NURS model, peer mentoring and tutoring enhances professional integration and socialization. They can maximize academic achievement, promote positive psychological outcomes, encourage self-efficacy and motivation, facilitate persistence behaviors, and enhance retention, assisting students maximally in achieving positive outcomes. Nurse educators can develop creative strategies for fostering peer mentoring and tutoring partnerships individually or as a component of a formally designed EP. Chapters 12 and 13 will provide examples.

> What types of peer mentoring and tutoring partnerships exist in your program?

MULTISERVICE INNOVATIONS FOR SUCCESS

Enrichment Programs

An EP is a formally designed multiservice program that aims to enrich the total nursing student experience by maximizing strengths, remedying weaknesses, promoting positive psychological outcomes, facilitating positive academic outcomes, and nurturing professional growth and development. Services may include several of the following: orientation, mentoring, tutoring, newsletters, career advisement and guidance, workshops, study groups, networking, transitional support, financial stipends, and referral. Services are best facilitated through a collaborative partnership in learning and professional development between nursing faculty, other professional nurses, and students. EPs are different from remedial programs; however, students and faculty alike often do not distinguish between the two. Misperceptions about EPs create barriers. Because remedial programs are often criticized and stigmatized, students may be reluctant to participate in EPs. Similarly, nursing faculty may not appropriately advocate and support EPs. Assuming that EPs are only appropriate for the academically weak or struggling student limits the immense possibilities that a well-designed EP can offer. Nurse educators should recognize that all students benefit from various forms of academic and emotional support throughout all stages of the educational process, especially during key transitional phases (82,107,108).

The most successful EPs offer a coordinated integration of proactive, ongoing, and transitional interventions that are free and available to all nursing students throughout the educational process. Proactive interventions are interventions implemented before the beginning of the semester and aim to prepare students academically, psychologically, and practically for the new semester, and focus on enhanced performance, satisfaction, and success. Ongoing interventions aim to maximize student success by the early identification of student strengths and weaknesses before academic difficulties, role conflicts, or stresses arise. Early identification of the at-risk student can prevent failure or withdrawal. Often students do not seek help until difficulty arises, and then it can be too late to improve an academically precarious situation. Therefore, nurse educators should be actively involved on an ongoing basis to assist students, especially because at-risk students often do not initiate adaptive and active help-seeking behaviors (62,109–112).

As students move from one phase of the educational process to the next, transitional interventions should be implemented (108). Transition from pre-professional to professional education (first nursing course) and one nursing course to the next level nursing course challenges students to embark on a new, unknown path in their journey toward becoming a registered nurse. Guidance at these transitional stages is crucial for self-efficacy, motivation, satisfaction, stress reduction, academic achievement, and retention. It is proposed that students who actively engage in EP services throughout the educational process will be exposed to more opportunities to interact with peers, students in various stages of the educational process, faculty, nurses, and college staff. This increased interaction has the potential to enhance professional integration. Additionally, it has the potential to positively influence self-efficacy and motivation. Students who perceive such interactions as beneficial will have more positive psychological outcomes (satisfaction and stress reduction) and maximized potential for positive academic outcomes. Consequently, persistence behaviors and retention will be enhanced.

The results of several studies using samples of EP study group participants indicated that the intervention (EP) group had lower failure rates, lower withdrawal rates, higher course success rates, and positive psychological outcomes (satisfaction). Social integration variables, such as faculty advisement and helpfulness, tutoring, and the EP, were perceived as highly supportive (46,47). High student satisfaction with the EP and perceptions that the EP supported retention emphasize the ongoing need for innovative strategies that enrich the nursing student experience. Additionally, the nursing and higher education literature strongly advocates retention programs that incorporate academic and nonacademic components. EP design, implementation, and evaluation should be a systematic and well-planned process. Chapter 13 presents the 11-step process that can guide EP development; a case exemplar is also provided.

> What multiservice enrichment innovations exist in your program? How are the services used by students in the first nursing course, your course, and other courses throughout the program?

Integrated Nursing Student Test Enhancement Program

An integrated nursing student test enhancement program (INSTEP) is an intensive multiservice program specifically aimed at enhancing test-taking preparation, skills, and outcomes throughout the curriculum both inside and outside class time. Services may include several of the following: a workshop series on test-taking preparation and skills, anxiety reduction workshops, independent and guided use of test-preparation software, mentoring, tutoring, test-prep study groups, in-class practice test questions, posttest structured reviews, posttest individual reviews, National Council Licensure Examination (NCLEX) review class, referral, and/or other test-related services. INSTEP may be incorporated within the nursing school's overall retention and success plan, and/or within a multiservice EP; however, INSTEP is distinguishable by its intense emphasis on test enhancement strategies (including psychological components) that focuses on high quality, integrated proactive and ongoing strategies throughout the program that is easily accessible, available, encouraged, and expected for all students by all faculty and administrators.

Although some schools may have a designated "retention or test-prep coordinator" for student-based activities (workshops, mentors, study groups, etc.), INSTEP requires full faculty involvement, necessitating planning, commitment, and coordination within and between faculty teaching various courses or course components. Skillfully blending undergraduate nursing content with test-taking skills, thoughtfully weaving together cognitive, psychomotor, and affective learning, complementing learning from other courses to prevent gaps, creating scaffolded learning outcome expectations at each curricular level that increases with complexity and depth, and integrating evidence-based teaching and learning activities takes well-planned cooperation and sharing within and between faculty in all courses. Consequently, curriculum meetings, a faculty retreat, or day(s) allocated for intensive work on test design, implementation, and evaluation strategies maximizes possibilities for swift, high-quality, evidence-based implementation further individualized to fit the special nuances of the school such as student population and curricular design. An outside expert consultant may provide valuable objective feedback to faculty and offer suggestions that may not be self-evident just by working exclusively within the group. At the curriculum level, techniques include mapping of concepts, content, teaching and learning strategies, objectives/goals, outcomes, and methods of evaluation. A generalized test blueprint that considers RN licensing exam content, concepts, format, diverse nursing roles, and levels of complexity guides number and types of questions for consistent implementation. For example, when the RN licensing exam increased the number and difficulty of pharmacology questions, faculty agreement about the increase on each unit exam by a predetermined percentage, taking into account the need to incorporate various levels of taxonomy and all phases of the nursing process, better prepares students for what to expect on the NCLEX exam. Routine appraisal of test questions using standardized item-analysis software and procedures provides faculty with objective quantitative feedback to guide the ongoing teaching and learning process and adapt INSTEP services and programs accordingly building upon student strengths and addressing/remedying weaknesses. (Further details about test questions are beyond the scope of this chapter; however, many reliable resources are available in the literature.)

In-class strategies may include integrating a certain number of practice test questions throughout the class at carefully placed transitional points to monitor student progress, increase attention, and provide immediate feedback to students and faculty. Use of clickers (a student response system) is one way to provide immediate individualized feedback about each question and comparatively in relation to the group's performance. One advantage is that students maintain anonymity with classmates yet the instructor has the option to identify weak students and reach out privately to students to address deficits or to provide positive reinforcement for good performance and/or improvements in performance. Adapting games such as *Jeopardy* (113) can create a lively, interactive, fun method for learning. In a warm, nurturing environment, INSTEP can help eliminate/reduce defeatist attitudes, self-handicapping behaviors, loneliness/isolation, and test anxiety by replacing them with empowering and realistic attitudes and behaviors, social integration, and group support. Concluding the class with several practice test questions by announcing a specialized time such as "It's TEA time" (test enhancement activity) alerts students that faculty set aside a special time for enhancing their success, thus creating a caring student-centered community atmosphere.

Students' perceptions are powerful. For example, a course instructor shared that she included a few test questions throughout the class and usually at the end but (when questioned) admitted that she never verbalized with students that she cared about their test success and carefully planned each class to include important example questions that should help prepare students. The instructor was angry that students wrote on her class evaluation that she did not seem to care about students and that she did not include any strategies to prepare them for nursing-type questions. The next semester, she implemented the suggestion about pointing out when she was integrating questions; student comments indicated that they now perceived that the faculty member cared, she was approachable for individual consultation, and they felt satisfied with the course. Student behaviors also changed; students were more interactive in class, sought individualized guidance more readily, and exam grades improved. Student perceptions changed dramatically, and this positively changed academic and psychological outcomes (stress reduction, satisfaction, resilient self-efficacy, and motivation).

Another critical element for INSTEP is consistency and security of tests and test-taking procedures. Student academic dishonesty (SAD) takes many forms, and faculty have legal and ethical obligations to prevent SAD, facilitate fair testing conditions, and confront SAD when it occurs. The acronym PROACTIVE can guide nurse educator actions. PROACTIVE communication refers to Policy, Responsibility, Ongoing action, Accountability, Commitment, Trust, Initiative, Values, and Expectations. (see Jeffreys & Stier [114] for action-oriented case exemplars and model).

Posttest reviews that are consistently agreed upon and applied throughout the curriculum reassures students that faculty work together and sincerely want to help students succeed. Consistently applied strategies decrease anxiety and increases self-efficacy and motivation. Diagnostic and prescriptive strategies may involve individual review with course instructor. The literature suggests several techniques for an organized posttest review individually, in small groups, and/or in the large classroom setting.

Test-taking difficulties present an obstacle to student success and retention by increasing the risk for poor academic outcomes, dissatisfaction, and stress. Successful academic outcomes will only result in continued persistence and nursing course retention if accompanied by positive psychological outcomes (satisfaction). Often, students are inefficacious, anxious, and/or uncertain about their test-taking skills, thus increasing the risk for poor academic and psychological outcomes. Overly confident (supremely efficacious) students are also at risk due to their unrealistic expectations, overestimates of ability, and lack of adequate test preparation. In a study on first-semester students, academic outcome was inversely related to perceived academic variable strength; students who perceived academic strengths as very high demonstrated higher failure rates (44,45).

Early, structured interventions to promote realistic self-appraisal and expectations can optimize test-taking preparation and success.

Because first-semester nursing students have the highest attrition rates and greatest difficulty with new format of nursing exams, the most intensive outside class interventions and most intensive encouragement incentives for service use should occur with this group. Students who successfully complete the first nursing course still need ongoing test-taking support outside class as they move through different courses, encounter new nursing roles and types of patient situations, and face higher levels of test questions. Examples of interventions outside class include the following:

- A general test-prep small-group workshop prior to the first exam is offered at various times to accommodate nontraditional student schedules and responsibilities.
- Subsequent series of follow-up small-group workshops that build on previous workshops are scheduled approximately one week prior to an exam, and incorporate targeted exam content areas.
- All workshops include self-appraisal, reflection, guided imagery, visualization, relaxation techniques, critical thinking in nursing, multiple choice question components, test-taking techniques, practice test questions with rationales, computer applications, time management in test-taking, mentoring, referral to test-taking resources, and evaluation.
- A programmed instructional guide for test-taking preparation throughout the semester using various computer and other educational resources.
- A learning contract to guide individual student's subsequent test-taking preparation plans, encouraging students to commit to weekly test-preparation activities independently and with a PMT.
- Individualized and small-group posttest review with instructor.
- Required and optional practice test questioning software programs that correspond with course and exam content areas.
- Interactive PMT-led study groups focused on test preparation.
- Individual mentoring and tutoring with PMT.
- Design of a "test-prep center"—a place for integrating various outside classroom test-preparation activities separately and/or within a Nursing Student Resource Center (NSRC) or nursing neighborhood (see section below and Chapter 14).

What INSTEP innovations exist in your program? How are the services used by students in the first nursing course, your course, and other courses throughout the program? How do they enhance professional integration and socialization, test success, satisfaction, and retention?

Nursing Student Resource Center or Nursing Neighborhood

An NSRC is a place that creates a caring, local nursing neighborhood of learners that holistically fosters professional growth, development, and socialization, through the careful integration of various strategies, thereby enhancing student persistence and retention through the attainment of positive academic and psychological outcomes. The well-designed NSRC or nursing neighborhood offers a place for effectively linking multiple strategies together. A NSRC is the heart or focus for specifically designed and coordinated resources and activities that are important in influencing student outcomes. The NSRC is a central place where learning, resources, support, peer interaction, professional socialization, and other activities enrich other learning experiences and settings separate from the classroom, clinical, and nursing skills laboratory. It is a place where students can seek help, support, and guidance through a coordinated effort between several activities and multimedia resources to enhance success, enrich learning, and promote positive academic and psychological outcomes. The philosophy behind designing a "center" is that creating a niche for nursing students will promote professional socialization, satisfaction, positive academic outcomes, persistence, and stress reduction. A center promotes active engagement of learners in various levels of the educational and professional development process that actively and purposely coordinates multidimensional and multimedia efforts and strategies to maximize learning and satisfaction and minimize stress. The center is where all points come together, that is, all phases and components of nursing education become integrated appropriately in a complementary fashion that seeks to elevate learning to a higher level (synthesis) between all components. This is enhanced by the positive influences of peers and students in more advanced levels in the educational and professional development process.

Incorporating EP services and/or INSTEP outside classroom activities within the nursing neighborhood or NSRC requires careful planning, conversion of old space, or creation of new space to accommodate students and services. For example, conversion of a computer laboratory adjacent to an already existing NSRC into a Nursing Student Test-Prep Center (NSTPC) provides easy access to students and helps facilitate optimal use of multidimensional educational and support strategies and resources aimed to enhance test-taking skills. Now the NSRC and NSTPC become part of the nursing neighborhood resources and all students should be invited into the neighborhood, join in neighborhood activities, and feel part of the neighborhood. Nursing test-taking resources include test-preparation software programs and books available for ongoing independent and guided student use. A NSTPC helps facilitate an ongoing and focused interaction between students in various levels of the educational process and career development process that is specifically aimed at test-taking preparation. An accessible and frequently used test-preparation center encourages students to become bound together by feelings of cooperation, support, and solidarity. Perspectives about appropriate goals, test-preparation activities, priorities, and persistence could be collectively shaped and guided by student role models and faculty. Additionally, students enrich their academic and professional growth by the increased use of current test enhancement resources in nursing. The interaction with student peers and more advanced students assists in encouraging use of effective test-taking preparation strategies and resources in a nonthreatening, relaxed environment conducive to learning and testing-taking (see Chapter 14).

KEY POINT SUMMARY

- Professional integration factors are those that enhance students' interaction with the social system of the college environment within the context of professional socialization and career development.
- Professional integration factors are at the center of the NURS model because it is believed that they are at the crossroads of the decision to persist, drop out, or stop out.
- Lack of professional integration increases the risk of attrition whereas strong professional integration increases professional commitment, persistence behaviors, and retention.
- Nurse educators are the key initiators and advocates of professional integration because they have the power to actively promote EPs, professional events, memberships, encouragement by friends in class, peer mentoring and tutoring, and other services.

APPLICATION STRATEGIES

EDUCATOR-IN-ACTION VIGNETTE

After teaching one year in an undergraduate nursing program, Professor Change concludes that student opportunities for professional integration and socialization are few, disconnected, and virtually invisible within the existing curriculum. Nursing program retention rates have declined; NCLEX pass rates on the first attempt have also decreased. During the curriculum committee meeting, Professor Change proposes that faculty work together to carefully plan and coordinate strategies to enhance professional integration and socialization throughout the curriculum. Furthermore, she suggests that strategies be purposely designed to complement each other so that professional integration and socialization and development are visible vertical threads that creatively combine cognitive, affective, and practical dimensions.

Consider the following faculty responses:

PROFESSOR ALWAYS: We have always had the curriculum this way. We have always had some students who either pass, fail, stop out, drop out, or graduate. It will always happen no matter what we do.

PROFESSOR SOLO: We all work individually on our own courses. Every teacher is responsible for including a professional development objective in the course outline.

PROFESSOR WAVER: Well, maybe we should think about doing something different, but maybe we should just leave things the way they are.

PROFESSOR SLOTH: That sounds like a lot of work. If students just worked harder, they would be more successful. We shouldn't be the ones doing extra work.

PROFESSOR CHALLENGER: What proof do you have to say that professional integration and socialization are insufficient? How do you know that more opportunities would make a difference?

Fortunately, two other nursing faculty members support Professor Change's idea and suggest that further exploration of this topic is warranted. Although Professor Change suggests a faculty development workshop with a featured guest speaker knowledgeable in this area, some faculty members are reluctant to allocate funds and their personal time to this event. Professor Change offers to provide faculty with several key articles and chapters concerning this topic prior to the next meeting. At the next meeting, Professor Change distributes a handout summarizing key points, a select bibliography of relevant nursing and higher education literature, and two books and three articles for quick reference. Additionally, she introduces two nursing students who were invited to discuss issues related to opportunities for professional integration and socialization within the curriculum. Students report:

DONNA: I am in my last semester of nursing. This is the first semester I was ever invited to attend a nursing conference by my instructor. I didn't even know there were so many nursing conferences available for students to attend. Professor Change arranged for me and two other students to attend for free in return for helping with the registration. Nurses were so friendly and treated us like part of the profession. It motivated me to try harder. I wish I had other opportunities earlier in nursing.

JERRY: Last semester I was thinking about dropping out of school. There are no other men in my clinical group and there were no male nurses on the hospital unit so I really felt out of place. Then I saw a male student in the library reading a nursing textbook so I asked him if he liked nursing. He was in his last semester and told me about some positive experiences and about dealing effectively with negative experiences. I decided not to drop out. Now I try to encourage other nursing students in the library whenever I see them.

Later, faculty agree that curricular concept mapping and strategy mapping will be conducted after attending a 3-hour faculty development workshop on "Promoting Achievement and Retention by Enhancing Opportunities for Professional Integration and Socialization in the Curriculum."

TOOLKIT RESOURCE BOX

Item 18—Active Promoter Assessment Tool: Student Professional Events and Memberships
Item 19—Active Promoter Assessment Tool: Positive and Productive Peer Partnerships
Item 22—Peer Mentoring and Tutoring
Item 25—Professional Integration and Socialization
Item 27—Enrichment Programs
Item 6—Enrichment Program Satisfaction Survey
Item 28—Nursing Student Resource Center (Nursing Neighborhood)
Item 7—Nursing Student Resource Center Satisfaction Survey
Items 1–4—Student Perception Appraisal Questionnaires—Pretests and Posttests

DISCUSSION QUESTIONS

1. What section of the chapter provided you with the most new information? Why? How will this new information influence your interaction with students and faculty?
2. Faculty unanimously vote to implement various INSTEP strategies during the next semester, including standardized test administration strategies to prevent SAD. A newly hired professor thinks, "I'm untenured and don't want to cause problems for myself with faculty or students so I just voted with everyone else. I don't intend to give away test questions in class and I don't intend to say something if I see something dishonest during my tests." Another professor thinks, "I don't have time to incorporate practice test questions within classes I've already squeezed some new content into class over the years. But I'm not going to be the only one who disagrees. Let everyone else do the extra work. My students always pass the class anyway unless they drop out before. Weeding out the weak ones keeps our NCLEX pass

rates up." What are the implications to students, other faculty, and the overall nursing program if faculty actions or inactions correspond with these two educator's thoughts? What could be done to prevent these consequences?

3. A faculty member disagrees with the proposal to use nursing student supplementary services fees (covered by student loans and financial aid) to pay a modest $20 fee per student for attendance at an upcoming professional conference that will be held at a nearby hospital. The professor says, "Students don't need to attend a conference now. We shouldn't waste student fees to pay for students who might fail or drop out anyway. They can attend plenty of conferences once they're a nurse if they want to. We should keep this money in the pot and award one graduating student a $500 savings bond." How would you respond? Why?

4. A faculty member says, "I can't believe some of the PMTs the new EP coordinator selected. Half of them have accents, like many of our students who usually end up failing or dropping out. I don't think I'm going to encourage my students to bother going to the NSRC; they can just study at home or come to see me if they have a question." What implications could this have on nursing student retention, achievement, self-efficacy, motivation, professional integration and socialization, satisfaction, and stress? How would you respond in a role as peer colleague, course coordinator/leader, chairperson, or dean?

5. How can the Snapshot Scenarios, Educator-in-Action Vignette, and Figure 6.1 be adapted to promote professional integration and socialization within your school?

REFERENCES

1. Nora, A. (1987). Determinants of retention among Chicano college students: A structural model. *Research in Higher Education, 26,* 31–60.
2. Pascarella, E. T., & Chapman, D. W. (1983). Validation of a theoretical model of college withdrawal: Interaction effects in a multi-institutional sample. *Research in Higher Education, 19,* 25–47.
3. Spady, W. (1970). Dropouts from higher education: Toward an empirical model. *Interchange, 2,* 38–62.
4. Tinto, V. (1975). Dropout from higher education: A theoretical synthesis of recent research. *Review of Educational Research, 45,* 89–125.
5. Wilson, S. B., Mason, T. W., & Ewing, M. J. M. (1997). Evaluating the impact of receiving university-based counseling services on student retention. *Journal of Counseling Psychology, 44*(3), 316–320.
6. Seidman, A. (2005). *College student retention: Formula for student success.* Westport, CT: American Council on Education, Praeger.
7. Braxton, J. M. (ed.) (2000). *Reworking the student departure puzzle.* Nashville, TN: Vanderbilt University Press.

8. Braxton, J. M., & McClendon, S. A. (2001). The fostering of social integration and retention through institutional practice. *Journal of College Student Retention: Research, Theory, & Practice, 3*(1), 57–72.

9. Palmer, R. T., & Young, E. M. (2009). Determined to succeed: Salient factors that foster academic success for academically unprepared black males at a black college. *Journal of College Student Retention: Research, Theory, and Practice, 10*(4), 465–482.

10. Davis, J. E. (1995). College in black and white: Campus environment and academic achievement of African American males. *Journal of Negro Education, 63*(4), 620–633.

11. Morales, E. E. (2010). Legitimizing hope: An exploration of effective mentoring for Dominican American male college students. *Journal of College Student Retention: Research, Theory, and Practice, 11*(3), 385–406.

12. Stott, A. (2004). Issues in the socialization process of the male student nurse: implications for retention in undergraduate nursing courses. *Nurse Education Today, 24,* 91–97.

13. McLaughlin, K., Muldoon, O. T., & Moutray, M. (2010). Gender, gender roles and completion of nursing education: A longitudinal study. *Nurse Education Today, 30,* 303–307.

14. Love, K. L. (2010). The lived experience of socialization among African American nursing students in a predominantly white university. *Journal of Transcultural Nursing, 21*(4), 342–350.

15. Campbell, E. T. (2009). Teaching Korean RN-BSN students. *Nurse Educator, 34*(3), 122–125.

16. Fleming, J. (2002). Who will succeed in college? When the SAT predicts black students' performance. *Review of Higher Education, 25*(3), 281–296.

17. Hinderlie, H. H., & Kenny, M. (2002). Attachment, social support, and college adjustment among black students at predominantly white universities. *Journal of College Student Development, 43*(3), 327–340.

18. Nora, A., & Cabrera, A. F. (1996). The role of perceptions of prejudice and discrimination on the adjustment of minority students to college. *Journal of Higher Education, 67*(2), 119–148.

19. Lee, J., Donlan, W., & Brown, E. F. (2011). American Indian/Alaskan Native undergraduate retention at predominantly white institutions: An elaboration of Tinto's theory of college student departure. *Journal of College Student Retention: Research, Theory, and Practice, 12*(3), 257–276.

20. Tucker-Allen, S., & Long, E. (1999). *Recruitment and retention of minority students: Stories of success.* Lisle, IL: Tucker Publications.

21. Bosher, S. D., & Pharris, M. D. (2009). *Transforming nursing education: The culturally inclusive environment.* New York, NY: Springer Publishing.

22. Gardner, J. (2005). A successful minority retention project. *Journal of Nursing Education, 44*(12), 566–568.

23. Campinha-Bacote, J. (2010). A culturally conscious model of mentoring. *Nurse Educator, 35*(3), 130–135.

24. Gilchrist, K. L., & Rector, C. (2007). Can you keep them? Strategies to attract and retain nursing students from diverse populations: Best practices in nursing education. *Journal of Transcultural Nursing, 18*(3), 277–285.

25. Seidman, A. (2007). *Minority student retention: The best of the journal of college student retention: research, theory, and practice.* Amityville, NY: Baywood.

26. Literte, P. E. (2010). Revising race: How biracial students are changing and challenging student services. *Journal of College Student Development, 51*(2), 115–134.

27. Fleming, S., & McKee, G. (2005). The mature student question. *Nurse Education Today, 25*, 230–237.

28. Mancuso, S. (2001). Adult-centered practices: Benchmarking study in higher education. *Innovative Higher Education, 25*(3), 165–181.

29. Chaves, C. (2006). Involvement, development, and retention: Theoretical foundations and potential extensions for adult community college students. *Community College Review, 34*(2), 139–152.

30. Hilberg, S., Joshi, A., & House, A. (2009). Washington state achievers program: Influence of the scholarship program on low-income college students' achievement and aspirations. *Journal of College Student Retention: Research, Theory, and Practice, 10*(4), 447–464.

31. Olenchak, F. R., & Hebert, T. P. (2002). Endangered academic talent: Lessons learned from gifted first-generation college males. *Journal of College Student Development, 43*(2), 195–212.

32. Bryan, E., & Simmons, L. A. (2009). Family involvement: Impacts on postsecondary educational success for first-generation Appalachian college students. *Journal of College Student Development, 50*(4), 391–406.

33. Smith, R. A. (2010). Feeling supported: Curricular learning communities for basic skills courses and students who speak English as a second language. *Community College Review, 37*(3), 261–284.

34. Sanner, S., & Wilson, A. (2008). The experiences of students with English as a second language in a baccalaureate nursing program. *Nurse Education Today, 28*, 807–813.

35. DeLapp, T., Hautman, M. A., & Anderson, M. S. (2008). Recruitment and retention of Alaska natives into nursing (RRANN). *Journal of Nursing Education, 47*(7), 293–297.

36. Martin, D. E., & Kipling, A. (2006). Factors shaping Aboriginal nursing students' experiences. *Nurse Education Today, 26*, 688–696.

37. Gonzalez, L. M., & Ting, S-M, R. (2008). Adjustment of undergraduate Latino students at a southeastern university. *Journal of Hispanic Higher Education, 7*(3), 199–211.

38. Brown, A. V. (2008). Effectively educating Latino/a students: A comparative study of participation patterns of Hispanic American and Anglo-American university students. *Journal of Hispanic Higher Education, 7*(2), 97–118.

39. Bond, M. L., Gray, J. R., Baxley, S., Cason, C. L., & Denke, L. (2008). Voices of Hispanic students in baccalaureate nursing programs: Are we listening? *Nursing Education Perspectives, 29*(3), 136–142.

40. Hernandez, J. C. (2000). Understanding the retention of Latino college students. *Journal of College Student Development, 41*(6), 575–588.

41. Kraemer, B. A. (1997). The academic and social integration of Hispanic students into college. *Review of Higher Education, 20*(2), 163–179.

42. Bean, J. P., & Metzner, B. (1985). A conceptual model of nontraditional undergraduate student attrition. *Review of Educational Research, 55*, 485–540.

43. Metzner, B., & Bean, J. P. (1987). The estimation of a conceptual model of nontraditional undergraduate student attrition. *Research in Higher Education, 27*, 15–38.

44. Jeffreys, M. R. (1993). *The relationship of self-efficacy and select academic and environmental variables on academic achievement and retention.* Unpublished doctoral dissertation, New York, NY: Teachers College, Columbia University.

45. Jeffreys, M. R. (1998). Predicting nontraditional student retention and academic achievement. *Nurse Educator, 23*(1), 42–48.

46. Jeffreys, M. R. (2001). Evaluating enrichment program study groups: Academic outcomes, psychological outcomes, and variables influencing retention. *Nurse Educator, 26*(3), 142–149.

47. Jeffreys, M. R. (2002). Students' perceptions of variables influencing retention: A pretest and post-test approach. *Nurse Educator, 27*(1), 16–19 [Erratum, 2002, 27(2), 64].

48. Bessent, H. (Ed.). (1997). *Strategies for recruitment, retention, and graduation of minority nurses in colleges of nursing.* Washington, DC: American Nurses Publishing.

49. Hesser, A., Pond, E., Lewis, L., & Abbott, B. (1996). Evaluation of a supplementary retention program for African-American baccalaureate nursing students. *Journal of Nursing Education, 35*(7), 304–309.

50. Ramsey, P., Blowers, S., Merriman, C., Glenn, L. L., & Terry, L. (2000). The NURSE Center: A peer mentor-tutor project for disadvantaged nursing students in Appalachia. *Nurse Educator, 25*(6), 277–281.

51. Escallier, L. A., & Fullerton, J. T. (2009). Process and outcomes evaluation of retention strategies within a nursing workforce diversity project. *Journal of Nursing Education, 48*(9), 488–494.

52. Sutherland, J. A., & Goodman, N. (2007). Affirming at-risk minorities for success (ARMS): Retention, graduation, and success on the NCLEX-RN. *Journal of Nursing Education, 46*(8), 347–353.

53. Rees, B. B. (2006). Can you have both retention and increased pass rates on the NCLEX-RN? *Teaching and Learning in Nursing, 1*, 18–21.

54. Miller, C. L., & Leadingham, C. (2010). A formalized mentoring program for LPN-to-RN students. *Teaching and Learning in Nursing, 5*, 149–153.

55. Sweet, S., & Fusner, S. (2008). Social integration of the advanced placement LPN: A peer mentoring program. *Nurse Educator, 33*(5), 202–205.

56. Colalillo, G. (2007). Mentoring as a retention strategy in a diverse, multicultural, urban associate degree nursing program. *Teaching and Learning in Nursing, 2*, 28–33.

57. Bagnardi, M., & Perkel, L. K. (2005). The learning achievement program: Fostering student cultural diversity. *Nurse Educator, 30*(1), 17–20.

58. Valencia-Go, G. (2005). Growth and access increase for nursing students: A retention and progression project. *Journal of Cultural Diversity, 12*(1), 18–25.

59. Robinson, E., & Niemer, L. (2010). A peer mentor tutor program for academic success in nursing. *Nursing Education Perspectives, 31*(5), 286–289.

60. Pascarella, E. T., & Terenzini, (1991). *How college affects students: Findings and insights from twenty years of research.* San Francisco, CA: Jossey-Bass.

61. Terenzini, P. T., Pascarella, E. T., & Blimling, G. S. (1996). Students' out-of-class experiences and their influence on learning and cognitive development: A literature review. *Journal of College Student Development, 37*(2), 149–162.

62. Alexitch, L. R. (2002). The role of help-seeking attitudes and tendencies in students' preferences for academic advising. *Journal of College Student Development, 43*(1), 5–19.

63. Herndorn, J. B., Kaiser, J., & Creamer, D. G. (1996). Student preferences for advising style in community college environments. *Journal of College Student Development, 37*(6), 637–647.

64. Baldwin, D., & Wold, J. (1993). Students from disadvantaged backgrounds: Satisfaction with a mentor-protégé relationship. *Journal of Nursing Education, 32*(5), 225–226.

65. Gasper, M. L. (2009). Building a community with your advisees. *Nurse Educator, 34*(2), 88–94.

66. Harrison, E. (2009). (Re)Visiting academic advising. *Nurse Educator, 34*(2), 64–68.

67. Lehna, C., Jackonen, S., & Wilson, L. (1996). Navigating a nursing curriculum: Bridges and barriers. *Association for Black Nursing Faculty Journal, 7(July/August)*, 98–103.

68. Peters, M. A. A. (2008). Defining the boundaries of the nurse faculty role. *Nurse Educator, 33*(5), 193–197.

69. Schultz, E. D. (1998). Academic advising from a nursing theory perspective. *Nurse Educator, 22*(2), 22–25.

70. Trent, B. A. (1997). Student perceptions of academic advising in an RN-to-BSN program. *Journal of Continuing Education in Nursing, 28*(6), 276–283.

71. Winters, C. E. (1990). Excellence in advisement: A strategy for declining nursing enrollments. *Journal of Nursing Education, 29*(5), 233–234.

72. Yoder, M. K., & Saylor, C. (2002). Student and teacher roles: Mismatched expectations. *Nurse Educator, 27*(5), 201–203.

73. Poorman, S. G., Webb, C. A., & Mastorovich, M. L. (2002). Students' stories: How faculty help and hinder students at risk. *Nurse Educator, 27*(3), 126–131.

74. Diekelmann, N. (1993). Spending time with students: Keeping my door open. *Journal of Nursing Education, 32*(4), 149–150.

75. Campbell, T. A., & Campbell, D. E. (1997). Faculty/student mentor program: effects on academic performance and retention. *Research in Higher Education, 38*(6), 727–742.

76. Milem, J. F., & Berger, J. B. (1997). A modified model of college student persistence: Exploring the relationship between Astin's theory of involvement and Tinto's theory of student departure. *Journal of College Student Development, 38*(4), 387–400.

77. Nora, A. (2001). The depiction of significant others in Tinto's "Rites of Passage": A reconceptualization of the influence of family and community in the persistence process. *Journal of College Student Retention: Research, Theory, & Practice, 3*(1), 41–56.

78. Leininger, M. M. (1995). *Transcultural nursing: Concepts, theories, research, and practice.* Blacklick, OH: McGraw-Hill College Custom Services.

79. Betts, V. T., & Cherry, B. (2002). Health policy and politics. In Cherry & Jacob (Eds.), *Contemporary nursing: Issues, trends, and management,* (2nd ed.). Philadelphia, PA: Mosby, 219–235.

80. Joel, L. A., & Kelly, L. Y. (2002). *The nursing experience: Trends, challenges, and transitions.* New York, NY: McGraw-Hill.

81. Gardner, E. A., & Schmidt, C. K. (2007). Implementing a leadership course and mentor model for students in the National Student Nurses' Association. *Nurse Educator, 32*(4), 178–182.

82. Vance, C. (2011). *Fast facts for career success in nursing: Making the most of mentoring in a nutshell.* New York, NY: Springer Publishing.

83. Vance, C., & Olson, R. K. (1998). *The mentor connection in nursing.* New York, NY: Springer Publishing.

84. Spickerman, S. (1988). Enhancing the socialization process. *Nurse Educator, 13*(6), 10–14.

85. Rendon, L. I. (1994). Validating culturally diverse students: Toward a new model of learning and student development. *Innovative Higher Education, 19*(1), 23–32.

86. Rendon, L. I., Jalomo, R. E., & Nora, A. (2000). Theoretical considerations in the study of minority student retention in higher education. In Braxton (Ed.), *Reworking the student departure puzzle,* (pp.127–156). Nashville, TN: Vanderbilt University Press.

87. Calder, W. B., & Gordon, W. (1999). Institutionalizing college networks for student success. *Journal of College Student Retention: Research, Theory, and Practice, 1*(4), 323–333.

88. Antonio, A. L. (2001). Diversity and the influence of friendship groups in college. *Review of Higher Education, 25*(1), 63–89.

89. Kuh, G. D. (2001). Organizational culture and student persistence: Prospects and puzzles. *Journal of College Student Retention: Research, Theory, & Practice, 3*(1), 23–40.

90. Skahill, M. P. (2002). The role of social support network in college persistence among freshman students. *Journal of College Student Retention: Research, Theory, & Practice, 4*(1), 39–52.

91. Morris, J., Reese, J., Beck, R., & Mattis, C. (2010). Facebook usage as a predictor of retention at a private 4-year institution. *Journal of College Student Retention: Research, Theory, and Practice, 11*(3), 311–322.

92. Karp, M. M., Hughes, K. L., & O'Gara, L. (2011). An exploration of Tinto's integration framework for community college students. *Journal of College Student Retention: Research, Theory, and Practice, 12*(1), 69–86.

93. Luo, J., & Jamieson-Drake, D. (2009). A retrospective assessment of the educational benefits of interaction across racial boundaries. *Journal of College Student Development, 50*(2), 115–134.

94. Buch, K., & Spaulding, S. (2011). The impact of a psychology learning community on academic success, retention, and student learning outcomes. *Teaching of Psychology, 38*(2), 71–77.

95. Callahan, K. M. (2009). Academic-centered peer interaction and retention in undergraduate mathematics programs. *Journal of College Student Retention: Research, Theory, and Practice, 10*(3), 361–389.

96. Goguen, L. M. S., Hiester, M. A., & Nordstrom, A. H. (2011). Associations among peer relationships, academic achievement, and persistence in college. *Journal of College Student Retention: Research, Theory, and Practice, 12*(3), 319–337.

97. Weaver, H. N. (2001). Indigenous nurses and professional education: Friends or foes? *Journal of Nursing Education, 40*(6), 252–258.

98. Yurkovich, E. E. (2001). Working with American Indians toward educational success. *Journal of Nursing Education, 40*(6), 259–269.

99. Steele, R., Lauder, W., & Caperchione, C. (2005). An exploratory study of the concerns of mature access to nursing students and the coping strategies used to manage these adverse experiences. *Nurse Education Today, 25,* 573–581.

100. Gardner, J. (2005). Barriers influencing the success of racial and ethnic minority students in nursing programs. *Journal of Transcultural Nursing, 16*(2), 155–162.

101. Jeffreys, M. R. (2007). Nontraditional students' perceptions of variables influencing retention: A multisite study. *Nurse Educator, 32*(4), 161–167.

102. Campbell, A. R., & Davis, S. M. (1996). Faculty commitment: Retaining minority nursing students in majority institutions. *Journal of Nursing Education, 35*(7), 298–303.

103. Bandura, A. (1986). *Social foundations of thought and action: A social cognitive theory.* Englewood Cliffs, NJ: Prentice-Hall.

104. Zimmerman, B. J. (1995). Self-efficacy and educational development. In A. Bandura (Ed.), *Self-efficacy in changing societies* (pp. 202–231). New York, NY: Cambridge University Press.

105. Martin, A. J., & Dowson, M. (2009). Interpersonal relationships, motivation, engagement, and achievement: Yields for theory, current issues, and educational practice. *Review of Educational Research, 79*(1), 327–365.

106. Lundberg, K. M. (2008). Promoting self-confidence in clinical nursing students. *Nurse Educator, 33*(2), 86–89.

107. Courage, M. M., & Godbey, K. L. (1992). Student retention: Policies and services to enhance persistence to graduation. *Nurse Educator, 17*(2), 29–32.

108. Schon, D. (1987). *Educating the reflective practitioner.* San Francisco: Jossey-Bass.

109. Chaney, B., Muraskin, L. D., Cahalan, M. W., & Goodwin, D. (1998). Helping the progress of disadvantaged students in higher education: The federal student support services program. *Educational Evaluation and Policy Analysis, 20*(3), 197–215.

110. Mattern, K. D., & Shaw, E. J. (2010). A look beyond cognitive predictors of academic success: Understanding the relationship between academic self-beliefs and outcomes. *Journal of College Student Development, 51*(6), 665–678.

111. Ofori, R. (2006). Measuring motivational orientations toward support-seeking: The development and predicative validity of the motives for tutorial support-seeking questionnaire. *Nurse Education Today, 26*, 228–239.

112. Barnard-Brak, L., Sulak, T., Tate, A., Lechtenberger, D. (2010). Measuring college students' attitudes toward requesting accommodations: A national multi-institutional study. *Assessment for Effective Intervention, 35*(3), 141–147.

113. Bayer-Hummel, T. (2010). The effects of *Jeopardy* as a test preparation strategy for nursing students. *Teaching and Learning in Nursing, 5*, 12–15.

114. Jeffreys, M. R., & Stier, L. (2003). Student academic dishonesty. In M. Oermann & K. Heinrich (Eds.), *Annual review of nursing education: Volume II* (pp. 255–281). New York, NY: Springer Publishing.

Academic and Psychological Outcomes

Entry into the nursing educational process assures an academic outcome, at least minimally, at the course level. That is, all students who begin a course will pass, fail, or withdraw. All nursing students will experience some degree of stress; however, not all students may experience satisfaction.

SNAPSHOT SCENARIO

Following the first nursing exam, Professor Narrows announces in class: "Students who failed the test must see me during office hours this week or next week. Those of you who passed just keep doing whatever you've been doing."

Students react differently to her announcement. Here are some excerpts of students' thoughts and feelings:

ALICE: Oh no. I will be so embarrassed to be seen in Professor Narrows's office. Everybody will know that I failed. If I don't show up, I might get failed. I feel so stressed about this.

OMAR: I passed, but I really wanted to do better on the exam. I think I'm not using the correct techniques for studying and answering nursing type questions. Professor Narrows made it clear that only failing students should go to office hours. I feel very unhappy about this, yet I do not want to just show up or challenge the professor.

DELIA: Is it really just about passing or failing? I want to be the best I can be. I am not confident about my study methods. I'm not satisfied with Professor Narrows's open-door policy that doesn't include me. It is really a closed-door policy. I should have messed up two more questions, and then I'd get the help I need.

CONNIE: My parents are both successful accountants and they can't understand why I only got an 82 on my first nursing test when I have an overall college GPA [grade point average] of 3.79. I wish I could talk to my professor about this. My parents are putting a lot of pressure on me and it is hard enough just to balance my nursing courses with living away from home for the first time.

ROSARIO: If other faculty see me sitting in Professor Narrows's office, I will be labeled as a weak student when I get to their class. This is so unfair. I just had an off day due to a personal crisis that is resolved, but this label will follow me around forever. I should just give up now and avoid the stigma.

HECTOR: My family is sacrificing so much for me to be in school. I'm not happy about how the nursing faculty is only available to help those who are failing. I owe it to my family and to my future patients to do more than just pass. I got an 85 this time, but I don't understand several of the questions I got wrong. I'm worried that if I don't straighten this out now, other content based on this will be even more complex and confusing.

JASMINE: I'm glad that Professor Narrows is willing to help me pass my exam. I didn't really study for this first test. I was waiting to see how much effort I needed to put in and what grade I got. Now that I got a 70 without studying and can tap Professor Narrows's brain for clues about the next exam and gain her sympathy, it will be much easier than I thought just to get by this course with the least effort possible.

BOBBY: This is very stressful. I got a 92 on this test because some of the beginning fundamentals material I already knew from my work as a nursing assistant. I'm not confident that I'll be able to handle more complex material for the next test because it covers new things that I know nothing about. It would be comforting to know that I could approach Professor Narrows about this but I don't want to take time away from my failing classmates.

LAVINIA: Well, I guess I'll have to continue cheating my way through the course. I could probably pass without cheating but I want to keep up my high GPA. It's great that I can avoid meeting with Professor Narrows. She might catch on that I don't really know my stuff if she tried to have a conversation with me about course content.

MARYBETH: I'm not really satisfied with the idea of becoming a nurse, but my husband really wants me to be a nurse and earn money. He puts a lot of pressure on me to do well and will be angry that I failed this test. I feel like I am just wasting my time and also wasting Professor Narrows's time when she could be helping someone who really wants to do better and become a nurse.

In contrast, Professor Broad emphasizes proactive inclusive enrichment (PIE) rather than exclusive remediation (ER). For example, Professor Broad implements a 2-hour interactive course orientation and discusses the course booklet titled "Your Enhanced Success—YES—Strategies to Enhance Critical Thinking and Success in Nursing," conducts several small group test-prep workshops 1 week prior to each exam, facilitates peer mentor-tutor-led study group formation beginning the first week, reaches out privately (via phone call, e-mail, and/or in person) to students who have notable difficulty in test-prep workshop, provides judicious positive feedback for students' improved efforts and outcomes, and encourages individual and/or small groups of students to stop by office during office hours prior to exam and after as needed, announcing, "everyone has the potential to enrich their nursing student experience by feeling more satisfied with the learning process, decreasing stress, and optimizing academic outcomes. They are all interrelated. I want each of you to enjoy learning, manage your stress effectively, and reach your potential in your career path. You are empowered to make choices that will enrich your experience. I am here to guide you in your journey so please feel free to stop by and see me during office hours."

What feelings and thoughts does each of the characters in the snapshot scenarios evoke? Why? How could each scenario influence student retention and success?

The general college experience involves multiple psychological and developmental opportunities and outcomes beyond course grades or GPA. The complex nursing educational experience offers unique professional, discipline-specific psychological and developmental opportunities and outcomes beyond course grades or GPA. Outcome expectations include learning, personal growth, and satisfaction. Students anticipate gaining more benefits than knowledge alone; therefore, any analysis of student outcomes should recognize various dimensions (1). Occasionally, academic outcome is the *only* variable considered in achievement and retention studies, thereby omitting the exploration of nonacademic outcomes that may greatly influence both achievement and retention.

As presented in the NURS model, student profile characteristics, student affective factors, academic factors, environmental factors, and professional integration factors interact and result in a range of academic and psychological outcomes. Outside and surrounding factors may also impact on academic and psychological outcomes. Academic outcomes are represented by the student's nursing course grade, cumulative GPA for nursing courses, and overall GPA. Psychological outcomes include satisfaction and stress. Both academic and psychological outcomes influence persistence and retention (2–4). Furthermore, academic and psychological outcomes interact and impact upon self-efficacy, motivation, persistence, and retention. As originally proposed by Bean and Metzner (5), nonacademic factors may compensate for low levels of academic success, and yet high levels of academic success result in persistence and continued enrollment only when accompanied by positive psychological outcomes. For nursing students, good academic performance results in retention only when accompanied by positive psychological outcomes for the nursing program and profession. In the NURS model, positive psychological outcomes include satisfaction and low (manageable) stress. In contrast, negative psychological outcomes include dissatisfaction and high stress. Although the constructs of satisfaction and stress seem dichotomous, in reality they are not. Even the use of a continuum of satisfaction or stress is insufficient in capturing the multidimensional and intertwining phenomenon of satisfaction and stress. This chapter will address pertinent issues surrounding academic outcomes and psychological outcomes (satisfaction and stress), present proposed relationships with other variables in the NURS model, and suggest implications for nurse educators.

> What academic and psychological outcomes are measured in your course? In your program? How are they measured? What are the results? How are results used to influence course(s) and the nursing program?

ACADEMIC OUTCOMES

The academic outcome most frequently measured in retention studies is GPA. Unfortunately, retention studies in higher education may not differentiate between majors, thereby compounding results. For example, a student may fail a course, yet have a GPA high enough to avoid probation or dismissal from the college or nursing program. The NURS model proposes that persistence and attrition decisions occur during and after each individual nursing course, and so course grade is included as an essential academic outcome measure. Looking at GPA alone is insufficient in determining progression within the nursing curriculum. Conducting discipline-specific retention studies allows for assessment of the particular nuances of a discipline.

Generalization in attrition research is difficult because institutional and program differences present extraneous variables (4,6). Whereas, the big picture may be college (institutional) retention, the NURS model allows for investigation at the course and program level. For this reason, course grade is included. Nursing course grade certainly impacts upon nursing major GPA and overall college GPA, which in turn influence attrition. For example, a student may successfully complete a nursing course yet still be dismissed from the college if other non-nursing courses lower overall GPA. Consequently, nursing course grade, nursing GPA, and overall GPA are all important academic measures to assess when seeking to identify at-risk students. Any low or failed academic outcome measure places a student at risk for attrition.

Established policies concerning progression in the nursing curriculum require minimum standards for nursing courses, non-nursing required courses, nursing GPA, overall GPA, minimum course grades for repeated courses and progression in the curriculum. Whether nursing program retention policies are the same as or different from general college policies can skew retention rate results for nursing when contrasted with other majors or the college in general. Such policy differences should be considered when comparing data. Policy differences may also affect retention indirectly through satisfaction and stress.

Course grades and GPA may seem to allow for direct comparison from course to course; however, methods of evaluation differ between courses and instructors, skewing a seemingly straightforward quantitative measure (calculation). Comparisons will always contain some degree of error. Because error is often overlooked when using academic outcome measures, further scrutiny and data analysis are warranted. Academic outcomes (course grades) may sometimes be collapsed into categories for the purpose of data analysis and descriptive statistics. For example, academic outcomes may be divided into pass, fail, and withdrawal. Theoretically, any student who achieves a passing grade can progress in the curriculum as expected. Students who withdraw or fail are at risk for nursing program attrition, either involuntarily or voluntarily, and are greatly influenced by nursing program progression policies. For example, a policy that requires students who withdraw or fail to reapply or file an appeal to continue in the nursing program discourages program retention. However, the need to assure client safety and maintain professional standards outweighs the risks of lenient retention policies. Screening reapplicants offers nurse educators an opportunity to proactively assist such at-risk students through the individual appraisal of student strengths and weaknesses and through the design of diagnostic and prescriptive support strategies for them. For some students, counseling and guidance recommending delayed continuation in the nursing program or alternate career options may be indicated (7–9).

Advantages of pass rate calculations include the ability to compare from year to year and to notice changes after intervention strategies are initiated. Even a moderate improvement in retention (course pass rates), with other variables kept constant, supports continuation of the retention strategies. Examining trends over time, as strategies are continued and/or expanded lends support for ongoing interventions. Frequently, academic outcome measures are the yardstick that funding agencies and institutions use to determine continued or canceled support. Therefore, it behooves nurse educators to exercise great care in determining what academic outcome measures will be appraised and to control for extraneous variables that might skew results, making them invalid or impractical.

A rise in course pass rates needs to be viewed in relation to achievement in subsequent courses, graduation, and RN licensing exam pass rate. In other words, high course pass rates as a result of low standards defeats the desired outcome of the NURS model, which addresses not only retention but emphasizes program success. Program success includes desired outcomes of graduation, passing the RN licensing exam, obtaining employment as a registered nurse, and/or enrolling in an advanced educational nursing program.

Academic outcomes are complex beyond a mere numerical calculation. A calculation does not tell educators if minimum or maximum effort was expended or if there were other factors that influenced academic outcomes. Furthermore, the course grade or GPA may have a different meaning to the nurse educator and the academic institution than to the individual student. The same academic outcome (nursing course grade, nursing GPA, or cumulative GPA) may hold different meanings for different students. For example, to the nurse educator and the academic institution, a B grade in nursing may mean "above average," "program retention," and "continued enrollment;" however, an "A-grade" student who exerted much energy, time, and commitment toward a course may be dissatisfied or distressed over a "B" grade. Another student who works full-time and is a single parent may feel satisfaction and (stress) relief after earning a "B" grade.

Table 7.1 contrasts student responses to several positive academic outcomes. To the institutional researcher, nurse educator, or college administrator, all of the academic outcomes would appear to lead to retention. Using just an academic outcome criterion measure, students would be viewed as low attrition risk; however, this conclusion is incorrect. Clearly, academic outcomes cannot be viewed without the understanding and exploration of psychological outcomes.

> What are your students' perceptions (feelings and thoughts) about their academic outcomes in your course, other nursing courses, non-nursing courses, and overall college? What are the academic outcomes that your students value? (pass grade, letter grade, GPA, amount of new knowledge and skills learned, etc.)?

PSYCHOLOGICAL OUTCOMES

Satisfaction

Student satisfaction strongly influences persistence and retention. Unmet expectations and unrealistic assumptions put the nursing student at risk for dissatisfaction and attrition (10,11). In this book, dissatisfaction refers

TABLE 7.1 Student Psychological Outcome Responses to Positive Academic Outcomes

POSITIVE ACADEMIC OUTCOME	POSITIVE PSYCHOLOGICAL OUTCOMES *(HIGH SATISFACTION OR SATISFACTION LOW STRESS, MANAGEABLE STRESS, OR STRESS RELIEF)*	NEGATIVE PSYCHOLOGICAL OUTCOMES *(LOW SATISFACTION OR DISSATISFACTION HIGH STRESS OR UNMANAGEABLE STRESS)*
B+ grade in nursing course	"Between working full-time, taking care of the kids, and going to school, I am so happy and relieved to get a B+ grade."	"I can't believe this B+ grade messes up my 4.0 GPA. I'm really dissatisfied and distressed."
75 (passing) grade in first nursing course	"After this first class, I know nursing is the career for me. I was stressed out in the beginning because I wasn't sure, but now I'm sure. I'll try to get higher grades next semester."	"I really thought nursing was different. I don't like it at all. I almost wish I failed so I would have an excuse to change my major. I feel more stressed now than if I failed."
A grade in nursing course	"I got the grade I deserved and I'm so relieved."	"It's too much stress between work, school, and family responsibilities."
"Pass" grade in clinical component	"I really worked hard in clinical and learned a lot. The instructor made some good comments and suggestions."	"All that work, time, and stress in clinical and all I get is a 'Pass.' What difference do the instructor's comments make?"
2.9 nursing course GPA	"I wish my nursing course GPA was higher. I tried my best so I just have to be satisfied."	"Only a 2.9. All I ever wanted to be was an pediatric nurse practitioner. I'll never get into an NP program now."
3.7 nursing course GPA	"Great, I made the dean's list this time. I can't wait to start critical care next semester."	"Now everyone will always expect me to excel. I feel so much pressure."
3.0 overall cumulative GPA	"Nursing really is different than other courses I've taken. My GPA dropped with nursing courses, but I love nursing. I'm learning so much so it's okay."	"Why does nursing have to be so different from other courses. My friends in other majors have higher GPAs and don't work half as hard as me."
3.2 overall cumulative GPA	"I really like going to this college. Everyone is so helpful. I feel welcome and included in many of the college and professional events."	"I hate this college. It's so hard to get help around here. I have never felt so out of place."

to the emotional discontent that arises from the discrepancy between expected academic, developmental, personal, and/or professional outcomes from the nursing educational process, and what actually occurs. Satisfaction refers to the emotional gratification that arises from the congruency between expected academic, developmental, personal, and/or professional outcomes from the nursing educational process and what actually occurs.

The nursing educational experience results in varying degrees of satisfying and/or dissatisfying outcomes. Perceived satisfaction varies among students and within students at different times. The impact of satisfaction on intent to persist, persistence behaviors, and retention may affect various student subgroups differently. Similarly, the impact of dissatisfaction on withdrawal cognitions (thoughts of withdrawal), dropout behavior, and attrition varies accordingly. The higher education literature addresses the impact of satisfaction on various student subgroups. Studies on retention have typically targeted beginning students due to high attrition rates; however, retention among other student populations must be emphasized as well (4). Studies among senior baccalaureate students have shown that dissatisfaction was a statistically significant predictor of attrition (12). Studies of minority student attrition and retention note the significance of satisfaction as a variable influencing academic achievement, persistence, and retention (13–19). Despite high levels of academic performance, minority students with low levels of satisfaction were at greater attrition risk than non-minority students. Some researchers report dissatisfaction and higher attrition rates among male nursing students than among female students (20,21). Other nursing authors note satisfaction as a factor influencing retention across student populations (11,22–26).

The overall college, individual departments, and specific academic programs influence student satisfaction, which in turn influences academic outcomes, persistence, and retention. Satisfaction with faculty, peers, and facilities affects overall college satisfaction (27–31). With the explosion of totally online or partially online (hybrid) courses, satisfaction with the online experience affects attrition and achievement (32,33). Satisfaction with particular student services can also impact on the overall college experience, thereby affecting academic outcomes, persistence, and retention (4,12,13,34–37). Satisfying and rewarding interactions in college lead to greater integration and persistence. Unpleasant or limited interactions lead to decreased persistence. Psychosocial outcomes such as satisfaction mediate performance (academic outcomes) and persistence outcomes (38). Working backwards in the NURS model, persistence or departure behavior is directly influenced by two dimensions of outcomes: academic and psychological. Satisfaction is also influenced by self-efficacy through self-perceptions of ability, effort expenditure, and motivation (16,39–42).

Through their psychological model of attrition, Eaton and Bean (6) propose that students who take an active approach and responsibility for learning are more satisfied. Students satisfied with their academic performance become more academically integrated and self-perceptions of future academic integration are positively influenced. In contrast, those who avoid responsibility for learning are more dissatisfied, often with the result of poor academic outcomes and lowered self-efficacy, whereby students envision a bleak academic future. This proposition has been empirically supported in nursing. Nursing students who participated consistently in enrichment program study groups led by peer mentor-tutors reported high satisfaction with nursing as a career choice, nursing courses, overall learning opportunities at the college, and specific enrichment program components. Such students took an active approach and responsibility for learning and self-selected participation in study groups; more positive academic outcomes (course pass rates) were noted among study group participants in comparison with student non-participants (43–45).

Satisfaction measures help identify responsiveness to student needs of the institution, program, or strategy. Student satisfaction is a complex, multidimensional construct. Because both general satisfaction and specific satisfaction variables can influence retention, it is helpful to assess both dimensions. General satisfaction in nursing includes nursing as a career, nursing courses, and learning opportunities at the college. Specific satisfaction items include the evaluation of specific retention strategy components or services. Despite positive academic outcomes, dissatisfaction with nursing as a career, nursing courses, and/or learning opportunities at the college adversely influences retention. If a student is truly dissatisfied with nursing as a career choice, then career guidance and referral to other programs is warranted. Nurse educators must recognize that not all students will or should be retained in nursing programs. Satisfaction with career choice but dissatisfaction with nursing courses presents a different case scenario, speaking to the need to view satisfaction on an individual item level, and not just use an aggregate measure of satisfaction.

Some of the purposes of a satisfaction scale are to provide a meaningful quantitative comparison over time and to identify differences between student subgroups. Each response category represents a different point on the satisfaction continuum; however, it must be remembered that satisfaction surveys provide ordinal data. Furthermore, positively packed scales can affect the quality of student responses (46), therefore adversely impacting on reliability and validity. Toolkit Items 6 and 7 present two satisfaction surveys used to assess general and specific satisfaction. Among several student samples, student responses were consistently diverse, suggesting that respondents were discriminating between items, lending support to the instruments' validity and reliability (43,44). Student responses in each of the general satisfaction items should be viewed both separately and together with other item responses. Specific satisfaction items delineating specific interventions or student services provide valuable information for guiding future strategies. Another benefit of administering a satisfaction survey is that students may perceive that faculty care enough to see if they are satisfied. This benefit is nullified if students do not perceive that faculty responded to their needs; students may even become dissatisfied. Therefore, it behooves nurse educators to carefully consider the direct and indirect impact or consequences of each survey item.

Nurse educators are in a powerful position to maximize satisfaction and minimize dissatisfaction. The NURS model can be used to systematically consider each factor as potentially influencing satisfaction. Student profile characteristics, student affective factors, academic factors, environmental factors, professional integration factors, and outside and surrounding factors can all affect and be affected by satisfaction. Satisfaction must be viewed together in context with academic outcomes and the other psychological outcome of the NURS model: stress. An ongoing bidirectional relationship exists between the two psychological outcomes in the NURS model: satisfaction and stress.

> To what degree are students satisfied with various aspects of your course, other courses, the nursing program, and the college? How is satisfaction measured? How are results used? What changes would you propose? Why? What are students most satisfied about in your course, other courses, the program, and the college? Least satisfied about?

Stress

The process of college is challenging and stressful. All college students experience stress to some degree as a result of the many developmental and life changes (2). The perception of an event or situation as stressful varies among students and within an individual student at different times. Through cognitive appraisal, a student perceives something to be stressful if its demands exceed the perceived ability to cope with the stressor. Coping is the process of managing the demands of the perceived stressful event or situation and the ensuing emotions (47). Ineffective coping places a student at risk for negative academic achievement, dissatisfaction, decreased persistence, and attrition. Perceived confidence for college-related tasks is a critical component in cognitive appraisal and coping; self-efficacy is a mediator of stress (48) (see Chapter 3).

Stress may range in a degree from mild to high and have positive or negative effects. There is a marked difference between manageable (positive) stress and unmanageable (negative) stress. A mild degree of stress is stimulating, impressing upon students the need for preparation, attentiveness, detail, and preciseness. Undoubtedly, high levels of stress negatively affect academic achievement, performance, and outcomes, thus adversely affecting student persistence and retention. Anticipatory efforts to manage and reduce stress are urgently needed.

Although the general college experience commonly produces some degree of stress, the nursing student is particularly at risk. It is well documented that the nursing educational process is highly stressful. Citations in the literature purport that nursing students experience greater stress throughout their educational process than do college students in general or even college students enrolled in other health professional programs (49–55). Enculturation into nursing is a developmental process (56) that presents new challenges that are especially stressful for beginning students. Nurse educators can play a significant role in recognizing sources of stress, anticipating stress, implementing prophylactic measures to prevent stress, assessing for stressors and stress levels, implementing strategies to reduce or manage stress, and evaluating outcomes.

The educational process of nursing students is unique and different from other types of educational experiences; there are specific stressors prevalent within the nursing educational experience. The rigors of nursing education include difficult courses, didactic courses, diversity within coursework, and clinical components (57). Unlike most college courses, nursing courses may include a theoretical, skills/simulation laboratory, and clinical laboratory component. More academic credits per course and more course contact hours may be an added stressor, especially to beginning nursing students. Additionally, more stress was observed among students enrolled in an accelerated tract (58–62) and among evening students (63) in comparison to students enrolled in traditional and day programs. Lengthy commutes to clinical sites, long hours, and nontraditional class schedules are added stressors to nontraditional students, especially those with dependent children (57,62). Lengthy clinical hours require both physical and emotional endurance that puts increased demands on students.

If the numerous uncertainties that prevail in clinical settings are stressful for registered professional nurses, the uncertainty surrounding the nursing student clinical experience is often overwhelming. In a "human lab," variables are not easily controlled; situations are dynamic, intense, and frequently unpredictable. Moreover, nursing students deal with the added demands of assuming responsibility for client safety, where inadequate preparation and performance can lead to serious outcomes and even death (51,52,59). Beginning students may lack the appropriate resources and effective coping strategies needed to deal with complex human experiences such as the pain and suffering of others (52,54). Other researchers (55,64) discovered that stress and anxiety also affected graduating students. Although practice in simulation labs reduces the threat of actual harm to a real patient, stressors such as learning new technology, performing new skills in front of a live audience with or without taping, videotaped performance for future grading and/or critique can influence students. Conclusively, stress is encountered throughout all stages of the nursing educational process.

Encountering new clinical rotations is another perceived stressor for nursing students. The uncertainty of a new site, experiences, peers, nursing skills, nursing staff, and instructor can all be stressful. For example, the community health experience may be stressful as students venture out of the somewhat familiar hospital environment into the unknown territory of a client's home; the home is the client's domain and the student lacks on-site professional support (65). Yonge, Myrick, and Hoase (66) noted nursing student stress associated with the preceptorship experience. Another general example includes stressors related to a pediatric clinical rotation (67). Certain clinical rotations may be increasingly stressful for particular student subgroups. Empirical evidence documents high stress levels among male nursing students during the obstetrical or maternal-child clinical rotation (68). Awareness of the transitional stress experienced as students encounter new clinical rotations should be acknowledged and addressed sensitively.

Other stressors that may affect specific subgroups of nursing students include perceived cultural incongruence, perceived (or fear of) discrimination and bias, acculturation stress, student-role incongruence (lack of fit between self and student role in comparison with peer norm reference role models, maternal-role stress, perceived multiple-role stress, and gender-role identity stress). Perceived cultural incongruence and perceived (or fear of) discrimination and bias are most prevalent among minority students in predominantly White institutions (69). Acculturation stress is more exacerbated by the new (challenging yet stressful) college experience; recent immigrants will experience higher levels of acculturation stress (70,71). In addition, coping with a foreign language medium of instruction is another source of stress (72,73). Academically weak students and/or low-efficacious students are especially at risk for student-role incongruence. Obviously, maternal-role stress targets individuals who assume both the maternal and student roles, whereas perceived multiple-role stress includes both men and women, particularly nontraditional students who may assume roles as caregiver, financial provider, employee, and student. With the increased numbers of single-parent fathers and fathers who assume active roles in child rearing, paternal-role stress must be given equal consideration. Caregiver stress may also include care of parents, grandparents, or other significant others. Stress related to gender-role identity may affect both female and male nursing students, however, differently. Pressures to abandon traditional female roles and to embrace a "womanist" or "feminist" identity can be perceived as a stressor (74). In contrast, male nursing students may experience stress related to conflict between traditional male role and nontraditional career choice and/or gender bias and discrimination (68,75–79). Any single or combination of stressors adversely influences student satisfaction with the learning environment and academic achievement, thus increasing attrition risk.

Minimal passing grades, fear of failure, academic uncertainty, high academic demands, overwhelming academic workload, test anxiety, and poor academic performance are all potential academic stressors that can result in even higher stress levels when compounded by unmet expectations and/or poor academic outcomes (50,51,80). High levels of test anxiety may adversely affect academic performance, and poor academic performance may intensify test anxiety. Among nursing students, test anxiety may be exacerbated by a rigorous nursing educational program that emphasizes test scores such as preadmission exams and the RN licensing exam (81–84). Even in controlled environments (such as a nursing skills laboratory or simulation laboratory) that aim to enhance learning opportunities in a nonthreatening environment, the testing and retesting of nursing skills can greatly increase stress, thereby decreasing learning and satisfaction (85). Test anxiety and other related academic stressors interact, adversely affecting academic achievement and retention.

Nurse educators are in a key position to recognize, reduce, and sometimes eliminate known stressors. The NURS model can be used to systematically appraise each factor as a potential stressor. Student profile characteristics, student affective factors, academic factors, environmental factors, professional integration factors, and outside and surrounding factors can all be potential stressors. Promoting stress management strategies for stressors that cannot be eliminated is equally important. Empirical studies of nursing students' process of seeking stress care to facilitate effective coping has been limited; however the unpredictability of clinical faculty can serve as a barrier to seeking stress care and help (65). Because help-seeking behaviors differ and may be influenced by cultural values and beliefs, nurse educators should anticipate stress surrounding help-seeking behaviors and actively offer stress management solutions (for example, teaching relaxation techniques such as guided imagery, deep breathing, visualization, and music therapy for use before an exam can help manage the stress associated with exams, or by assisting a student who is a single parent to develop acceptable time management strategies, task prioritization, and task delegation in order to manage multiple role conflict [maternal- or paternal-role stress]). A multidimensional test-prep center that offers proactive test-taking workshops (focused on content, skills, and anxiety reduction), peer mentor-tutors for weekly group and individualized test prep practice, and computerized programs with National Council Licensure Examination (NCLEX)-type questions and rationale is another strategy aimed at enhancing academic outcomes and satisfaction and reducing stress. (See Chapter 6 and the Intensive Nursing Student Test Enhancement Program [INSTEP].)

> What level and types of stress do students in your course, other courses, and the overall program experience? How do they affect academic outcomes (grades, learning, persistence, graduation, licensure)? How do they affect satisfaction? How do you know about the level and type of stress students experience? What stress management resources and strategies are available to students in your course, other courses, and the program? How are they used, perceived, and evaluated? What else can be done?

INTERACTION BETWEEN ACADEMIC AND PSYCHOLOGICAL OUTCOMES

There is an ongoing, complex, and multidimensional interaction between academic and psychological outcomes in the NURS model that influences persistence, retention, and other factors. Entry into the nursing educational process assures an academic outcome, at least minimally, at the course level. That is, all students who begin a course will pass, fail, or withdraw. Incomplete grades are excluded because most colleges have policies that predetermine progression of incomplete (I) grades to either a passing grade or failing grade. Nursing major GPA and overall GPA will be affected by pass and fail grades; official withdrawals are invisible in GPA calculations. All nursing students will experience some degree of stress; however, not all students may experience satisfaction. Academic and psychological outcomes are a complex, multidimensional component of the nursing student retention process. Outcome factors continually interact with each other and with the other factors in the NURS model.

KEY POINT SUMMARY

- Two dimensions of outcomes directly influence student persistence, retention, and departure: academic and psychological.
- Academic outcomes are represented by the student's nursing course grade, cumulative GPA for nursing courses, and overall GPA.
- Good academic performance results in retention only when accompanied by positive psychological outcomes.

- Positive psychological outcomes include satisfaction and low (manageable) stress; negative psychological outcomes include dissatisfaction and high stress.
- Outcome factors continually interact with each other and with the other factors in the NURS model, influencing persistence.

APPLICATION STRATEGIES

EDUCATOR-IN-ACTION VIGNETTE

As part of the Writing Across the Curriculum initiative, Professor Glass continues with the low-stakes written "reflection" component in the first introductory nursing fundamentals and medical–surgical nursing course. After mid-semester, she asks students to first reflect and then write about "How have your perceptions about nursing changed since the beginning of the semester?" (Or how they have remained the same?). Although students respond diversely, Professor Glass identifies several students with varying levels of satisfaction and stress. She sees this as an important opportunity to intervene and promote positive psychological and academic outcomes. Professor Glass returns the written assignment the next week with constructive comments written for each student. Common themes will be addressed generally in class. Select written excerpts and instructor-written responses and actions follow:

MARILYN: I realize now that nursing is a profession. Nurses have great responsibility for patients' health status. Most of my patients in clinic were so appreciative of the care I provided. I know for sure that nursing is the right career for me.

ANALYSIS: Marilyn has a high level of satisfaction for nursing.

Professor Glass writes, "Yes, nurses have much responsibility and make quite a difference in patients' lives. Keep up your positive attitude, commitment, motivation, and hard work." Intermittently, Professor Glass asks Marilyn about her perceived progress in clinical and continues to encourage her diligent efforts, recognizing that all students can benefit from encouragement and sincere interest.

DERRICK: I didn't think nurses had so many responsibilities and so many patients. In the beginning, I thought that nurses just carried out doctors' orders. I learned that nurses perform physical assessments, plan patient care, make important decisions, and are under a lot of stress. Nursing is not at all what I expected. The nursing program involves more study time and is very stressful.

ANALYSIS: Derrick mentions stress both in the nursing profession and in his student role. There is a mismatch between his previous expectations and current perceptions. Derrick may be at risk for undesirable academic and psychological outcomes (unmanageable stress and dissatisfaction).

Professor Glass writes, "Nursing is more complex than many people initially realize; however it can be quite a rewarding profession. I would like to talk with you about the nursing profession and share some ideas for maximizing study strategies and reducing stress."

Professor Glass meets with Derrick. He is appreciative of strategies for enhancing time management, study skills, and stress management. Derrick reports being "somewhat satisfied" with nursing as a career choice since he sometimes "feels like an outsider." He admits that he had been thinking about dropping out of the nursing program despite his B+ course average. Professor Glass links him with a nursing program alumnus who has volunteered to mentor a student. As the alumnus describes satisfying professional experiences, vast opportunities in nursing, and past struggles, Derrick views nursing in a different light and becomes more satisfied with his career choice.

TOOLKIT RESOURCE BOX

Item 6—Enrichment Program Satisfaction Survey
Item 7—Nursing Student Resource Center Satisfaction Survey
Item 21—Who Are At-Risk Students?
Items 1–4—Student Perception Appraisal Questionnaires—Pretests and Posttests
Item 5—Educational Requirements Subscale

DISCUSSION QUESTIONS

1. A faculty member teaching in a community college says, "My clinical group students are all achieving course averages ranging between 80 and 92. They are also meeting all the objectives in clinical and are completing their care plans satisfactorily. I am so relieved that I don't need to worry about students dropping out this semester." How would you respond to this teacher?

2. A colleague says, "If academic outcomes are good, the student will be satisfied and stress will decrease. Dissatisfied students are just troublemakers who want to complain because they didn't meet the grade. Stressed-out students wouldn't make good nurses anyway because the real-life hospital setting is full of stress." How would you respond?

3. Which part of the chapter provided you with the most new information? How will this affect your future teaching, advisement, and interaction with students?

4. Which three students in the snapshot scenarios would you intervene with first? Why? How would you intervene? What strategies would you use with each situation? Why?

5. Compare and contrast an ER approach versus a PIE approach. What are the advantages and disadvantages of each strategy? (see Snapshot Scenario).

REFERENCES

1. Toutkoushian, R. K., & Smart, J. C. (2001). Do institutional characteristics affect student gains from college? *Review of Higher Education, 25*(1), 39–61.

2. Bean, J. P., & Eaton, S. B. (2000). A psychological model of student retention. In, Braxton, J. (ed.), *Reworking the student departure puzzle* (pp.48–61). Nashville, TN: Vanderbilt University.

3. Bean, J. P., & Eaton, S. B. (2001). The psychology underlying successful retention practices. *Journal of College Student Retention: Research, Theory, & Practice, 3*(1), 73–90.

4. Seidman, A. (2005). *College student retention: Formula for student success.* Westport, CT: American Council on Education, Praeger.

5. Bean, J. P., & Metzner, B. (1985). A conceptual model of nontraditional undergraduate student attrition. *Review of Educational Research, 55*, 485–540.

6. Eaton, S. B., & Bean, J. P. (1995). An approach/avoidance behavioral model of college student attrition. *Research in Higher Education, 36*, 617–645.

7. Jeffreys, M. R. (2007). Tracking students through program entry, progression, graduation, and licensure: Assessing undergraduate nursing student retention and success. *Nurse Education Today, 27*, 406–419.

8. Myton, C. L., Allen, J. K., & Baldwin, J. A. (1992). Students in transition: Services for retention and outplacement. *Nursing Outlook, 35*(1), 227–230.

9. Urwin, S., Stanley, R., Jones, M., Gallagher, A., Wainwright, P., & Perkins, A. (2010). Understanding student nurse attrition: Learning from the literature. *Nurse Education Today, 30*, 202–207.

10. Yoder, M. K., & Saylor, C. (2002). Student and teacher roles: Mismatched expectations. *Nurse Educator, 27*(5), 201–203.

11. O'Donnell, H. (2011). Expectations and voluntary attrition in nursing students. *Nurse Education in Practice, 11*, 54–63.

12. Mohr, J. J., Eiche, K. D., & Sedlacek, W. E. (1998). So close, yet so far: Predictors of attrition in college seniors. *Journal of College Student Development, 39*(4), 343–354.

13. Constantine, M. G., & Watt, S. K. (2002). Cultural congruity, womanist identity attitudes, and life satisfaction among African American college women attending historically black and predominantly white institutions. *Journal of College Student Development, 43*(2), 184–193.

14. Mayo, J. R., Murguia, E., & Padilla, R. V. (1995). Social integration and academic performance among minority university students. *Journal of College Student Development, 36*(6), 542–552.

15. Solis, E. (1995). Regression and path analysis models of Hispanic community college students' intent to persist. *Community College Review, 23*(3), 3–15.

16. Zell, M. C. (2010). Achieving a college education: The psychological experiences of Latina/o community college students. *Journal of Hispanic Higher Education, 9*(2), 167–186.

17. Torres, V., & Hernandez, E. (2010). Influence of an identified advisor/mentor on urban Latino students' college experience. *Journal of College Student Retention: Research, Theory, and Practice, 11* (1), 141–160.

18. Seidman, A. (2007). *Minority student retention: The best of the Journal of College Student Retention: Research, Theory, and Practice.* Amityville, NY: Baywood.

19. Bosher, S. D., & Pharris, M. D. (2009). *Transforming nursing education: The culturally inclusive environment.* New York, NY: Springer Publishing.

20. McLaughlin, K., Muldoon, O. T., & Moutray, M. (2010). Gender, gender roles and completion of nursing education: A longitudinal study. *Nurse Education Today, 30,* 303–307.

21. Stott, A. (2004). Issues in the socialization process of the male student nurse: implications for retention in undergraduate nursing courses. *Nurse Education Today, 24,* 91–97.

22. Ujvarine, A. S., Zrinyi, M., Toth, H., Zekanyne, I. R., Szogedi, I., & Bethlehem, J. (2011). The role of faculty and clinical practice in predicting why nurses graduate in Hungary. *Nurse Education Today, 31,* 94–101.

23. Dorsey, L. E., & Baker, C. M. (2004). Mentoring undergraduate nursing students: Assessing the state of the science. *Nurse Educator, 29*(6), 260–265.

24. Copeland, K. J., & Levesque-Bristol, C. (2011). The retention dilemma: Effectively reaching the first-year university student. *Journal of College Student Retention: Research, Theory, and Practice, 12* (4), 485–515.

25. Reason, R. D. (2009). An examination of persistence research through the lens of a comprehensive conceptual framework. *Journal of College Student Development, 50*(6), 659–682.

26. Harrison, E. (2009). (Re)Visiting academic advising. *Nurse Educator, 34*(2), 64–68.

27. Liegler, R. M. (1997). Predicting student satisfaction in baccalaureate nursing programs: Testing a causal model. *Journal of Nursing Education, 36*(8), 357–364.

28. Martin, A. J., & Dowson, M. (2009). Interpersonal relationships, motivation, engagement, and achievement: Yields for theory, current issues, and educational practice. *Review of Educational Research, 79*(1), 327–365.

29. Jaeger, A. J.,& Hinz, D. (2009). The effects of part-time faculty on first semester freshmen retention: A predictive model using logistic regression. *Journal of College Student Retention: Research, Theory, and Practice, 10* (3), 265–286.

30. Strayhorn, T. L. (2010). Majority as temporary minority: Examining the influence of faculty-student relationships on satisfaction among White undergraduates at Historically Black Colleges and Universities. *Journal of College Student Development, 51*(5), 509–524.

31. Luo, J., & Jamieson-Drake, D. (2009). A retrospective assessment of the educational benefits of interaction across racial boundaries. *Journal of College Student Development, 50*(2), 115–134.

32. Angelino, L. M., Williams, F. K., & Natvig, D. (2007). Strategies to engage online students and reduce attrition rates. *Journal of Educators Online, 4*(2), 1–14.

33. Bambara, C. S., Harbour, C. P., Davies, T. G., & Athey, S. (2009). Delicate engagement: The lived experience of community college students enrolled in high-risk online courses. *Community College Review, 36*(3), 219–238.

34. Baldwin, D., & Wold, J. (1993). Students from disadvantaged backgrounds: Satisfaction with a mentor-protégé relationship. *Journal of Nursing Education, 32,* 225–226.

35. Cameron-Buccheri, R., & Trygstad, L. (1989). Retaining freshman nursing students. *Nursing and Health Care, 10*(7), 389–393.
36. Metzner, B. S. (1989). Perceived quality of academic advising: The effect on freshman attrition. *American Educational Research Journal, 26,* 422–442.
37. Davidson, W. B., Beck, H. P., & Milligan, M. (2009). The college persistence questionnaire: Development and validation of an instrument that predicts student attrition. *Journal of College Student Development, 50*(4), 373–390.
38. Napoli, A. R., & Wortman, P. M. (1998). Psychosocial factors related to retention and early departure of two-year community college students. *Research in Higher Education, 39*(4), 419–455.
39. Greene, B. A., & Miller, R. B. (1996). Influences on achievement: Goals, perceived ability, and cognitive engagement. *Contemporary Educational Psychology, 21,* 181–192.
40. DeWitz, S. J., Woolsey, M. L., & Walsh, W. B. (2009). College student retention: An exploration of the relationship between self-efficacy beliefs and purpose in life among college students. *Journal of College Student Development, 50*(1), 19–34.
41. Friedman, B. A., & Mandel, R. G. (2010). The prediction of college student academic performance and retention: Application of expectancy and goal setting theories. *Journal of College Student Retention: Research, Theory, and Practice, 11* (2), 227–246.
42. Betz, N. E. (2007). Career self-efficacy: Exemplary recent research and emerging directions. *Journal of Career Assessment, 15*(4), 403–422.
43. Jeffreys, M. R. (2001). Evaluating enrichment program study groups: Academic outcomes, psychological outcomes, and variables influencing retention. *Nurse Educator, 26*(3), 142–149.
44. Jeffreys, M. R. (2002). Students' perceptions of variables influencing retention: A pretest and post-test approach. *Nurse Educator, 27*(1), 16–19 [Erratum, 2002, 27(2), 64].
45. Jeffreys, M. R. (2003). Strategies for promoting nontraditional student retention and success. In Oermann, M., & Heinrich, K. (Ed.). *Annual review of nursing education: Volume I,* (pp. 61–90). New York, NY: Springer Publishing.
46. Beltyukova, S. A., & Fox, C. M. (2002). Student satisfaction as a measure of student development: Towards a universal metric. *Journal of College Student Development, 43*(2), 161–172.
47. Lazarus, R. S., & Folkman, S. (1984). *Stress, appraisal, and coping.* New York, NY: Springer Publishing.
48. Solberg, V. S., & Villarreal, P. (1997). Examination of self-efficacy, social support, and stress as predictors of psychological and physical distress among Hispanic college students. *Hispanic Journal of Behavioral Sciences, 19*(2), 182–201.
49. Beck, D. L., Hackett, M. B., Srivastava, R., McKim, E., & Rockwell, B. (1997). Perceived level and sources of stress in university professional schools. *Journal of Nursing Education, 36*(4), 180–186.
50. Courage, M. M., & Godbey, K. L. (1992). Student retention: Policies and services to enhance persistence to graduation. *Nurse Educator, 17*(2), 29–32.
51. Kirkland, M. L. S. (1998). Stressors and coping strategies among successful female African American baccalaureate nursing students. *Journal of Nursing Education, 37*(1), 5–12.

52. Sprengel, A. D., & Job, L. (2004). Reducing student anxiety by using clinical peer mentoring with beginning nursing students. *Nurse Educator, 29*(6), 246–250.
53. Lambert, V. A., & Nugent, K. E. (1994). Addressing the academic progression of students encountering mental health problems. *Nurse Educator, 19*(5), 33–39.
54. Meadows, L. C. (1998). Integrating self-care into nursing education. *Journal of Nursing Education, 37*(5), 225–227.
55. Gibbons, C., Dempster, M., & Moutray, M. (2009). Surveying nursing students on their sources of stress: A validation study. *Nurse Education Today, 29,* 867–872.
56. Leininger, M. M., & McFarland, M. R. (2002). *Transcultural nursing: Concepts, theories, research, and practice* (3rd ed.). New York, NY: McGraw-Hill.
57. Burris, R. F. (2001). Teaching student parents. *Nurse Educator, 26*(2), 64–65, 98.
58. Youssef, F. A., & Goodrich, N. (1996). Accelerated versus traditional nursing students: A comparison of stress, critical thinking ability and performance. *International Journal of Nursing Studies, 33*(1), 76–82.
59. Hegge, M., & Larson, V. (2008). Stressors and coping strategies of students in accelerated baccalaureate nursing programs. *Nurse Educator, 33*(1), 26–30.
60. Stuenkel, D., Nelson, D., Malloy, S., & Cohen, J. (2011). Challenges, changes, and collaboration evaluation of an accelerated BSN program. *Nurse Educator, 36*(2), 70–75.
61. Weitzel, M. L., & McCahon, C. P. (2008). Stressors and supports for baccalaureate nursing students completing an accelerated program. *Journal of Professional Nursing, 24*(2), 85–89.
62. Seldomridge, L. A., & DiBartolo, M. C. (2007). The changing face of accelerated second bachelor's degree students. *Nurse Educator, 32*(6), 240–245.
63. O'Connor, P. C., & Bevil, C. A. (1996). Academic outcomes and stress in full-time day and part-time evening baccalaureate nursing students. *Journal of Nursing Education, 35*(6), 245–251.
64. Mozingo, J., Thomas, S., & Brooks, E. (1995). Factors associated with perceived competency levels of graduating seniors in a baccalaureate nursing program. *Journal of Nursing Education, 34*(3), 115–122.
65. Shipton, S. P. (2002). The process of seeking stress-care: coping as experienced by senior baccalaureate nursing students in response to appraised clinical stress. *Journal of Nursing Education, 41*(6), 243–256.
66. Yonge, O., Myrick, F., & Haase, M. (2002). Student nurse stress in the preceptorship experience. *Nurse Educator, 27*(2), 84–88.
67. Oermann, M., & Lukomski, A. (2001). Experiences of students in pediatric nursing clinical courses. *Journal of the Society of Pediatric Nurses, 6*(2), 65.
68. Patterson, B. J., & Morin, K. H. (2002). Perceptions of the maternal-child clinical rotation: The male student nurse experience. *Journal of Nursing Education, 41*(6), 266–272.
69. Reynolds, A. L., Sneva, J. N., & Beehler, G. P. (2010). The influence of racism-related stress on the academic motivation of Black and Latino/a students. *Journal of College Student Development, 51*(2), 135–149.
70. Fuertes, J. N., & Westbrook, F. D. (1996). Using the social, attitudinal, familial, and environmental (S.A.F.E.) acculturation stress scale to assess the adjustment needs of Hispanic college students. *Measurement and Evaluation in Counseling and Development, 29,* 67–76.

71. Smart, J. F., & Smart, D. W. (1995). Acculturative stress: the experience of the Hispanic immigrant. *The Counseling Psychologist, 23*, 25–42.
72. Suliman, W. A., & Tadros, A. (2011). Nursing students coping with English as a foreign language medium of instruction. *Nurse Education Today, 31*, 402–407.
73. Jeong, S. Y-S., Hickey, N., Levett-Jones, T., Pitt, V., Hoffman, K., Norton, C. A., & Ohr, S. O. (2011). Understanding and enhancing the learning experiences of culturally and linguistically diverse nursing students in an Australian bachelor of nursing program. *Nurse Education Today, 31*, 238–244.
74. Constantine, M. G., Robinson, J. S., Wilton, L., & Caldwell, L. D. (2002). Collective self-esteem and perceived social support as predictors of cultural congruity among black and Latino college students. *Journal of College Student Development, 43*(3), 307–316.
75. Baker, C. R. (2001). Role strain in male diploma nursing students: A descriptive quantitative study. *Journal of Nursing Education, 40*(8), 378–380.
76. Streubert, H. J. (1994). Male nursing students' perceptions of clinical experience. *Nurse Educator, 19*(5), 28–32.
77. Wang, H., Li, X., Hu, X., Chen, H., Gao, Y., Zhao, H., & Huang, L. (2011). Perceptions of nursing profession and learning experiences of male students in baccalaureate nursing program in Changsha, China. *Nurse Education Today, 31*, 36–42.
78. Keogh, B., & O'Lynn, C. (2007). Male nurses' experiences of gender barriers: Irish and American perspectives. *Nurse Educator, 32*(6), 256–259.
79. Anthony, A. S. (2004). Gender bias and discrimination in nursing education: Can we change it? *Nurse Educator, 29*(3), 121–125.
80. Brown, M. L. (1987). The effects of a support group on student attrition due to academic failure. *Journal of Nursing Education, 26*(8), 324–327.
81. Gallagher, P. A., Bomba, C., & Crane, L. R. (2001). Using an admissions exam to predict student success in an ADN program. *Nurse Educator, 26*(3), 132–135.
82. Siktberg, L. L., & Dillard, N. L. (2001). Assisting at-risk students in preparing for NCLEX-RN. *Nurse Educator, 26*(3), 150–152.
83. Waltman, P. A. (1997). Comparison of traditional and non-traditional baccalaureate nursing students on selected components of Meichenbaum and Butler's model of test anxiety. *Journal of Nursing Education, 36*(4), 171–179.
84. Cunningham, H., Stacciarini, J-M. R., & Towle, S. (2004). Strategies to promote success on the NCLEX-RN for students with English as a second language. *Nurse Educator, 29*(1), 15–19.
85. Delgado, C., & Mack, B. (2002). A peer-reviewed program for senior proficiencies. *Nurse Educator, 27*(5), 212–213.

The Outside Climate: Forecast, Impact, and Action

Nurse educators are in a key position to survey the existing outside surrounding climate, to forecast climate conditions favorable or unfavorable to student persistence, to evaluate the impact of select factors on student subgroups, and to determine appropriate actions.

SNAPSHOT SCENARIO

PROFESSOR NUMBERS: Our quantitative data indicate that 17% of our students withdrew from a nursing course this semester and that 8% of our students did not register for next semester despite their academic eligibility to do so. Obviously, the money allocated for the new nursing student retention and success program is being wasted. The program isn't working. We're still losing students.

PROFESSOR PONDER: I wonder why these students withdrew or did not register. Does it really mean our new retention program isn't working? Isn't there some more information we need?

PROFESSOR LIGHT: When I attended a conference last month, two researchers presented survey results as to why students did not persist from one semester to the next. The reasons were enlightening, and we recognized that there are outside surrounding factors (OSF) over which students and faculty have no control that can influence persistence and retention. Let me share their handout listing sample-student responses on the qualitative comment section.

A: Two years ago, I was thrilled to pursue my dream to become a nurse when I received a scholarship earmarked for former military personnel. I completed two semesters successfully, and last April, I received notice that I would be put on active military duty. Recent worldwide events make this necessary. I'm disappointed to discontinue my nursing education now but I intend to continue when I return from overseas.

B: Over the spring break, I traveled to help out as a volunteer for Habitat for Humanity. When I got there, an unexpected severe tornado tore through a nearby community, leaving many homeless and without food, water, and other basic supplies. It was impossible to travel back. Transportation was halted for over 1 week. I stayed an additional 2 weeks and helped out. I missed too much nursing coursework and clinical, so I needed to withdraw. The college agreed to refund my tuition after the semester is over. Once I receive the money back, I plan to register for next semester.

C: When I heard on the news about the civil unrest and violence in my native country, I was devastated and scared. I tried communicating with my family, but I could only reach my youngest sister. My parents, two younger brothers, and several cousins, aunts, and uncles were missing. I needed to leave school temporarily. Fortunately, I was able to locate my family in a shelter across the border of a neighboring country. Unfortunately, immigration problems, transportation difficulties, and a flare-up with malaria prevented me from returning for 5 months.

PROFESSOR PONDER: I guess that we should get more details about why students stop out or drop out. The first student mentioned that a scholarship helped get the journey started. I wonder if there are some OSF that encourage persistence?

PROFESSOR LIGHT: At this same conference, another group of researchers presented their study on why students choose nursing and why students stay. Here is one of their students' comments.

D: My chiropractor was telling me about the latest Institute of Medicine (IOM) report indicating that the role of registered nurses and advanced practice nurses like nurse practitioners would be much expanded in the future. I was intrigued by the proposed reimbursement changes and high value placed on nurses for making a difference in improving our nation's health. Nurse practitioners will be prepared at the doctoral level. I like that advanced practice nurses will have the title "doctor," just like other autonomous health professionals who have recently changed their educational requirements, such as physical therapists and audiologists. I decided that I would like to become a pediatric nurse practitioner. I shared this goal with my physician and chiropractor. Now, whenever I see them, they ask me about my progress, offer encouragement, and tell me how favorable the health care environment is for nurses. I also keep up with postings on the ANA [American Nurses Association] website and read the local nursing magazine. There are many jobs available and so many options. I also like that new TV show about a nurse. She is intelligent, professional, respected by physicians, and an assertive advocate for patients. All these things keep me motivated.

PROFESSOR PONDER: I wonder what other types of OSF influence student persistence and retention? I wonder if there is anything faculty can do to help students?

Despite students' positive academic and psychological outcomes, and despite other background, affective, academic, environmental, and professional integration factors favorable for student success, students may still drop out or stop out. Models proposed to explain attrition in higher education have generally focused on variables (or interventions) within the specific domain of the academic institution. Frequently, models incorporated student background characteristics and/or students' personal environmental factors in an attempt to identify at-risk students prospectively or to explain failed retention efforts retrospectively. It has been important to examine these factors in student persistence research, theory, and practice; however, a different explanation for attrition and variation in persistence behaviors must also be considered. OSF exist that can exert great influence on student persistence. The NURS model seeks to acknowledge the importance of these factors with specific application for nursing student retention.

OSF exist outside of the academic setting and the individual student's personal environment that can influence retention. They include world, national, and local events; politics and economics; the health care system; nursing professional issues; and job certainty. Together, OSF interact to create an outside climate that has the power to influence student persistence, retention, and success. These factors may affect students at any point in the model and may be unpredictable. They may affect student retention positively or negatively. In the NURS model, a cloud illustration is used to signify the possible uncertainties that continually exist and surround nursing student persistence, retention, and success (see Figure 1.2). The peeking sun represents a favorable climate conducive for retention; the lightning represents adverse climate conditions. Students' motivation to overcome hardships and obstacles and persist in the program may be heightened when OSF are more favorable or appealing. In contrast, it may be lessened when OSF are perceived to be overwhelming obstacles to success.

OSF have the power to affect all undergraduate nursing students, but in potentially different ways. Some OSF may result in a wide range of voluntary student choices whereas other OSF may lead to a predetermined involuntary result. Nurse educators are in a key position to survey the existing outside surrounding climate to forecast climate conditions favorable or unfavorable to student persistence, to evaluate the impact of select factors on student subgroups, and to determine appropriate actions. The purpose of this chapter is to enhance awareness of OSF on student retention, highlight the potential significance of select factors, stimulate further inquiry, and suggest implications for nurse educators.

WORLD, NATIONAL, AND LOCAL EVENTS

World, national, and local events usually happen unpredictably and can have a positive or negative effect on nursing student persistence, retention, and success. Local events occur near the student's nursing program residence, such as neighborhood, town, city, county, state, province, or region. Local events may become national and world events if they are either publicized nationally and globally or if they have an effect on a nation or the world. Such effects may include changes in policy, resource allocation, government, priorities, and philosophy. National events occur within the student's country of residence/attendance while in the nursing program, and world events are those occurrences outside of the student's country of residence/attendance while in the nursing program.

Some events, such as natural disasters, are beyond human control yet can have tremendous impact on nursing student retention. For example, a local flood, tornado, hurricane, earthquake, or other natural disaster may result in financial loss, homelessness, stress, and other losses, requiring nursing students to withdraw from school. Other local accidental disasters such as fires, explosions, train derailments, plane crashes, building collapses, or partial bridge collapses can also result in losses or obstacles that necessitate student withdrawal. Nonaccidental tragic events resulting from terrorist or other criminal acts may have local, national, and worldwide impact both directly and indirectly. Reallocation of local and national funds to assist in the aftermath of disasters and tragedies may necessitate smaller budget allocation for public higher education, scholarships, student stipends, or financial aid, thus potentially creating adverse effects on future student persistence and retention.

Wars, threats of war, or impending war can result in drafting or activation of soldiers in reserve units. A student in the military or military reserve may be required to stopout if called into active duty during time of national crisis. Recent immigrants, refugees, or asylees may be personally affected by wars or civil unrest in their former residence or place of origin. For example, a nursing student whose family is missing after a war incident in another country may need to return and search for lost family members. Similarly, students may withdraw from school following a natural disaster, accidental disaster, or other world event that directly or indirectly affects them emotionally.

Positive local events can exert great positive influence on nursing student retention, and may have direct and immediate effects on student retention or indirect and delayed effects. Additionally, the effects may be instrumental (concrete) or motivational (abstract). A substantial donation to the nursing school for resources and scholarships, new grant funding for nursing student stipends, or tuition-work exchange program at the local hospital present favorable conditions that can cause direct, immediate, and positive effects on student retention. Both instrumental and motivational support would result through the enhancement of the surrounding climate favorable for optimizing student success. The addition of a new hospital wing, a local hospital reaching "Magnet" status, or worldwide recognition of a local hospital's expertise are examples of events leading to possible direct and indirect positive effects. Motivation to persist would be enhanced with the indirect, long-term focus on locally enhanced opportunities for highly satisfying, rewarding careers in nursing.

Local, national, and world events that involve nurses are yet another indication of how nursing student persistence can be influenced. News media publicity showcasing the heroic acts of nurses rendering assistance during times of crisis is one example. Reporting the positive difference a nurse made in the life of a local "everyday" person, a national celebrity, or world-respected leader may altruistically motivate current nursing students to persist. On the other hand, nurses may also gain local, national, or worldwide attention when guilty of malpractice, drug abuse, insurance fraud, abandonment, or murder. A publicized local event involving a patient death and an impaired nurse does much damage to nursing image. A nurse shot to death in an emergency room or other acts of violence against nurses at the workplace is disturbing and frightening, thus potentially influencing nursing student retention through decreased motivation, ambivalence over career selection, and fear.

Threat of a nursing strike or an actual nursing strike at a local hospital shows discontent over professional issues ranging from unsafe working conditions, patient overcrowding, unsafe staffing, poor salary and benefits, lack of nursing governance, dissatisfaction, and/or lack of professional respect. A favorable outcome settlement for nurses may represent hope and professional unity to undergraduate nursing students, thus favorably influencing persistence. On the other hand, some students may become discouraged by the dissatisfaction experienced by many working nurses. The manner in which news media coverage portrays the event and the outcome can greatly skew the event in the eyes of nursing students and the public.

Consequently, nurse educators are challenged to keep actively informed of current events, forecast the potential impact of events on nursing student retention (professional nursing and the public), and demonstrate visionary leadership actions in context with the event(s). Proactive action rather than retrospective reaction is the recommended approach for obtaining the best results. Openly discussing the event, encouraging students to reflect on it, presenting alternative perspectives, and offering constructive suggestions for effectively dealing with an event empowers students to take appropriate actions that facilitate persistence behaviors.

What recent world, national, and local events occurred that did or could influence nursing student persistence? How have you addressed these events in your nursing course? In your nursing program?

POLITICS AND ECONOMICS

Politics refers to the process of influence used for decision making and allocation of resources (1). Economics refers to the financial investment in specific resources used for particular purposes. Both politics and economics critically impact upon nursing student retention. In the NURS model, politics and economics are labeled as one OSF to recognize the virtually inseparable relationship between them, as specifically pertinent to nursing student retention. Politics and economics foster the development of policies that can directly or indirectly influence nursing student persistence and retention.

Most definitely, national policies that support the growing need for nurses are an impetus for nursing student recruitment and retention. The Nurse Reinvestment Act (2) is one example of a legislative measure in the United States aimed at resolving the severe nursing shortage crisis. The Nurse Education, Practice, and Retention Grants and the Loan Repayment and Scholarship Program will provide both financial and motivational incentives for nursing student persistence. The Nurse Faculty Loan Program aims to increase the number of prepared nursing faculty, thus providing an indirect and more distant effect on student retention. However, in the future the program could have potentially more impact on nursing student persistence, retention, and success by having more full-time and well-prepared nursing faculty. Although such measures are a step in the right direction, the American Nurses Association (ANA) notes that the promise of meeting the health care needs amidst the growing nursing shortage will not be met without a substantial funding increase for the Health Resources and Services Administration's (HRSA) Nursing Workforce Development programs (3).

Current financial aid policies and scholarship incentives for disadvantaged students usually stipulate full-time enrollment and demonstrated financial need. Frequently, older students with family and employment responsibilities are unable to pursue educational endeavors full-time and have substantial financial strain. Similarly, middle-class full-time students also report severe financial strain, which discourages persistence (4–6). Across all income and ethnic groups, the net price (out of pocket or loan) expense of attending a post-secondary institution was higher in 2007–2008 than in 1999–2000 with increasing amounts of loan debt accumulation (7). Loan attainment can positively or negatively influence retention. Among Black students, loan attainment positively influenced degree attainment; however, loan attainment negatively influenced degree attainment among Asian, Latino, and White students (8). In addition, the modest increase in federal direct student aid aimed to assist community college persistence and degree attainment could not meet the demands of a 40% tuition increase and over 2 million new student enrollees (9). In other words, it became financially more challenging for students to attain college degrees nationwide. The nursing literature worldwide also reported financial strain and economic changes adversely influencing student retention (10–12).

Publicly supported career ladder programs offer an incentive to those employed in health care agencies; however, second-career students employed elsewhere are excluded. The current nursing applicant pool reflects a great number of nontraditional, second-career students who may not be able to meet the criteria for full-time student status and/or financial need requirements, yet still experience financial strain. The perception that one is excluded from incentive measures could be construed as an obstacle for student persistence. Therefore, new policies that accommodate the part-time, nontraditional college student are urgently needed to promote persistence. Current financial aid policies, loans, and other financial incentives must be transformed to enhance college access and success (13).

Visionary nurse educators must remain updated about politics, policy, and economics; forecast the potential impact of proposed policies on nursing student retention; evaluate the actual and potential impact on student subgroups; and demonstrate commitment to active political involvement. Commitment may range from philosophical support of a nursing organization's position on current and/or proposed policies to more personal political action initiatives, such as running for political office. The danger of inaction is the assumption that the status quo is acceptable. Silence and inactivity often assumes support, whereas, action demands sincere thought, commitment, effort, ingenuity, energy, enthusiasm, and deliberate activity.

How have/could current changes in politics and economics influence nursing student persistence? How have you addressed these changes in your nursing course? In your nursing program? What else can/should be done?

HEALTH CARE SYSTEM

The health care system is the combination of resources, financing, organization, and management that results in the delivery of health services (14,15). The health care system presents favorable and unfavorable conditions within the current and future outside surrounding climate. The existence (or nonexistence) of national health insurance, socialized medicine, private health insurance, no health insurance, and/or government-subsidized health benefits for all (or select) citizens and residents offers different types of environments for current nursing student education and later nursing student employment. Additionally, the emphasis (or lack of emphasis) of the health care system on primary preventive care (health promotion and illness prevention) helps shape the present and future of nursing practice and societal health. A health care system that is truly consistent with the World Health Organization's (WHO) position that health is not merely the absence of disease but the state of physical, mental, and social well-being and that health care is a human right, not a privilege (16) must emphasize primary health care. Such a health care system demands qualified nurses in sufficient numbers and must provide incentives for current and future nurses. The recent IOM "Future of Nursing" report highlights the important role nurses have in future health of the nation and the elimination of health disparities (17).

Whether the health care system embraces the full scope of professional nursing practice or restricts it is an important consideration. For example, a health care system that favors replacing registered nurse positions with unlicensed assistive personnel de-values or minimizes the scope of nursing practice. Such an action would be detrimental to societal health overall, let alone the severe long-term effects on cost and quality of health care. Similarly, a health care system that favors downsizing by eliminating positions held by experienced nurses and/or advanced practice nurses is counterproductive to patient and employee satisfaction, and adversely impacts on nursing student retention through decreased motivation and morale.

In contrast, a health care system that embraces professional nursing practice seeks to provide quality patient care by maximizing the quality of nursing practice, thereby enhancing positive client outcomes, patient satisfaction, and nurse–employee satisfaction (18). For example, a health care system promoting nurses as CEOs or facilitating the development of Magnet hospitals presents a favorable outside climate that can motivate nursing student persistence. A health care system that directly reimburses nurses acknowledges that nurses have provided unique, valuable services to society; nursing services that are not reimbursed or itemized on a bill makes professional nursing invisible. Direct reimbursement to advanced practice nurses through Medicare is a beginning step for the recognition of nursing services (19). Reimbursement pay equity for nurse practitioners, mentioned in the IOM report, takes recognition to the next level. Controversy over proposed health care reform from the public, politicians, and multidisciplinary health care providers corresponds with change that challenges the status quo. Such controversy in changing times creates an uncertain environment. Uncertainty and controversy can be frightening, but when viewed optimistically, it offers renewed hope for expanded opportunities, recognition, and tangible rewards.

Nurse educators must not only be astutely aware of the political and economic dynamics that shape the health care system but recognize how the current and projected health care system will potentially impact on nursing students, nursing practice, and societal health care needs of the future. The changing health care system can influence the popularity or desirability of becoming a nurse, and hence influence persistence and retention. Addressing nursing students' concerns, questions, dissatisfaction, confusion, and/or ambivalence regarding the health care system proactively opens discussion and acknowledges the favorable and unfavorable conditions within the health care system environment. Candid dialogue directed towards stimulating creative nursing student involvement in the development, implementation, and evaluation of strategies to improve the health care system acknowledges the imperfections of any health care system yet offers the option for change through active and committed involvement.

> How can/will proposed and recent changes in the health care system influence nursing student persistence? How have you addressed these events in your nursing course? In your nursing program? What else can/should be done?

NURSING PROFESSIONAL ISSUES

Nursing professional issues are numerous and can be any topic or matter that is directly relevant to the nursing profession. They include entry into practice, credentialing, nursing image, nursing shortage, professional self-image, public nursing image, burnout, reality shock, salaries, workplace conditions, malpractice, educational mobility, career advancement, satisfaction, and organizations. Several of these topics will be highlighted and relationships to actual and/or potential impact on nursing student retention in the United States will be proposed.

Continued controversy over entry into practice is often confusing to students, nurses, and the public (20,21). Academically well-prepared college-bound high school students may be discouraged from nursing as a career because it appears that it is unnecessary for nurses to pursue a full, four-year college education. The availability of various nearby nursing educational programs may influence student selection or consideration of nursing as a career option. For example, an academically well-prepared high school student may never consider nursing as a career option if the only nearby program is offered in a community college. Nursing student retention is affected through a less academically prepared and a more academically diverse nursing student applicant pool.

Positive images of nurses on local, national, or worldwide levels can be motivating to potential and currently enrolled nursing students, especially if the nurses portrayed are similar to students in age, cultural identity, and/or gender. Some examples include movie releases or TV shows featuring nurses in a positive way. Nursing recruitment advertisements and commercials targeting diverse student populations and portraying vast career opportunities broaden the applicant pool but also motivate currently enrolled nursing students.

Nursing students are greatly influenced by nursing professional self-image. Nurse educators, nurses in affiliating agencies, and preceptors all have the potential to make a positive or negative impact on nursing student retention. Statements to students by nurses on the clinical unit, such as, "I'm just a nurse, so I don't know...," "Don't become a nurse...," or "You're too smart to be a nurse...," all have potentially adverse effects on nursing student retention and the nursing profession. Diplomatically confronting nurses with poor professional self-image may be an unpopular nurse educator task; however, it is important. Seeking continual opportunities for student exposure to outstanding nurse role models of different gender, age, and cultural backgrounds is an equally important nurse educator responsibility.

The nursing shortage has been well publicized and can have various impacts on nursing student retention (18). Patient safety issues, mandatory overtime, lack of whistleblower legislation, nurse dissatisfaction, low nurse morale, unsafe work environments, lack of respect, complexity of health care needs, high patient acuity levels, the aging patient population, the aging practicing nurse population, low nurse retention rate, high dropout of new nurses from nursing, and poor salary and job benefits all contribute to the nursing shortage. Certainly, many of these issues present an unfavorable outside climate unless students are mainly motivated by altruistic reasons (to help humanity) or if unfavorable conditions are outweighed by the high probability of employment following graduation and licensure.

Nurse educators must recognize the challenges facing the nursing profession today and be able to forecast the impact of these challenges on future nursing practice and nursing student retention. Ongoing dialogue, coursework on professional issues, and strategies to promote positive professional integration provide students with opportunities to explore the nursing profession from various perspectives. Such guided opportunities should encourage student active involvement in strategy design, implementation, and evaluation aimed at advancement of the nursing profession. Active involvement in the nursing profession throughout the nursing educational experience is strongly recommended (22).

> How did/could recent events and publicity about nurses and nursing influence nursing student persistence? How have they been addressed in your nursing course? In your nursing program? What else can/should be done?

JOB CERTAINTY

Job certainty has been included as a variable within other conceptual models of college student attrition (23). Proponents of adult learning theory attest to the marked influence of educational endeavors, motivation, and commitment in relation to immediate career goals (24,25). Historically, nursing enrollment has fluctuated according to nursing shortages, supply, and demand. Recent welfare-to-work initiatives, displaced homemakers, high divorce rates, increasing single-parent families, prevalence of mid-life career changes, large employee layoffs, and a fluctuating world economy contribute to a greater emphasis on job certainty. Loan repayment initiatives, financed career ladder programs, and full tuition for post-graduation work agreements offer incentives that promote post-graduation job certainty. The NURS model acknowledges the powerful influence that job certainty has on nursing student retention due to both practical effects and motivational effects. It is proposed that a high degree of job certainty correlates with higher student motivation and effort expenditure to overcome obstacles; therefore, nursing student persistence, retention, and success will be enhanced. Many students will be driven by practical reasons such as economic advancement, financial independence, employee health benefits, or even escape from unwanted domestic/family relationships. During periods of nursing shortages, especially when there is an economic recession and job cuts in the corporate world, there may be an increased motivation to persist and complete the nursing program swiftly.

While nursing students today and in the near future may be certain that nursing jobs exist (3,17), students may be overwhelmed by the diversity of job opportunities and choices. Recognizing that graduating nursing students who become licensed then become part of the OSF, nurse educators must focus efforts on a smooth transition into the nursing workforce. Collaborative partnerships with employers of nurses can assist in this process (18). Preparing students at the onset in their first nursing course and subsequently reinforcing and expanding on professional nursing job issues in other courses will help.

> What types of nursing jobs are being obtained by your recent nursing graduates? How does/could this influence the persistence behaviors of currently enrolled students? How have these issues been addressed in your nursing course? In your nursing program? What else can/should be done?

KEY POINT SUMMARY

- OSF exist outside the academic setting and the individual student's personal environment.
- OSF include "world, national, and local events;" "politics and economics;" "the health care system;" "nursing professional issues;" and "job certainty."

- Together, OSF interact to create an outside climate that has the power to positively or negatively influence student persistence, retention, and success.

APPLICATION STRATEGIES

EASY APPLICATION ACTION STEPS

Determining Incidence of Negative OSF on Student Attrition

1. List relevant components within each category of OSF (see chapter headings) that could have a negative impact on persistence and retention.
2. Using the list, survey nonpersisters (students who withdrew or did not register for subsequent semester) about the influence of OSF on their stopout or dropout.
3. Aggregate data, noting themes that emerge from qualitative comment section.

Determining Incidence of Positive OSF on Student Persistence and Retention

1. List relevant components within each category of OSF (see chapter headings) that could have a positive impact on persistence and retention.
2. Using the list, survey persisters (students who completed the semester and/or registered for subsequent semester) about the influence of OSF on their decision to persist.
3. Aggregate data, noting themes that emerge from qualitative comment section.

EDUCATOR-IN-ACTION VIGNETTE

During a postclinical conference, Professor Change notices that two students (Veronica and Jamie) who usually are quite talkative, energetic, enthusiastic, and conscientious seem distracted and do not participate in the group discussion. She asks them if they have anything to add to the group discussion topic or if they would like to discuss another topic. At first, neither student answers. Then Veronica says, "When Jamie and I gave our report about our patients to the nurse, we felt rather discouraged." When Professor Change asks for further elaboration, Jamie says, "I asked the nurse whether the patient had any difficulty or questions about her new medications yesterday. The nurse said to me, 'I'm just a nurse here for 8 hours, so I don't know about medications given yesterday. My advice is that don't become a nurse. Get out while you can. This is

the most horrible job. You must be smart enough to do something else.'"
Veronica adds, "The same nurse said something similar to me. When I
said I liked nursing, she said I would quickly change my mind when I got
my first job. I now wonder if I'm really wasting my time, money, energy,
and college degree on nursing?" Several other students report positive
experiences and interactions with other nurses and yet several students
confirm having had similar negative experiences in the past.

Professor Change clarifies the issues of concern, writes them on the
dry-erase board, and invites further discussion from the whole group.
The group's main issues center on quality patient care, nursing self-image,
satisfaction, motivation, and opportunities in professional nursing. Professor Change assists students in identifying ways to prioritize issues
and develop strategies accordingly. The students collaborate and plan
strategies to promote and publicize positive nursing image and opportunities in professional nursing—especially to motivate students. Additionally, they discuss and plan strategies for predicting, preventing, and
dealing effectively with negative nursing image. Several student com-
ments/ideas and educator actions are presented below:

HILDA: We should tell the nurse how her comments make us feel. With such
a nursing shortage, shouldn't nurses be happy that there are nursing students interested in providing quality patient care? Why isn't she happy?

ACTION: Professor Change institutes a role play in which students take turns
expressing their feelings after a nurse makes inappropriate remarks. Her
constructive comments assist students in developing assertive, professional communication techniques. Professor Change offers to meet with
the nurse privately to explore issues related to her negative behavior and
to offer strategies for promoting a satisfying and rewarding professional
nursing practice.

JAMIE: Maybe it would be a good idea to post positive stories about professional nursing practice on the Nursing Student Club (NSC) bulletin board
and webpage. We could feature a new story every month.

ACTION: Professor Change assists NSC officers to select stories from professional nursing publications. Stories are posted on the bulletin board and
are accessible via a website link on the NSC webpage. At the monthly NSC
meeting, students are invited to discuss the motivational stories.

VERONICA: I guess I focused on the negative today and felt discouraged.
There isn't time to hear positive stories from the nurses while we are on
the unit. Other nurses before were encouraging and nice to me but right
now I need more positive stories and feelings to keep going.

ACTION: Professor Change invites several local nursing alumni to share
motivational stories and participate in a roundtable luncheon discussion
with students.

TOOLKIT RESOURCE BOX

Items 1–4—Student Perception Appraisal Questionnaires—Pretests and Posttests

---

DISCUSSION QUESTIONS

1. Which category of OSF has the greatest adverse influence on student persistence and retention? Why?
2. Which category of OSF has the greatest positive influence on student persistence and retention? Why?
3. What are the OSF that most influenced student persistence and retention at your school in the last 3 years? What strategies were implemented in response to these OSF?
4. How can the Educator-in-Action Vignette be adapted for use with students? With new full-time and part-time (adjunct) faculty?
5. When you read the snapshot scenarios at the beginning of the chapter, what visual images popped into your head? What race, gender, age, weight, religion, and other physical, mental, and professional attributes did you visualize/imagine for each student and faculty member? Why? What thoughts and feelings did you experience as you read each snapshot scenario? How will these images, thoughts, and feelings influence your future role with diverse student populations?

REFERENCES

1. Mason, D. J., & Leavitt, J. K. (1998). *Policy and politics in nursing and health care.* (3rd ed.). New York, NY: Saunders.
2. United States House of Representatives. (2002). *H.R. 3487 – Nurse Reinvestment Act.* Retrieved from http://thomas.loc.gov
3. American Nurses Association. (2011). *Funding for nursing workforce development.* Retrieved from http://www.nursingworld.org
4. Crawford, L. A., & Olinger, B. H. (1988). Recruitment and retention of nursing students from diverse cultural backgrounds. *Journal of Nursing Education, 27*(8), 379–381.
5. Nora, A., Cabrera, A., Hagedorn, L. S., & Pascarella, E. (1996). Differential impacts of academic and social experiences on college-related behavioral outcomes across different ethnic and gender groups at four-year institutions. *Research in Higher Education, 37*(4), 427–451.
6. Padilla, R. V., Trevino, J., Gonzalez, K., & Trevino, J. (1997). Developing local models of minority student success in college. *Journal of College Student Development, 38*(2), 125–135.
7. U. S. Department of Education, National Center for Education Statistics. (2011). *The condition of education, 2011,* Washington, DC: Author.

8. Museus, S. D. (2010). Understanding racial differences in the effects of loans on degree attainment: A path analysis. *Journal of College Student Retention: Research, Theory, and Practice, 11* (4), 499–527.

9. Kennamer, M. A., Katsinas, S. G., & Schumacker, R. E. (2011). The moving target: Student financial aid and community college retention. *Journal of College Student Retention: Research, Theory, and Practice, 12* (1), 87–103.

10. Steele, R., Lauder, W., & Caperchione, C. (2005). An exploratory study of the concerns of mature access to nursing students and the coping strategies used to manage these adverse experiences. *Nurse Education Today, 25,* 573–581.

11. Urwin, S., Stanley, R., Jones, M., Gallagher, A., Wainwright, P., & Perkins, A. (2010). Understanding student nurse attrition: Learning from the literature. *Nurse Education Today, 30,* 202–207.

12. Glogowska, M., Young, P., & Lockyer, L. (2007). Should I go or should I stay? A study of factors influencing students' decisions on early leaving. *Active Learning in Higher Education, 8*(1), 63–77.

13. College Board. (2008). *Fulfilling the commitment: Recommendations for reforming federal student aid.* (Report from the Rethinking Student Aid Study Group). Retrieved from http://www.collegeboard.com

14. Barton, P. L. (1999). *Understanding the U. S. health services system.* Chicago, IL: Health Administration Press.

15. Roemer, M. I. (1991). *National health systems of the world, Vol. I.* New York, NY: Oxford University Press.

16. World Health Organization. (1947). *Constitution.* Geneva: WHO.

17. Institute of Medicine. (2010). *The future of nursing: Leading change, advancing health.* Washington, DC: Author.

18. Kimball, B., & O'Neil, E. (2002). *Health care's human crisis: The American nursing shortage.* Princeton, NJ: Robert Wood Johnson.

19. Wong, S. T. (1999). Reimbursement to advanced practice nurses (APNs) through Medicare. *Image: Journal of Nursing Scholarship, 31*(2), 167–172.

20. Joel, L. A., & Kelly, L. Y. (2002). *The nursing experience: Trends, challenges, and transitions.* New York, NY: McGraw-Hill.

21. Neal, L. J. (2003). Elder RNs perspectives on nursing education: Lessons learned. *Nurse Educator, 28*(1), 18–22.

22. Fitzpatrick, J. J. (2000). 2000: The millennium of the student. *Nursing and Health Care Perspectives, 21*(1), 3.

23. Bean, J. P., & Metzner, B. (1985). A conceptual model of nontraditional undergraduate student attrition. *Review of Educational Research, 55,* 485–540.

24. Brookfield, S. D. (1986). *Understanding and facilitating adult learning.* San Francisco, CA: Jossey-Bass.

25. Knowles, M. (1984). *The adult learner: A neglected species.* Houston, TX: Gulf.

Drop Out, Stop Out, or Go On?

*The decision to remain in a course, persist in the nursing program,
graduate, take the RN licensing exam, and enter the nursing workforce and/
or begin a more advanced nursing program occurs during and at the
conclusion of each nursing course.*

SNAPSHOT SCENARIO

Consider the following students' thoughts and feelings, their possible impact on student retention and success, and implications for nurse educators:

PATTI PERPLEXED: I didn't know that I could withdraw from a course without penalty if I withdrew by a certain date. No one ever told me. In high school, I just had to stay in a course and struggle to either fail or pass. Why didn't I know this before I failed this nursing course?

WILLIE WEASLEY: I thought that I could just keep withdrawing until I was passing the course by mid-semester. I withdrew from the pediatric course for the third time because I had a 67 average by the nonpenalty withdrawal date. Now I got a letter from the dean saying that I am dismissed from the program unless I follow a special procedure to ask the departmental committee to give me another chance. Why didn't I know about this? I would have quit my second job during the second time and passed without difficulty. I'll have to weasel my way through this one but it won't be easy.

HELEN HESITANT: My teacher announced in class that the nonpenalty withdrawal date was next week and that if anyone was having difficulty, an option could be to withdraw and take the course next semester. I hesitate to talk with the professor about it because I have so many personal problems going on right now. I don't want the faculty to think poorly of me.

OTIS OPTIMISTIC: I don't really know where I stand in this course or what will happen next, but I'm optimistic that everything will turn out okay. I'll just take my chances and see what happens.

PETER PESSIMISTIC: Nothing ever works out for me. Everything is so complicated and confusing. I used to get good grades in biology, but I only got a 79 on this first test. I won't bother reading the progression policies because I'm probably not going to make it anyway.

TRUDY TREMBLE: I'm so scared to tell my parents that I want to drop out. They sacrificed so much so I could go to college. I am scared to take care of patients. I don't even like the scenarios and tasks in the simulation lab.

DORA DREAMER: I was watching that movie *Grease* and then fell asleep at the part where the girl dropped out of beauty school and that famous male singer was leading the chorus singing "beauty school dropout." I dreamed that I dropped out of nursing school and Florence Nightingale was leading a chorus of my friends and family singing "nursing school dropout." I must be strange that dropping out crept into my thoughts and dreams. What's wrong with me?

FRANNY FRET: I am so worried about starting this new nursing course. I just got divorced and I don't know if I'm going to adjust well, or need extra time to help my three children adjust or if I will actually get the child support I so desperately need to pay the bills. I'm worried that if I stop nursing school now, I will never go back and will just end up going back to my abusive relationship or end up on public assistance.

FRIEDA FULLER: I thought I needed to fill up my schedule with 21 credits because full-time tuition costs the same whether you take 12 credits or more. So I took critical care, nursing research, physics, advanced biostatistics, French literature, microbiology, and sculpture to get my money's worth and experiment. I figured I would just divide up my time and try everything a little bit and then drop three courses by mid-semester. Now I am just barely passing anything, so I don't know which three to drop. Sculpture takes a lot of time but it's the only one I'm passing. What should I do?

WANDA WONDER: I wonder if it is normal to have doubts about whether I can make it in nursing? I wonder if I am doing well enough in this course? I wonder if I need to get an A grade to be a safe nurse?

Attrition may be voluntary or involuntary; however, retention is strictly voluntary. The decision to remain in a course, persist in the nursing program, graduate, take the RN licensing exam, and enter the nursing workforce and/or begin a more advanced nursing program occurs during and at the conclusion of each nursing course. Engaging in activities associated with course progress, remaining in a course past the college withdrawal date, and registering for a subsequent course all involve a decision to persist. Student profile characteristics, student affective factors, academic factors, environmental factors, professional integration factors, academic outcomes, psychological outcomes, and outside surrounding factors interact and influence retention decisions (see Figure 1.2).

Retention decisions are the determined resolution to persist in the nursing curriculum and educational pathway toward becoming a registered nurse. Ideally, they should be made after careful consideration, purposeful deliberation, and thoughtful weighing of benefits and costs. To ensure retention, the values or benefits of pursuing nursing education, graduation, licensing, and entry into professional nursing practice and/or advanced nursing program must outweigh the costs of nursing program attendance. Careful consideration of factors supporting success and of factors restricting success must be realistically appraised. Unfortunately, student expectations and perceptions may be unrealistic, thus increasing the risk for limited option appraisal, myopic views, and misguided decisions. Additionally, students are frequently indecisive and ambivalent, vacillating between persistence, stopout, or dropout.

Nurse educators are in a strategic position to make a difference by facilitating the process of systematic decision making and enhancing opportunities for retention and success. Awareness of the intricate complexities of retention decisions is a necessary precursor for taking effective action. This chapter will briefly introduce select background information and main concepts surrounding retention decisions. Implications for nurse educators will be proposed.

> **What do you think is the role of the nurse educator in assisting students in the decision-making process to persist, stopout, or dropout? Why?**

BACKGROUND

Attempts to understand decisions concerning persistence and voluntary attrition has mainly centered on students' perceived reasons for withdrawal via post-hoc studies. Data from autopsy attrition studies, however, should be viewed cautiously for several reasons. First, students are called upon to account for their attrition but may be unaware of the underlying reasons that may have contributed to their decision. Second, students may feel the need to cope with their dropout decision by rationalizing it and providing the most socially acceptable response. Moreover, they may be reluctant to criticize the institution (1). With time, students' perceptions concerning withdrawal decisions may become clouded and assume less importance, therefore adversely affecting validity.

Several valuable benefits concerning autopsy attrition data should be noted nonetheless. First, it is important to differentiate between voluntary and involuntary attrition, especially when evaluating the impact of specific retention strategies on attrition rates. Students who withdraw for nonacademic reasons can be considered separately in data analysis when evaluating postintervention attrition rates. For example, a student who withdraws due to an unplanned pregnancy does not provide valid data concerning the effectiveness of an educational support intervention to prevent attrition. The decision to withdraw was not influenced by the nursing program, educational support intervention, or academic institution. Including this student in the evaluation of the intervention would incorrectly lower the intervention's success rate.

Second, data can provide additional and valuable insight into the overall student's learning experience. For example, students who withdrew from a nursing course were surveyed to gain insight into why students withdrew. The questionnaire (Toolkit Item 8) was mailed after the end of the semester and asked students to respond anonymously. Consistent with other autopsy attrition studies and mailed questionnaires, the response rate was poor. Data was not robust enough to conduct statistical analyses; however, respondents did provide interesting information. Most cited several academic and nonacademic underlying factors (see Toolkit Item 8) that influenced withdrawal decisions, with the most influential factor usually nonacademic.

The comment section added richness to the data. Several students indicated that after settling other interfering life situations, they would return to the nursing program and expected to be successful. Students who consider themselves as stopping out are different from dropouts, who have no intention of reentering the nursing program. Notably, several students wrote that they thanked faculty for their concern; other students wrote that they felt encouraged about reenrolling because they believed that faculty "cared" enough to send a letter and questionnaire (2). However, as mentioned above, autopsy attrition data do need to be interpreted cautiously, especially with small samples.

Several researchers proposed a psychological approach to understanding attrition decisions. Mashburn (3) suggested that dropout decisions are preceded by a psychological process that involves level of student satisfaction and withdrawal cognitions, which include thoughts of quitting, intentions to search for other options (transfer), and dropout intentions. Low satisfaction combined with high withdrawal cognitions resulted in higher dropout rates. In contrast, students with low satisfaction and low withdrawal cognitions demonstrated lower dropout rates. Eaton and Bean (4–6) purported a relationship among attitudes, intentions, and behaviors. Stress, coping, self-efficacy, avoidance/approach behaviors, satisfaction, and intent to leave were all important contributors to attrition decisions. (See Chapter 7 for more details on satisfaction.)

Although asking students why they decided to discontinue their education provides valuable information, it does not explain why other students decide to persist. Optimally, it is advantageous to examine closely the factors perceived as supportive or restrictive among students who persist. In one college, persisters were surveyed at the end of the semester and asked to rate the supportiveness or restrictiveness of select variables on their retention in a nursing course that semester (7). As a group, students perceived faculty advisement and helpfulness, the enrichment program, tutoring, personal study skills, and friends in class as "greatly supportive." The most restrictive variables included family responsibilities, family crises, financial status, family financial support for school, family emotional support, financial aid, and child-care arrangements. Conclusively, environmental variables greatly influenced retention, with professional integration variables perceived as supportive.

> When was the last time students in your course and/or program were surveyed about factors that restricted or supported their retention? When was the last time students in your course and/or program were surveyed about why they withdrew from a nursing course or dropped out of the program? What were the results?

CROSSROADS IN DECISION MAKING

As presented in the NURS model, professional integration factors are at the crossroads of the decision to persist, drop out, or stop out. Here, "crossroads" means a critical turning point in the student's decision-making process. Professional integration factors represent factors can enhance students' interaction with the social system of the college environment within the context of professional socialization and career development (see Chapter 6). These factors include nursing faculty advisement and helpfulness, professional events, memberships in professional organizations, encouragement by friends in class, peer mentoring and tutoring, and enrichment programs. Such factors offer many advantages, resources, and support for students in the decision-making process. Lack of professional integration factors isolates students, hinders realistic option appraisal, and limits thoughtful decision making.

Although nurse educators have a legal responsibility for communicating nursing program policies concerning course withdrawals and progression criteria, they also have an ethical responsibility to assist students in the decision-making process. Proactive interventions that take into account cultural and other individual differences in decision-making will be most effective (8–12) (see Chapters 3 and 10). Nurse educators may need to initiate dialogue before misperceptions arise, before students are confronted with overwhelming obstacles, and before they make haphazard decisions. Figure 9.1 presents a systematic approach to the decision-making process that can serve as a beginning guide for student self-reflection, proactive group discussion, family/significant other consideration, and nurse educator intervention. Appraisal of options, strengths, supports, weaknesses, obstacles, benefits, costs, and

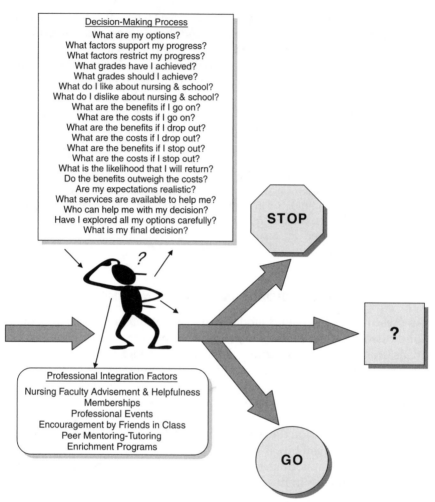

FIGURE 9.1 Crossroads in decision making: A systematic approach.

expectations should be systematically considered before arriving at a decision.

Good academic performance only results in retention decisions when accompanied by positive psychological outcomes for the nursing program and profession. Additionally, academic strengths cannot compensate for weak environmental factors, although strong environmental supports may compensate for weak academic factors (13,14). Students with weak environmental supports are increasingly at risk for attrition, despite academic strengths and past successes. Professional integration factors have the power to tip the scale in favor of retention and success because of their unique potential for enhancing academic outcomes, satisfaction, and stress management via a holistic and integrated approach. Nurse educators can make a tremendous positive difference in the overall student experience and thus enhance retention. Part II presents several strategies for making a difference.

> What professional integration factors do you currently use to enhance nursing student retention? What proactive strategies are in place to assist students in the decision-making process?

KEY POINT SUMMARY

- Student profile characteristics, student affective factors, academic factors, environmental factors, professional integration factors, academic outcomes, psychological outcomes, and outside surrounding factors interact and influence retention decisions.
- Retention decisions are the determined resolution to persist in the nursing curriculum and educational pathway toward becoming a registered nurse.
- Professional integration factors are at the crossroads of the decision to persist, drop out, or stop out.
- Options, strengths, supports, weaknesses, obstacles, benefits, costs, and expectations should be systematically considered before arriving at a decision.
- Nurse educators have an ethical responsibility to assist students in the decision-making process.

APPLICATION STRATEGIES

EASY APPLICATION ACTION STEPS

Publicizing Policies and Options Proactively

1. Proactively publicize college and departmental policies, responsibilities, rights, and procedures concerning nursing student withdrawal, failure, progression, retention, and graduation during orientation and at the beginning of a course (website, handouts, bulletin board postings, course outlines, etc.).
2. Discuss positive strategies and resources to optimize student success, beginning with an open acknowledgment that deliberations and decision making about studying, nursing, persistence, time management, and so on occurs consciously and unconsciously before, during, and at the end of a course.
3. At mid-semester and/or close to nonpenalty withdrawal date and near registration time, remind students about realistic self-appraisal and

options, inviting all students to meet individually to discuss options and future career path.

Assisting At-Risk Students With Persistence Decision Making

1. Privately reach out to at-risk students by e-mail, letter, phone call, or in person to discuss options and future career path.
2. Discuss and individually implement decision-making process illustrated in Figure 9.1.
3. Refer students to ancillary student services as needed.

EDUCATOR-IN-ACTION VIGNETTE

Nurse educators are in a strategic position to facilitate the process of systematic decision making and enhancing opportunities for retention and success. After the second exam, three students (Cindy, Paolina, and Maxine) have averages below 70 in the nursing course; a minimum 75 grade is required for passing. The nonpenalty course withdrawal date is next week. Two additional exams, two quizzes, and a final exam remain. Professor Bridges requests to meet with each failing student privately. As another reminder to previous announcements, she offers to meet with students concerning course progress and career decision making. Rosita schedules a meeting with Professor Bridges. Another student, Dawn, stops in during office hours. Professor Bridges asks students to review the steps of the decision-making process (Figure 9.1). Excerpts of student responses, educator actions, and resulting decisions follow below:

CINDY: I know I have not been keeping up with the reading or studying the way I should. My grades reflect the amount of time I've been putting into nursing. I will need to get at least an 80 on all of the exams and at least a 78 on the quizzes in order to pass the course. If I withdraw now, I will have to repeat all of the coursework and clinical completed so far. It's better that I stay in the course and work hard. I really want to be a nurse.

Professor Bridges discusses positive study and time-management strategies with Cindy. Together, they develop a weekly schedule for reading, review, and study. Cindy is referred to the Nursing Student Resource Center for additional support.

DECISION: Continue.

PAOLINA: I will need to get at least a 90 on all of the exams and at least an 86 on the quizzes in order to pass the course. I'm taking two advanced chemistry courses, Spanish, and art history. Those courses require a lot of time and I am struggling to pass them too. All I do is study or go to class.

If I withdraw from any class, I will not be a full-time student, so I will lose my financial aid and health insurance. I can't afford to withdraw.

Professor Bridges encourages Paolina to discuss her future career goals. Paolina admits that she is really interested in being a pharmacist but thinks that pharmacy school will be too expensive. She indicates that her parents think it is more appropriate for her to become an associate degree nurse and start earning money in 2 years to help support her seven younger brothers and sisters. She dislikes nursing, especially the clinical component. Professor Bridges arranges for Paolina to meet with a career counselor individually and then with her parents present.

DECISION: Drop out (of nursing). Paolina changes her major and applies for a student loan and on-campus work.

MAXINE: I do not work or have other responsibilities. I only need at least 76 on all of my future exams and quizzes. I've always wanted to be a nurse. When I study in my group and with my tutor, I know everything. My anxiety gets in the way and I change many of my answers. I'm so close to passing that I don't want to drop out but I am afraid of failing.

Professor Bridges determines, after some discussion, that Maxine does comprehend course material. She further explores the issue of test anxiety, suggests several strategies to reduce test anxiety, and refers Maxine to test anxiety reduction workshops.

DECISION: Continue.

ROSITA: My second test grade dropped by 30 points. I really like nursing and I'm usually a good student. My husband was just diagnosed with terminal cancer with a 6-month prognosis. I am devastated. I feel that I want to spend every moment with him, yet I don't know what will happen if I drop the course.

Professor Bridges offers emotional support and invites Rosita to talk more about her feelings. Rosita appreciates the opportunity to talk about her husband. When finished, Professor Bridges provides her with information concerning readmission into the nursing program and counseling services.

DECISION: Stop out.

DAWN: I don't want to mess up my 4.0 average. My last grade was only an 86. I was thinking about withdrawing and taking the class next semester, but, I don't want to be behind my classmates. Tell me what to do.

Professor Bridges assists Dawn to appraise her academic situation, goals, and career progress by going through each step of the decision-making process. She asks Dawn to write "pros and cons" for each step on the dry-erase board. Together they compare and contrast pros and cons for stopping out or continuing. Professor Bridges does not make the decision, but patiently guides Dawn through the process.

DECISION: Continue.

Professor Bridges actively seeks to promote persistence and retention by meeting with the at-risk enrolled nursing students periodically. Follow-up correspondence via e-mails, letters, and phone calls are conducted with students who stop out.

TOOLKIT RESOURCE BOX

Item 8—Student Withdrawal Questionnaire
Item 20—Decision-Making Appraisal Tool for Dropout, Stopout, or Persistence

---

DISCUSSION QUESTIONS

1. What are the reasons for students to persist, stop out, or drop out of the first nursing course, your course, other nursing courses, and the nursing program? What are the predominant reasons? What demographic characteristics are predominant (if any) among the stated reasons for persistence, stopouts, or dropouts? How are data collected? What changes to data collection would you suggest? Why?
2. Review Figure 9.1. How could this be adapted for use with your students? With your faculty colleagues?
3. Review the snapshot scenarios at the beginning of the chapter. What proactive strategies could you implement to prevent each situation? What strategies would you implement to address each student's statement? Why?
4. Which Educator-in-Action Vignette at the end of the chapter captivated you the most? Why?
5. Professor Numbers says, "Gathering reasons for withdrawal in each nursing course this semester will never result in any statistically significant findings. The response rate for mailed questionnaires in autopsy attrition studies is low, making validity of findings questionable. It is better to just aggregate data via the tracking pathway and document numbers of students who pass, fail, or withdraw. We can even collapse the failing students and the withdrawing students together because their progress is impeded along the ideal trajectory pathway. We can do some more sophisticated statistical analyses than just frequency and percent; the qualitative comments section on the withdrawal

questionnaire can never be collapsed to create meaningful quantitative data." How would you respond? Why?

REFERENCES

1. Braxton, J. M., Brier, E. M., & Hossler, D. (1988). The influence of student problems on student withdrawal decisions: An autopsy on "autopsy" studies. *Research in Higher Education, 28*(3), 241–253.
2. Jeffreys, M. R. (2000). *Nursing student withdrawal data.* Unpublished material.
3. Mashburn, A. J. (2000). A psychological process of student dropout. *Journal of College Student Retention, Research, Theory, & Practice, 2*(3), 173–190.
4. Eaton, S. B., & Bean, J. P. (1995). An approach/avoidance behavioral model of college student attrition. *Research in Higher Education, 36*, 617–645.
5. Bean, J. P., & Eaton, S. B. (2000). A psychological model of college student retention. In J. M. Braxton (ed.). *Rethinking the departure puzzle: New theory and research on college student retention* (pp. 48–61). Nashville, TN: Vanderbilt University Press.
6. Bean, J. P. (2005). Nine themes of college student retention. In A. Seidman (ed.). *College student retention: Formula for success* (pp. 215–244). Westport, CT: Praeger.
7. Jeffreys, M. R. (2002). Students' perceptions of variables influencing retention: A pretest and post-test approach. *Nurse Educator, 27*(1), 16–19 [Erratum, 2002, 27*(2), 64].
8. Brown, L. L., & Kurpius, S. E. R. (1997). Psychosocial factors influencing academic persistence of American Indian college students. *Journal of College Student Development, 38*(1), 3–12.
9. Nora, A., Cabrera, A., Hagedorn, L. S., & Pascarella, E. (1996). Differential impacts of academic and social experiences on college-related behavioral outcomes across different ethnic and gender groups at four-year institutions. *Research in Higher Education, 37*(4), 427–451.
10. Seidman, A. (2005). *College student retention: Formula for success.* Westport, CT: Praeger.
11. Jeffreys, M. R. (2007). Tracking students through program entry, progression, graduation, and licensure: Assessing undergraduate nursing student retention and success. *Nurse Education Today, 27*, 406–419.
12. Jeffreys, M. R. (2010). *Teaching cultural competence in nursing and health care: Inquiry, action, and innovation* (2nd ed.). New York, NY: Springer Publishing.
13. Bean, J. P., & Metzner, B. (1985). A conceptual model of nontraditional undergraduate student attrition. *Review of Educational Research, 55*, 485–540.
14. Metzner, B., & Bean, J. P. (1987). The estimation of a conceptual model of nontraditional undergraduate student attrition. *Research in Higher Education, 27*, 15–38.

Making a Difference: Spotlight on Retention and Success Strategies

Part II presents strategies for promoting retention and success. Chapters describe the process of designing, implementing, and evaluating specific strategies. Topics include culturally congruent nursing faculty advisement and helpfulness, expanding the web of inclusion through professional events and memberships, promoting positive and productive peer partnerships, enrichment programs (EPs), and nursing student resource centers (NSRC). Case exemplars, illustrations, and tables are included to assist in creatively adapting described strategies. Consistent with Part I, practical application is further emphasized in the numerous action-oriented "Application Strategies" that follow the chapter summaries.

The main purpose of Chapter 10 is to describe the process of developing a culturally congruent approach to faculty advisement and helpfulness. The process includes self-assessment, literature review, consultation and collaboration, student assessment, analysis, plan, communication, and interaction. Culturally congruent and culturally incongruent faculty actions, student perspectives and their influence on academic outcomes, psychological outcomes, and retention are examined.

Chapter 11 discusses creative strategies for expanding the web of inclusion by enhancing student opportunities for participation in professional events and memberships. Barrier recognition, solutions, strategies, and incentives are proposed.

Chapter 12 describes strategies for promoting positive and productive peer partnerships (purposeful affiliations, alliances, and connections among peers that result in constructive, generative, creative, and desirable outcomes). Carefully patterned and interwoven student-centered interactive experiences throughout the nursing curriculum can be structured to promote positive and productive peer partnerships. Recommendations for barrier recognition, solutions, strategies, and incentives are presented.

Nurse educators can make a difference in nursing student retention and success through a carefully designed EP. Chapter 13 describes the process of designing, implementing, and evaluating such a program. An illustrative case exemplar, using the prenursing enrichment program (PEP), complements each step of the process.

The well-designed NSRC offers a place for effectively linking multiple strategies. The main purpose of Chapter 14 is to describe the process of designing, operating, and evaluating a NSRC. Key definitions, concepts, decisions, and considerations are discussed. Several checklists are provided to assist in planning and practical application.

Current and future enrollment trends predict a more academically and culturally diverse nursing student population, suggesting that nursing student persistence, retention, and success will be even more complex in the future. Nurse educators will always be in the most strategic position to influence retention positively. Unfortunately, the predicted nursing faculty shortage; the declining number of nurses who will be adequately prepared for the educator role; the growing need to defend, define, and redefine the "scholarship of teaching," compounded by the substantial gaps in nursing student retention research impose grave obstacles for the future. Chapter 15 proposes future directions and suggests a positive vision for tomorrow.

Faculty Advisement and Helpfulness: A Culturally Congruent Approach

Consideration of the student as a whole person demands a culturally congruent approach to advisement and helpfulness.

SNAPSHOT SCENARIO

At a nursing faculty meeting, Professor Glass introduces the topic of "culturally congruent faculty advisement and helpfulness" by sharing a personal experience. "I used to think of myself as being a helpful advisor to all students; however, this opinion changed recently. I realized that I made a cultural mistake with one of my students. This mistake set up obstacles for future communication and caused her obvious stress. I apologized immediately, but later I always felt a gap was present. I realized that the increased number of new immigrant nursing students from diverse countries meant that I could not use the same approach with all students. I was also concerned that I may have offended others unintentionally. The next week in class, I asked students to reflect on their experiences with nursing faculty so far and anonymously write down helpful faculty actions, unhelpful faculty actions, student expectations about faculty advisement and helpfulness, and any cultural customs relevant to faculty–student interactions. Responses were amazing."

Professor Glass read several student comments that contrasted student perceptions, cultural values and beliefs, and student experiences with faculty.

A: My advisor always stares right into my eyes during the registration advisement session. I get so uncomfortable that I feel as though I can't even speak.

B: My advisor hardly ever looks me in the eye so I don't think she even sees me as a person.

C: When nursing faculty greet me in the hall or library and offer to help me during office hours, it makes me feel like they care.

D: My advisor was right behind me in the cafeteria line and didn't even acknowledge my greeting or say hello.

E: Every time I see my advisor at the college or during her office hours, she smiles and greets me by name, beginning with some small talk first to get me comfortable and then asking me how I am doing. In my culture, it is considered impolite to get right to the point directly in business. Some other faculty are so direct, short, and business-like all the time so I don't feel comfortable asking questions.

F: My advisor has no clue about time management or what I need. Whenever I see her, she begins with 2 minutes of small talk or short stories like something new at the college, the weather, an ANA [American Nurses Association] conference, and so on, and I could go on and on. She is not very business-like and this is a waste of time. I was always taught at home to be direct and business-like with professors; small talk is a time waster. This really irritates me and I can't get beyond this to feel comfortable trusting her responses to career questions.

G: When my advisor changed her office hours to Friday afternoons, she offered to set an alternate meeting time with me instead of making me change advisors. That made me feel as though she really cared about me and respected my religious beliefs.

H: Thank you for asking about our [students'] feelings, experiences, and concerns. Even if you do something other than what I expect, I will now feel as though you are trying to treat us as individuals and respect our cultural values and beliefs.

Other faculty members begin discussing similar experiences and concerns about providing culturally congruent advisement and helpfulness.

PROFESSOR PONDER: I never really thought too much about it but I guess sometimes I do feel lost in knowing how to best advise, teach, and interact with students who are culturally different from me. I hope I did not hurt anyone's feelings by doing the wrong thing.

PROFESSOR NUMBERS: We must be doing something right because we still make the average numbers on the state board-licensing exam.

PROFESSOR WINGER: I just use common sense and wing it, just like I did in the clinical setting with culturally different patients. No one's complained so far.

PROFESSOR BOOKE: The higher education and nursing literature notes the significant role that faculty advisement can play in students' decisions to drop out, stop out, or stay in school and graduate. I read that faculty advisement and helpfulness inside and outside the classroom is very influential, especially with minority students in predominantly White universities, first generation college students, and older students. In general, students are considered a vulnerable population and may be hesitant to complain because of feared academic or other penalties. Among many cultures, confronting an advisor or teacher is culturally inappropriate behavior so complaining would be unheard of. Just because no one complains doesn't mean students are happy, satisfied, and receiving the best advisement to enhance their academic performance.

Professor Ponder thinks, "In my advanced practice nursing program, I never took any courses that addressed curriculum, principles of teaching, the advisor role, or cultural issues. How can I become a better advisor for a diverse student population?"

Faculty advisement and helpfulness is the active involvement of nursing faculty in student's academic endeavors, career goals, and professional socialization. It is manifested through faculty actions such as encouraging realistic educational and career goals, promoting positive feelings of self-worth, verbalizing belief in the student's ability to succeed, listening to problems and concerns, expressing interest in academic progress, showing optimism, offering assistance, and presence. Presence means caring about the student as a whole person, being available as a resource person, and making appropriate referrals when needed.

Consideration of the student as a whole person demands a culturally congruent approach to advisement and helpfulness. The inclusion of cultural values and beliefs (CVB) in the Nursing Undergraduate Retention and Success (NURS) model recognizes that a student's CVB unconsciously and consciously guide thinking, decisions, and actions that ultimately affect nursing student retention (see Figure 1.2). The NURS model proposes that high levels of cultural congruence will serve as a bridge to promoting positive academic and psychological outcomes, thus enhancing persistence behaviors and retention (see Chapter 3). Cultural congruence is the degree of fit between the student's values and beliefs and those of their surrounding environment, that is, nursing education within the educational institution and the nursing profession. The term "cultural congruent nursing care" was first coined and defined by Leininger (1) to describe nursing care with clients that is meaningful, beneficial, and satisfying; however, the definition can be adapted to the educational setting. In this book, a culturally congruent approach to faculty advisement and helpfulness refers to those faculty actions that are tailored to fit with the student's CVB in order to promote, facilitate, or support academic endeavors, career goals, and professional socialization.

A culturally congruent approach to faculty advisement and helpfulness requires faculty commitment and active engagement in the ongoing process of developing cultural congruence and becoming "culturally competent" faculty advisors and helpful teachers. The main purpose of this chapter is to describe the process of developing a culturally congruent approach to faculty advisement and helpfulness. The process includes self-assessment, literature review, consultation and collaboration, student assessment, analysis, plan, communication, and interaction.

Self-Assessment

> **What thoughts and feelings do you have about diverse student populations? What thoughts and feelings do you have about the faculty advisor role, help-seeking behaviors, and faculty helpfulness?**

Because faculty may be "unconsciously incompetent" in providing nursing advisement and help, the first step is self-assessment. According to Purnell (2), one is unconsciously incompetent when one is not aware of cultural differences or when one unknowingly carries out actions that are not culturally congruent. Cultural blindness, cultural imposition, and culturally incongruent actions can cause cultural pain to others (3). The major aim of self-assessment is raising consciousness and self-awareness.

Here, self-assessment is a process in which the nurse educator systematically appraises various dimensions that can impact upon the achievement of cultural congruent advisement and helpfulness. A systematic assessment can be initiated using the dimensions described in Chapter 3, listed in Table 3.1, and illustrated in Figure 10.1 (see Toolkit Item 16). The

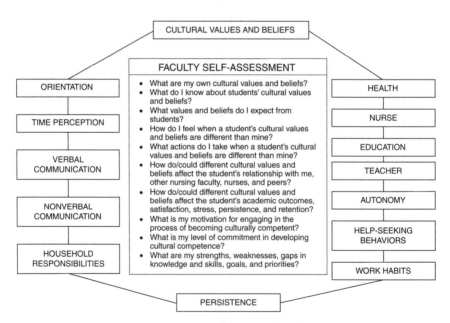

Note: Multidimensional cultural values and beliefs (CVB) surround and encompass all aspects of a systematic faculty self-assessment. See Table 3.1 for CVB category examples.

FIGURE 10.1 Cultural values and beliefs: Faculty self-assessment.

realization that there are multidimensional variables influencing student–faculty interaction is overwhelming, yet these variables are essential to evaluate before developing a cultural congruent approach. In addition to raising consciousness and self-awareness, self-assessment can help identify areas of strengths and weaknesses and should be compared with a student's own self-assessments and expectations.

Although the faculty member may be immersed within the "culture" of nursing education and be familiar with long-held nursing education CVB, it is important to be aware that unconscious and conscious CVB in nursing education and in one's own values and belief systems, many of which were developed long before entering the nursing culture, may influence practices, behaviors, and actions. For example, a nursing faculty member whose traditional cultural values favor direct eye contact for all communication and who views lack of eye contact suspiciously will need to be consciously aware of his or her underlying values and beliefs and aim to consciously avoid distrusting students based solely on this nonverbal cue.

Awareness of one's knowledge about different CVB, especially the CVB that most directly affect nursing student retention (through academic and psychological outcomes) must be explored (see Table 3.1). Although Table 3.1 presents a snapshot approach of selected CVB that may impact upon nursing student retention, it does allow for a quick comparison of different CVB. One benefit of this approach is that it evokes the awareness that there may be CVB in various cultures that the nurse educator is unaware of. The realization that one is not and cannot be "culturally competent" all of the time is often a powerful awakening. Becoming conscious of one's incompetence can be a humbling experience but frequently sparks a desire for obtaining cultural knowledge. Cultural awareness, desire, and knowledge are essential for the process of cultural competence (4–6).

Cultural knowledge is a thorough educational foundation about various CVB with the goal of comprehending and empathizing with others' perspectives. The nurse educator must assess one's cultural desire or motivation for engaging in the process of becoming culturally competent. Reflecting on the feelings one experiences and the actions taken when student's CVB are different from one's own CVB can further one's insight. Because the process of cultural competence is ongoing, nurse educators should examine their commitment toward achieving this goal. True commitment requires time, energy, persistence, extra effort to overcome obstacles, and willingness to learn from mistakes. Commitment is essential in achieving positive outcomes in student retention (7,8).

Nurse educators must appraise the multidimensional factors influencing undergraduate nursing student achievement, retention, and success, or full understanding will not truly be achieved. Furthermore, they need to evaluate how CVB can influence persistence behaviors (9–18). Nurse educators should reflect on the last time an updated review of the literature, workshop, or conference on student retention and success was completed. Again, appraisal of one's desire for updated knowledge and commitment in relation to other faculty responsibilities and available time should be critically determined.

Similarly, self-expectations of the advisor role and helpfulness toward students should be examined. Faculty often overlook the significant role that their attitudes and behaviors can have on student satisfaction and retention (11,19–23). Although the developmental advisement approach is strongly supported in the literature as offering the most benefits to enhance student academic and psychological growth and development, not all nursing faculty may value, support, or practice developmental advisement. In a developmental approach, student–faculty relationships encourage open communication, shared responsibility and power, caring, mentoring, total student development, self-direction, active help-seeking behaviors, and decision making. Developmental advisement is more focused on the "process" of learning whereas prescriptive advisement is grade-oriented, focused on the attainment of a prescribed product. Prescriptive advisement views the faculty advisor as the authority person who dispenses information and prescribes the measures needed for students to complete their curriculum requirements (24,25).

Developmental advisement necessitates a commitment on the part of both faculty member and student; the advisor–advisee relationship changes over the educational process. Although the developmental approach is advocated in the NURS model, students may inwardly view faculty advisement and helpfulness differently. Not all students may value a developmental advisement approach. Often student perceptions and expectations about the faculty advisement role are different from that of the faculty (26–34). Additionally, expectations about "helpfulness" can be different from that of faculty (11,35). The mismatch between student and faculty expectations and perceptions creates another barrier, whereby, students can become disappointed and dissatisfied; poor psychological outcomes for the nursing program increase the risk for attrition. Consequently, faculty members should appraise their knowledge about student expectations and perceptions. Lack of knowledge or limited knowledge in this area identifies targets for further self-development. However, one must have the desire to obtain such knowledge and be committed to its pursuit amidst other faculty responsibilities. Finally, self-assessment should conclude with a listing of strengths, weaknesses, gaps in knowledge, goals, commitment, and priorities.

What are your strengths, weaknesses, gaps in knowledge, goals, commitments, and priorities?

Literature Review

Next, a review of the nursing and higher education literature should be conducted. A review of the literature in psychology, anthropology, and sociology may also prove fruitful. Materials should be reviewed for gathering background information or updating previously gathered information about CVB, cultural competence, student retention, advisement, faculty helpfulness, help-seeking behaviors, and faculty–student interactions. Priority areas, weaknesses, or gaps in knowledge previously identified in the self-assessment can guide the review. Choice of a relevant conceptual framework can be instrumental to an organized review. For example, the NURS model can structure a systematic approach to the review and organization of retention literature. After gathering general background information, it may be appropriate to begin targeting specific student cultural groups, especially those with whom there is frequent interaction. The dimensions targeted in Chapter 3 (Table 3.1), and Figure 10.1 can provide a guide for organizing specific information; however, it is vital to individually appraise each student and avoid stereotypical assumptions.

When was the last time you conducted a review of the literature concerning nursing student retention and success, advisement, and cultural competence? What books, book chapters, websites, journal articles, dissertations, and other scholarly resources can help you develop a culturally congruent approach to faculty advisement and helpfulness?

Consultation and Collaboration

Once sufficient background information has been reviewed and synthesized, collaboration with others should be initiated. Sufficient background knowledge is a precursor for successfully optimizing consultation and collaboration. The nurse educator will now have a mutually shared conceptual and empirical knowledge base with colleagues and experts that will promote deeper dialogue and added benefits. Consultation with experts in specific cultures, cultural competency, advisement, and student retention is helpful. Collaboration with colleagues (other nursing faculty) can help coordinate efforts and avoid unnecessary duplication. Consultation and collaboration can occur formally and informally via conferences, e-mail, webinars, telephone, and meetings.

A major benefit of collaboration among faculty is that nurse educators can become aware of each other's expertise and interests. Other goals include learning from others, avoiding pitfalls, and gaining insight into special program-specific considerations. Still another plus is broadening information sources and soliciting conceptual and/or instrumental support from others.

What resources and expertise currently exists among your nursing colleagues and in your college? What is the climate like for mutual collaboration? What else is needed?

Student Assessment

What do you know about your students' perceptions about faculty advisement and helpfulness? What do you know about your students' cultural values and beliefs?

The ability to gather relevant and valid cultural information is an essential component in the development of cultural competence (4). Moreover, a systematic appraisal of CVB is a precursor to determining the needs and priorities within a cultural context (36). Promoting student self-assessment of cultural values and beliefs must be initiated in a positive supportive environment that embraces diversity. Students will need to feel comfortable exploring their own CVB in the context of the nursing educational setting and secondly will need to feel comfortable in sharing CVB with others, especially faculty. The literature suggests that students of different cultural backgrounds than faculty often feel isolated and reluctant to share differences for fear of reprimand, discrimination, or misunderstanding (11,12,15,16,37–50).

Encouraging students to explore their own CVB concerning such dimensions as listed in Table 3.1 will enhance awareness of cultural similarities and differences with peers, clients, and faculty. This awareness will aid in the development of cultural competence in professional settings with clients, peers, other health care professionals, and ancillary workers. Asking about students' expectations concerning faculty advisement and helpfulness in the classroom, clinical setting, college skills laboratory, and informal settings will publicize and emphasize the fact that faculty care and have the desire to help students. Student's perception that an instructor or advisor is asking about student needs is helpful in and of itself and creates a caring environment. Perceptions that faculty sincerely care about students and openly apologize for (cultural) mistakes is more important than flawless, superficial, and distant interactions with students.

Student assessment may be done formally using survey tools; however, the development of valid and reliable survey tools that are free of cultural bias and social desirability response bias is a complicated and lengthy process (51). A previous review of literature may reveal already existing survey tools with adequate estimates of reliability and validity that can be used or adapted with permission. Use of a survey tool that has not been tested for validity and reliability not only provides questionable results but can impact adversely on student perceptions if items are offensive, misinterpreted, unclear, insulting, or culturally inappropriate. Such unwanted outcomes create dissatisfaction, added stress, and negatively influence retention.

Another formalized assessment approach may be the use of focus groups consisting of select small groups of students (52,53). Dialogue with students, using a set of predetermined questions to guide the discussion and allow for comparison between student groups, will allow for unsolicited comments, solicited comments, and qualitative data that can add richness not achievable via a quantitative or close-ended survey questioning. Focus groups that are guided by peer mentors or faculty who are not in a teaching role may ease fear of penalty or adverse consequences. A systematic assessment can be initiated using the dimensions listed in Table 3.1 and illustrated in Figure 10.2 (see Toolkit Item 17). Student responses can then be compared with those of faculty.

In the classroom, clinical setting, or college laboratory, a simple technique may be to survey students anonymously on the first day. After an introduction, the instructor can express interest in meeting student needs through advisement and helpfulness and can ask students to write several ways that they believe the instructor can be helpful during the semester.

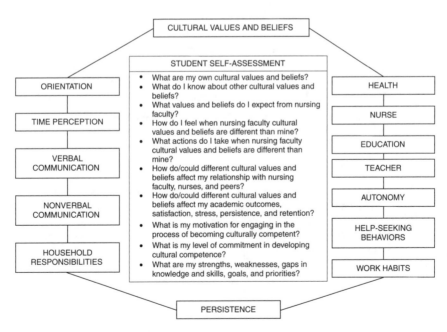

Note: Multidimensional cultural values and beliefs (CVB) surround and encompass all aspects of a systematic student self-assessment. See Table 3.1 for CVB category examples.

FIGURE 10.2   Cultural values and beliefs: Student self-assessment.

It may also be beneficial to ask students to write anything that they experienced in the past that was not helpful or anything that they would perceive to be inappropriate or not helpful. This strategy can also be adapted to ask questions about faculty helpfulness in an informal setting.

Advisement and helpfulness should be developmental, that is, changing over time as student needs and expectations change, and so student assessment should be ongoing throughout the course and throughout the program at regularly scheduled intervals. For example, mid-semester, a classroom instructor may want to ask students to write comments again as before and compare with group's previous responses. Over time, common trends or themes may emerge, especially in a particular clinical setting or classroom course component. A systematic program appraisal can provide an overview of successful strategies and outcomes (54).

> To what degree do your students perceive faculty advisement and helpfulness as supportive or restrictive to their retention and success?

Analysis

Insight into students' perceptions is important in meeting needs of adult learners (55). A systematic analysis of students' self-assessment should identify realistic versus unrealistic expectations, areas of untapped or underutilized advisor role, trends among the students surveyed, group similarities, individual differences, and perceived student needs. A thorough and objective analysis to determine the gap between student and faculty expectations, perceptions of what is important, and level of cultural congruence should be estimated. Mismatches need priority attention. The analysis should list strengths and congruency as well as weaknesses, gaps, and incongruency. Analysis of findings may be enhanced through the review of relevant literature to explain findings, elaborate major points, and offer suggestions.

> What mismatches exist between faculty and student expectations concerning faculty advisement and helpfulness? What mismatches exist because of cultural incongruency? What strategies will reduce or eliminate existing mismatches? What strategies can be implemented proactively to prevent mismatches in the future?

Plan

Next, a written action plan is developed. Individual faculty can review student comments for areas of unrealistic or unclear expectations and then plan to address this in a group setting to clarify advisor and faculty role. Similarly, faculty can verbally and positively respond to realistic, clear, and important expectations in faculty–student interactions. Relevant issues reported in the literature and/or uncovered through consultation and collaboration should be incorporated. Another strategy may be to develop, distribute, and discuss an academic advising guide delineating responsibilities as an advisee and responsibilities of the advisor (28). The advisor guidebook of the National Academic Advising Association can provide some foundational information generalizable to multidisciplinary college students (56).

A plan for a faculty development workshop or series of workshops in enhancing cultural congruent advisement and helpfulness is central to promoting retention through positive psychological outcomes. Inadequate planning of effective advisement strategies appropriate for various students throughout the educational process supports the need for faculty development workshops (8,11,16,27,28,42,47,57–64). Nursing education goes beyond a single nurse educator. It is the whole nursing educational experience that impacts positively or negatively in the minds of students. One experience of cultural pain can do much to undermine the efforts of other faculty members who strongly advocate and consciously implement culturally congruent approaches.

The plan for faculty development should recognize that some faculty may fail to recognize the need for a workshop or may demonstrate reluctance to participate. Even if a workshop or series of workshops is mandatory, this does not necessarily mean that faculty will change values, beliefs, and traditions in favor of culturally congruent advisement and helpfulness. However, it is important to remember that all faculty members and students have CVB that may potentially be congruent or incongruent with each other and/or traditional nursing education values (Table 3.1). Both faculty and students may belong to multiple cultural groups, and the boundaries between cultural groups and affiliations are often unclear (15,65). Therefore, formalized educational experiences concerning culture are necessary for all individuals, regardless of age, ethnicity, gender, sexual orientation, lifestyle, religion, socioeconomic status, or geographic location (66–69).

Tables 10.1, 10.2, and 10.3 provide case examples contrasting culturally incongruent and culturally congruent student–faculty interactions and the resulting outcomes. These case examples can be incorporated into a plan to initiate discussion with faculty and students. Such dialogue may help promote inner reflection or self-awareness of one's CVB, cultural imposition, ethnocentric tendencies, and potential impact of cultural pain on nursing student retention. Using case examples can point out that despite the intent to help, one's actions may not always be helpful. In fact, they may be counterproductive, causing pain, conflict, dissatisfaction, and stress for the student. Planning communication strategies to convey

TABLE 10.1 Examples of Culturally Incongruent and Culturally Congruent Advisement Approaches

ADVISEMENT SITUATION	CULTURALLY INCONGRUENT	CULTURALLY CONGRUENT
Shari arrives for academic course advisement accompanied by her husband. She states that she prefers having her husband with her. Shari's husband asks several questions concerning the nursing curriculum. Her CVB view decision making as a process involving her husband. Nonverbal communication cues (relaxed facial expression and relaxed body posture) suggest comfort with each other's presence during the advisement session.	Professor ignores students' CVB and does not actively explore preferred advisement style. Professor imposes her own CVB by stating, "I will be glad to answer any questions that Shari has. Shari, if you want to be a professional nurse, you must learn to be assertive, speak for yourself, and make decisions on your own." *Result*: Shari and her husband experience cultural pain and feel embarrassed. Because they view the professor as an authority figure, they do not want to confront her. Instead, they remain quiet. Later, Shari and her husband decide that she should drop out of the nursing program.	Professor recognizes the importance of Shari's CVB. Professor states, "It is nice to see such strong family support. I hope that I will be able to answer your questions. If you would like to move your chairs into a more comfortable arrangement, please feel free to do so. I want to help you in the best way possible, so please let me know if something I say or do makes you uncomfortable or is unclear." *Result*: Shari and her husband feel that the professor genuinely cares about Shari holistically and is sincerely interested in accommodating their needs.
Dana, a 25-year-old unmarried part-time student visits the nursing advisor for registration. She has her three small children with her. She expresses concern over getting daytime courses that coincide with the college child-care services. Her CVB place family responsibilities over all other responsibilities. Single parenting is not viewed negatively in her culture.	Professor holds traditional nursing values and beliefs as well as own CVB that are congruent with nursing CVB. Professor states, "When I went to school, we weren't concerned about things like that. None of us were married and none of us had children. School was the priority. Nursing is hard work and should be a priority." *Result*: Dana feels discouraged and experiences hurt, anger, and pain.	Professor acknowledges the importance of Dana's concerns, and compliments her beautiful children and her motivation to pursue her nursing degree. Professor offers to call the child-care guidance counselor to assist her with the child-care aspect. *Result*: Dana feels satisfied that the advisor respects and understands her values and beliefs.

(continued)

TABLE 10.1   Examples of Culturally Incongruent and Culturally Congruent Advisement Approaches (*continued*)

ADVISEMENT SITUATION	CULTURALLY INCONGRUENT	CULTURALLY CONGRUENT
Iris experiences a personal crisis during the last semester before graduation. The stress associated with the crisis situation interferes with her ability to complete assignments and tests successfully. Iris's CVB stigmatize psychological stress. Talking about one's personal feelings is taboo. Indirect verbal communication and periods of silence for reflection are the preferred communication patterns. Iris asks the advisor for help in improving her grades.	Professor values a direct approach that aims to encourage verbalization of feelings. Professor states, "You obviously are under a lot of emotional stress. I think you should talk about your feelings with me or a college counselor." *Result*: Iris experiences cultural pain and distress because her emotional stress is outwardly recognizable. She feels stigmatized and reluctant to talk about feelings. This results in negative psychological feelings associated with school.	Professor recognizes that students may view stress differently and that different advisement approaches may be needed. Professor states, "Last month I had a student whose grades dropped following a personal crisis. Sometimes students experience stress related to outside issues or events. Some students have benefited from speaking with a counselor about their feelings" (pause). *Result*: Iris does not feel stigmatized and is satisfied with the advisor's approach.

faculty commitment and holistic caring about culturally diverse students is necessary to avoid misunderstandings and to enhance the quality of faculty–student interactions.

Communication

How do you communicate to students that culture and students matter?

Communicating that "culture matters" and that "students matter" requires an integrated, well-planned approach. Multimedia strategies to promote open communication, clarify misperceptions about the faculty advisor role, convey caring and helpfulness, and develop student–faculty partnerships in achieving cultural congruency should be proactive and ongoing. For example, communication can be initiated in new student

TABLE 10.2 Faculty Helpfulness in the Classroom, Clinical Setting, and Nursing Skills Laboratory: Examples of Culturally Incongruent and Culturally Congruent Approaches

SITUATION	CULTURALLY INCONGRUENT	CULTURALLY CONGRUENT
Classroom Lou performed excellently on an exam, achieving the highest grade. Lou has group orientation rather than individual orientation, therefore is uncomfortable with individual praise.	Professor intends to be helpful, acknowledge strong performance, and motivate other students. Professor verbally praises Lou's performance in the classroom, announcing her name and exceptional performance. *Result*: Lou is embarrassed and feels ashamed over being singled out in the class.	Professor intends to be helpful and acknowledges strong performance and motivates other students yet is aware of CVB that impact upon a cultural congruent approach. Professor verbally acknowledges the outstanding performance demonstrated by several students without mentioning their names. *Result*: Lou feels satisfied and comfortable with the knowledge that her performance and that of others in the group has been appreciated.
Clinical During clinical postconference, one student (Jane) assertively questions the clinical instructor's statement about a medication. Jane's CVB openly encourage assertiveness and equally view teachers and learners as co-participants in the teaching-learning process. Several students with different CVB are obviously uncomfortable by the perceived confrontation.	Professor's CVB consider the preservation of group harmony and "saving face" as a priority. She sees the discomfort of two other students in the group and aims to help the group avoid conflict. Professor's response is to evade answering Jane's question and dismiss the postconference early. *Result*: Jane is still confused and feels stressed about the medication. She is dissatisfied with the professor's actions.	Professor recognizes differences between an individual versus group orientation. Although her own CVB are group orientation, the professor realizes that Jane's behavior is appropriate. Professor answers Jane's question and uses this opportunity to discuss various differences in communication patterns, values, and beliefs among different cultures. *Result*: Jane and the other students receive clarification about the statement and receive new information about culture and values clarification, enhancing academic outcomes and promoting positive psychological outcomes.

(continued)

TABLE 10.2   Faculty Helpfulness in the Classroom, Clinical Setting, and Nursing Skills Laboratory: Examples of Culturally Incongruent and Culturally Congruent Approaches (*continued*)

SITUATION	CULTURALLY INCONGRUENT	CULTURALLY CONGRUENT
Nursing skills laboratory		
After a detailed skills laboratory class on injections, it is now Lee's turn to administer an intramuscular injection into the skills laboratory mannequin for the first time. Lee's CVB view the teacher as an authority figure. Less than perfect performance would poorly reflect on the teacher and cause embarrassment for the teacher in front of the other students. Lee is fearful that she will not demonstrate the skill perfectly and feels that she must "save face" yet Lee does not want to refuse the professor's request to "inject." Anxiously, she asks if she can first practice with her peers.	Professor wants to help all students equally and aims to "treat all students alike." Professor insists that Lee administer the injection. *Result*: Lee feels increasingly anxious and pressured that she must perform the injection perfectly. Additionally, she feels cultural pain because she believes that she initiated conflict with an authority figure. Lee attempts the injection but when she forgets to aspirate, she becomes even more anxious and experiences cultural pain because she has now "embarrassed her teacher." Lee feels much dissatisfaction and stress; she questions her ability to complete the nursing program.	Professor recognizes that Lee's anxiety may not be related to lack of academic readiness, but due to underlying CVB. Professor reassures Lee that she does not expect perfection on the first attempt, however still notes nonverbal cues of anxiety (facial tension, shaking hands, flushed appearance). Professor pairs Lee with a strong student who has already performed the injection and allows privacy for several practice injections. *Result*: Lee does not feel pressured to "save face" and can relax enough with her peer to perfect her skill prior to observation by the instructor. After demonstrating the injection to the professor accurately, Lee experiences satisfaction.

orientations, on initial assignment to an advisor, on the first day of class/ clinical via verbal, written, and other media format. Slides, PowerPoint presentations, videos, case examples, and other multimedia approaches can be used to supplement previous information and initiate discussions in large groups, small groups, or individual settings with students. The faculty advisor role, teacher's role, and student rights and responsibilities can be delineated and described in student newsletters, handout materials, student handbook, welcome letters to new students, course outlines, bulletin board postings, e-mail list serves, and webpages. Messages that openly celebrate diversity encourage others to appreciate and embrace the diversity among students, faculty, clients, and society in general. Such

TABLE 10.3 Faculty Helpfulness Beyond Class: Examples of Culturally Incongruent and Culturally Congruent Approaches

SITUATION	CULTURALLY INCONGRUENT	CULTURALLY CONGRUENT
Outside		
Maria walks across the campus with her father and encounters her former nursing instructor. Maria's CVB place parents, elders, teachers, and nurses as highly respected individuals. Family and traditions are priorities; education is secondary. She formally introduces her father and instructor.	Professor values casual, informal interaction with students, thinking that this is helpful for all students. She states, "Oh, just call me Cathy. There's no need to be so formal." *Result*: Maria and her father experience cultural pain and embarrassment. Maria's father is concerned that Maria will abandon her traditional CVB. Maria feels pulled between her traditional CVB and pursuit of a nursing career.	Professor is comfortable with casual, informal interaction with students, yet respects alternative values. Professor does not attempt to impose her values; rather she graciously thanks Maria for the formal introduction and responds formally. *Result*: Maria and her father experience positive psychological outcomes (satisfaction).
Office hours		
During office hours, several students asked the instructor's help for completing a written paper assignment. Pat does not understand how to complete a written paper assignment, however, his CVB are not congruent with self-initiated actively help-seeking behaviors.	Professor holds CVB that value assertiveness, active help-seeking behaviors, and confrontation with authority. Professor states to her colleague, "I keep my office door open so students can stop by and ask for help. If students don't ask for help, they deserve the grade they get." *Result*: Pat still does not understand the assignment, fails the paper, resulting in poor academic outcomes and poor psychological outcomes.	Professor recognizes that help-seeking behaviors vary culturally and consciously makes an effort to follow-up on students who do not seek help. Professor requests that Pat meet during office hours to discuss the written paper assignment, stating, "When students share their questions and feedback concerning papers and the class, it helps me a great deal. Could you please help me by stopping by to talk about the paper?" *Result*: Pat receives the necessary help needed and passes the assignment. Positive academic and psychological outcomes occur.

messages permit the open sharing and exchange of cultural information that is a necessary precursor to mutually satisfying interactions with culturally different individuals.

> What new strategies can you implement in your course to communicate that culture and students matter? In your program? In off-campus clinical settings? On your campus?

Interaction

> When was the last time you entered a culturally different world or felt like the "outsider"? How did you feel, think, and act? Why?

It is not sufficient for educators to have read about cultures, attended workshops, professed commitment to cultural competence, or surveyed students; faculty must take action and enter a new phase in the journey of achieving cultural competence. Campinha-Bacote (4) calls this interaction phase "cultural encounter." Leininger (70) however defines cultural encounter as a situation in which someone meets or briefly interacts with a culturally different individual. Such a brief encounter fails to allow deep understanding or insight into the culture (70). In this book, cultural interaction refers to the ongoing, planned, and unplanned situations in which faculty and students with various, different CVB have shared experiences or interactions. The faculty member committed to the goal of developing cultural competence and providing culturally congruent advisement and helpfulness will make a concerted effort to actively initiate and engage in cultural interactions throughout the educational process and possibly beyond graduation and into the student's entry into the nursing profession.

Cultural interaction leads to greater insight into the student's culture on the individual level. Interactions offer the opportunity to recognize the cultural variations that exist among individuals, families, and groups (70). Through ongoing interactions, the discovery that cultural variations exist and impact differently on faculty–student interactions, persistence, and all dimensions of culture helps prevent stereotyping of individuals based on perceived cultural group affiliation. Cultural interaction fosters the exchange of CVB, thus facilitating personal growth, professional growth, and the development of cultural competence for educators and students.

An initial interaction that values, appreciates, and embraces diversity will do much for encouraging the further exchange of information, values, beliefs, and ideas as well as promoting positive psychological outcomes (satisfaction and decreased stress) associated with the educational experience.

Entering a culturally different or unknown world can be intimidating or stressful for fear making a mistake or inadvertently doing something "wrong." Such fears are a barrier to initiating and engaging in substantive cultural interactions with students. Acknowledging ahead of time that mistakes may occur is important; however, learning from one's mistakes and moving forward is even more important. A "cultural mistake" can make one more consciously competent next time when encountering a similar or even different situation.

Cultural competency must never be taken for granted. One cannot really ever be totally culturally competent, but one can exert conscious effort into achieving cultural congruence. Insight can be enhanced by self-reflection and reflection-in-action (71). Reflection calls for ongoing self-assessment, updated knowledge, consultation, collaboration, student assessment, analysis, plan, communication, and cultural interactions.

> Prior to reading this chapter, when was the last time you reflected on your cultural congruence as an advisor and/or helpful teacher? When will you reflect in the future?

KEY POINT SUMMARY

- Faculty advisement and helpfulness are manifested through faculty actions such as encouraging realistic educational and career goals, promoting positive feelings of self-worth, verbalizing belief in the student's ability to succeed, listening to problems and concerns, expressing interest in academic progress, optimism, offering assistance, and presence.

- A culturally congruent approach to faculty advisement and helpfulness refers to those faculty actions that are tailored to fit with the student's cultural values and beliefs (CVB) in order to promote, facilitate, or support meaningful, beneficial, and satisfying academic endeavors, career goals, and professional socialization.

- The process of developing cultural congruence and becoming "culturally competent" faculty advisors and helpful teachers includes self-assessment, literature review, consultation and collaboration, student assessment, analysis, plan, communication, and interaction.

APPLICATION STRATEGIES ▬▬▬▬▬▬▬▬▬

EASY APPLICATION ACTION STEPS

Developing a Culturally Congruent Approach to Faculty Advisement and Helpfulness

1. List ideas for each step of the process (self-assessment, literature review, consultation and collaboration, student assessment, analysis, plan, communication, and interaction).
2. Develop a timeline for implementation and evaluation.
3. Implement, evaluate, and modify accordingly.

EDUCATOR-IN-ACTION VIGNETTE

Without appropriate background knowledge, individual appraisal, and sensitivity, educators' actions may adversely impact upon students' academic and psychological outcomes, persistence, and retention. In contrast, culturally sensitive actions incorporated within clearly defined boundaries for advisement and helping behaviors have the most potential for promoting positive academic and psychological outcomes, persistence, and retention. Consider the possible effects on students and other faculty colleagues in the situations described in the dialogue scenarios.

Scenario 1

PROFESSOR SOLO: I do everything for my students all by myself. Why refer students with personal crises, financial aid questions, health issues, test anxiety, library search problems, or academic difficulty to some stranger over in another part of campus? I was a psychiatric nurse for many years at the state mental health clinic. I've heard it all. There's nothing I can't handle.

PROFESSOR BEST: Well, it really isn't about what you can handle or what your clinical expertise is. It should be about what's best for the student. Although I worked as a mental health nurse and at the student health center for many years, my hired position and job description as a tenure-track college professor defines my teaching and advisor roles, hours, and expectations. I'm not hired as a registered nurse; I'm hired as a college professor and am expected to carry out my role like my colleagues in other departments. That includes referring students to the appropriate college resources and guiding them as needed. I don't want students to become dependent on me. Besides, specific departments and resources have updated expertise to answer a specific need. In addition, some students would feel uncomfortable sharing personal information with me and then seeing me in class or the clinical setting. At the beginning of the semester, I share a handout about student resources around the college and encourage the students to use them as appropriate during the semester, and I follow up as needed with students.

Scenario 2

PROFESSOR HUGGS: I love helping our students. Many of our minority, middle-aged, and immigrant students have so many obstacles and challenges facing them. When they are successful on an exam or perform well in clinical, I just give them the hugs they don't get from their families. Of course, I only hug students when they deserve it. For the men, I just give them a pat on the back when they do well. A handshake would be so impersonal.

PROFESSOR LAW: I have three major concerns here. First, you may be making many stereotypical assumptions about your students. Second, perceptions about nonverbal communication, touch, space, and distance vary culturally. Even handshakes may have different positive or negative interpretations within different cultures related to gender and socioeconomic or other status differences. Third, there are boundaries between students and faculty advisors that are there for many ethical and legal reasons. For example, the college policy concerning sexual harassment defines acceptable and unacceptable behaviors. Your behaviors could be misinterpreted on many levels.

Scenario 3

PROFESSOR QUICK: That Native American student with the big backpack—I forgot her name—but she always looks down at the floor when she's talking to me and takes a long time to respond when I ask a question. She must be drinking or on drugs and not doing her work. When she finally responds, I just can't trust her because she avoids looking directly at me. I don't have time for this when I have so many other students who just know exactly what they want from me and spit it right out.

PROFESSOR LIGHT: The student's name is Jessica. She is in my clinical course and is excelling in her academic and clinical work. In the clinical postconference discussion focused on communication patterns, she shared that she has many traditional Cherokee traditions, values, and communication styles. Among many traditional Native American groups, silence is expected to enhance understanding and exemplifies respect for the other person. Avoidance of eye contact also indicates respect and that the person is paying close attention to what is being said. Nonverbal and verbal communication patterns, values, and meanings vary so much culturally. I have an excellent journal article that highlights some of these issues that I will share with you. It taught me to be more aware of cultural differences and similarities. To best meet the needs of our students, we should work together to embrace diversity and consciously prevent ethnocentrism, stereotypes, discrimination, cultural imposition, and cultural pain. Whether cultural misunderstandings are intentional or not—cultural pain still hurts and can last a long time after a cultural mistake occurs.

Scenario 4

PROFESSOR MATCH: I decided it would be quicker and best to pair up some of my first-semester students with former students of the same background, especially for the ESL [English as a second language] students. I can't understand why my students don't seem to appreciate my help in doing this.

PROFESSOR FRANK: Well, it might be because you were offering help that wasn't wanted or because you mismatched students and created cultural pain. For example, you told a Puerto Rican student who has a current GPA of 4.0 and a previous masters' degree in biology to be tutored by a second-semester international student from Nigeria with a 2.5 GPA; you then told them to join the National Black Nurses Association so they would feel less alone in a foreign country. Both students felt extremely hurt, although the Nigerian student was very reluctant to talk about it. Then, you paired an international student from Taiwan with a recent immigrant from the Philippines stating, "You can speak to each other in your native language since you are from the same country." Neither of those students challenged your suggestion because they wanted to "save face" and not be confrontational; however, another student overheard what happened, became upset, and told me about it. Beside the fact that the two students are from different countries and speak different primary languages, there are also many different languages and dialects spoken within the Philippines as well as in Mainland China that are different from that in Taiwan. In another case, you paired two students from the same country who spoke the same language however they were not really compatible study partners because one student was in an unhappy and abusive arranged marriage to a wealthy U.S. citizen and the other financially struggling student was in a happy marriage to a man from her native country; she was worried that he might be deported in a few months due to visa and work restrictions. This created an uncomfortable, embarrassing, stressful, and fearful situation for both students so that is when I discovered them crying in the study lounge. They did not want to challenge your authority as a teacher.

Scenario 5

PROFESSOR PONDER: I was lost with how to help Lena improve her grades. I decided to refer her to you because you offered to help me in the past and you shared some valuable literature with faculty on cultural competence.

PROFESSOR BOOKE: As I conversed with Lena, I discovered that she had difficulty with multiple-choice questions because she had never been exposed to them in her primary and secondary education. I mentioned a few NCLEX [National Council Licensure Examination] review books but then realized that she was economically disadvantaged and might be reluctant to accept charity either due to pride or due to religious reasons. I then called her to my office next week after class and asked her if she would help me out by using an NCLEX review book given to me free by the publisher, return it at the end of the semester, and give me feedback so I could make decisions about which books to recommend to students. I also did this with several other students and several books so that no one would feel stigmatized and all be helping me (but also learning how to successfully answer nursing type questions).

TOOLKIT RESOURCE BOX

Item 16—Cultural Values and Beliefs: Faculty Self-Assessment

Item 17—Cultural Values and Beliefs: Student Self-Assessment

Item 29—Culturally Congruent Approach to Nursing Faculty Advisement and Helpfulness

Item 23—Promoting Positive Help-Seeking Behaviors

Item 24—Appraising Teaching Strategies: Potential Effect on Diverse Populations

Item 26—Strategy Mapping Across the Curriculum

Items 1–4—Student Perception Appraisal Questionnaires—Pretests and Posttests

DISCUSSION QUESTIONS

1. Identify three areas in the chapter that provided you with the most learning. Discuss what you learned that was new and how this will impact on your role as a nurse educator when teaching, advising, and interacting with academically and culturally diverse male and female students representing various ages, ethnicities, religious affiliations, socioeconomic levels, immigration status, and first languages.

2. Review the first advisement situation in Table 10.1. What are your thoughts and feelings? How would you handle the advisement session? Now, discuss your thoughts, feelings, and advisement actions when the characters of "Shari and her husband" are substituted with each of the following: (a) a gay couple, Robert and Mark; (b) a lesbian couple, Mary Ellen and Loretta; (c) an Orthodox Jewish married couple, Ruth and David; (d) a multiracial married couple, Amina and Kareem; (e) a couple with an apparent age gap of 20 years; (f) a clergyman and his wife; (g) student Maribel and her husband George who was recently released

from prison; (h) student Bob and his wife on leave from active military duty; (i) an obese couple; (j) a couple using canes for ambulation; and (k) a 19-year-old couple living together in off-campus housing. Did you discover any differences in your initial thoughts and feelings with the different couples presented? Why? How can awareness of your thoughts and feelings influence future interactions with diverse student populations?

3. Professor Overly states, "I came in on my day off to meet with two single-parent students to review their exam paper because they could not make my office hours due to their children's soccer practice. Then they didn't show up. That's not the first time it's happened. Although I have a 3-day teaching schedule and schedule our required 3-hour weekly office hours broken up over the 3 days, I find that I am commuting in to campus 5 days a week to meet with students who have such horrendous work schedules and family lives. Sometimes they show up; other times they don't. I know that's to be expected of the Latino students who have a relaxed view of time and put family first but even some of the poor Whites and others do it. Many students end up dropping out or failing anyway but I still want to be there for them. I even spend an hour or more with some students while they review their old exams. It must pay off because after doing this a few semesters, my subsequent students are getting high scores on my exams. Because I am spending so much time advising students, I have not been able to update my exams so I just keep using the old ones. It must be working because now everyone does well in my class. After they leave my class, they get other instructors who don't do all this and then they end up failing. All faculty should be like me, but they're not. I am trying to figure out ways to help my former students who are now in other classes." What are some of the major issues and concerns in this scenario? How should they be addressed?

4. What did you learn from the Educator-in-Action Vignette? How can the vignette be adapted for use with faculty in your program?

5. A faculty colleague suggests that it is too late to change tenured faculty but that culturally congruent faculty advisement and helpfulness should be incorporated into a formal orientation and mentoring program for new faculty advisors. How would you respond?

REFERENCES

1. Leininger, M. M. (1991). *Culture care diversity and universality: A theory of nursing,* (p. 49). New York, NY: National League for Nursing.
2. Purnell, L. D. (2008). Purnell's model for cultural competence. In L. D. Purnell & B. J. Paulanka (ed.), *Transcultural health care: A culturally competent approach* (3rd ed.) (pp. 19–55). Philadelphia, PA: FA Davis.
3. Leininger, M. M., & McFarland, M. R. (2002). *Transcultural nursing: Concepts, theories, research, and practice* (3rd ed.). New York, NY: McGraw-Hill.

4. Campinha-Bacote, J. (2003). *The process of cultural competence in the delivery of healthcare services: A culturally competent model of care* (4th ed.). Cincinnati, OH: Transcultural C.A.R.E. Associates.

5. Campinha-Bacote, J. (2007). *The process of cultural competence in the delivery of healthcare services: The journey continues.* Cincinnati, OH: Transcultural C.A.R.E. Associates.

6. Campinha-Bacote, J. (2010). A culturally conscious model of mentoring. *Nurse Educator, 35*(3), 130–135.

7. Campbell, A. R., & Davis, S. M. (1996). Faculty commitment: Retaining minority nursing students in majority institutions. *Journal of Nursing Education, 35*(7), 298–303.

8. McLaughlin, B. N. (2008). Retention issues: What can we do? *Teaching and Learning in Nursing, 3,*83–84.

9. Ackerman-Barger, P. W. (2010). Embracing multiculturalism in nursing learning environments. *Journal of Nursing Education, 49*(12), 677–682.

10. Bond, M. L., Gray, J. R., Baxley, S., Cason, C. L., & Denke, L. (2008). Voices of Hispanic students in baccalaureate nursing programs: Are we listening? *Nursing Education Perspectives, 29*(3), 136–142.

11. Bosher, S. D., & Pharris, M. D. (2009).*Transforming nursing education: The culturally inclusive environment.* New York, NY: Springer Publishing.

12. Flinn, J. B. (2004). Teaching strategies used with success in the multicultural classroom. *Nurse Educator, 29*(1), 10–12.

13. Gardner, J. (2005). Barriers influencing the success of racial and ethnic minority students in nursing programs. *Journal of Transcultural Nursing, 16*(2), 155–162.

14. Gilchrist, K. L., & Rector, C. (2007). Can you keep them? Strategies to attract and retain nursing students from diverse populations: Best practices in nursing education. *Journal of Transcultural Nursing, 18*(3), 277–285.

15. Kuh, G. D., & Love, P. G. (2000).A cultural perspective on student departure. In, J. M. Braxton (Ed.) (2000). *Reworking the student departure puzzle.* Nashville, TN: Vanderbilt University Press, 196–212.

16. Nnedu, C. C. (2009). Recruiting and retaining minorities in nursing education. *Association of Black Nursing Faculty Journal, 20*(4), 93–96.

17. Olinger, B. H. (2011). Increasing nursing workforce diversity: Strategies for success. *Nurse Educator, 36*(2), 54–55.

18. Pijl-Zieber, E. M., & Hagen, B. (2011).Towards culturally relevant nursing education for aboriginal students. *Nurse Education Today, 31*(6), 595–600.

19. Creasey, G., Jarvis, P., & Gadke, D. (2009). Student attachment stances, instructor immediacy, and student-instructor relationships as predictors of achievement expectancies in college students. *Journal of College Student Development, 50*(4), 353–372.

20. Komarraju, M., Musulkin, S., & Bhattacharya, G. (2010).Role of student-faculty interactions in developing college students' academic self-concept, motivation, and achievement. *Journal of College Student Development, 51*(3), 332–342.

21. Lundquist, C, Spalding, R. J., & Landrum, R. E. (2002). College student's thoughts about leaving the university: The impact of faculty attitudes and behaviors. *Journal of College Student Retention: Research, Theory, and Practice, 4*(2), 123–134.

22. Shelton, E. N. (2003). Faculty support and student retention. *Journal of Nursing Education, 42*(2), 68–76.

23. Strayhorn, T. L. (2010). Majority as temporary minority: Examining the influence of faculty-student relationships on satisfaction among White undergraduates at Historically Black Colleges and Universities. *Journal of College Student Development, 51*(5), 509–524.
24. Alexitch, L. R. (2002). The role of help-seeking attitudes and tendencies in students' preferences for academic advising. *Journal of College Student Development, 43*(1), 5–19.
25. Herndorn, J. B., Kaiser, J., & Creamer, D. G. (1996).Student preferences for advising style in community college environments. *Journal of College Student Development, 37*(6), 637–647.
26. Baldwin, D., & Wold, J. (1993). Students from disadvantaged backgrounds: Satisfaction with a mentor-protégé relationship. *Journal of Nursing Education, 32*(5), 225–226.
27. Gasper, M. L. (2009).Building a community with your advisees. *Nurse Educator, 34*(2), 88–94.
28. Harrison, E. (2009). (Re)Visiting academic advising. *Nurse Educator, 34*(2), 64–68.
29. Lehna, C., Jackonen, S., & Wilson, L. (1996).Navigating a nursing curriculum: Bridges and barriers. *Association for Black Nursing Faculty Journal, 7*(July/August), 98–103.
30. Peters, M. A. A. (2008). Defining the boundaries of the nurse faculty role. *Nurse Educator, 33*(5), 193–197.
31. Schultz, E. D. (1998). Academic advising from a nursing theory perspective. *Nurse Educator, 22*(2), 22–25.
32. Trent, B. A. (1997). Student perceptions of academic advising in an RN-to-BSN program. *Journal of Continuing Education in Nursing, 28*(6), 276–283.
33. Winters, C. E. (1990). Excellence in advisement: A strategy for declining nursing enrollments. *Journal of Nursing Education, 29*(5), 233–234.
34. Yoder, M. K., & Saylor, C. (2002). Student and teacher roles: Mismatched expectations. *Nurse Educator, 27*(5), 201–203.
35. Poorman, S. G., Webb, C. A., & Mastorovich, M. L. (2002). Students' stories: How faculty help and hinder students at risk. *Nurse Educator, 27*(3), 126–131.
36. Leininger, M. M. (1978). *Transcultural nursing: Theories, concepts, and practices.* New York, NY: John Wiley & Sons.
37. Barbee, E. L., & Gibson, S. E. (2001). Our dismal progress: The recruitment of non-whites into nursing. *Journal of Nursing Education, 40*(6), 243–244.
38. Bessent, H. (1997). *Strategies for recruitment, retention, and graduation of minority nurses in colleges of nursing.* Washington, DC: American Nurses Publishing.
39. Campinha-Bacote, J. (1998). Cultural diversity in nursing education: Issues and concerns. *Journal of Nursing Education, 37*(1), 3–4.
40. Colosimo, R., & Xu, Y. (2006). Research on shame: Implications for English as a second language nursing students. *Home Health Care Management and Practice, 19*(1), 72–75.
41. Kirkland, M. L. S. (1998). Stressors and coping strategies among successful female African American baccalaureate nursing students. *Journal of Nursing Education, 37*(1), 5–12.
42. Labun, E. (2002). The Red River College Model: Enhancing success for native Canadian and other nursing students from disenfranchised groups. *Journal of Transcultural Nursing, 13*(4), 311–317.

43. Literte, P. E. (2010). Revising race: How biracial students are changing and challenging student services. *Journal of College Student Development, 51*(2), 115–134.
44. Love, K. L. (2010).The lived experience of socialization among African American nursing students in a predominantly white university. *Journal of Transcultural Nursing, 21*(4), 342–350.
45. Manifold, C., & Rambur, B. (2001).Predictors of attrition in American Indian nursing students. *Journal of Nursing Education, 40*(6), 279–281.
46. Reynolds, A. L., Sneva, J. N., & Beehler, G. P. (2010). The influence of racism-related stress on the academic motivation of Black and Latino/a students. *Journal of College Student Development, 51*(2), 135–149.
47. Tucker-Allen, S., & Long, E. (1999). *Recruitment and retention of minority students: Stories of success.* Lisle, IL: Tucker Publications.
48. Villaruel, A. M., Canales, M., & Torres, S. (2001). Bridges and barriers: Educational mobility of Hispanic nurses. *Journal of Nursing Education, 40*(6), 245–251.
49. Weaver, H. N. (2001). Indigenous nurses and professional education: Friends or foes? *Journal of Nursing Education, 40*(6), 252–258.
50. Yurkovich, E. E. (2001). Working with American Indians toward educational success. *Journal of Nursing Education, 40*(6), 259–269.
51. Jeffreys, M. R., & Smodlaka, I. (1996). Steps of the instrument-design process: An illustrative approach for nurse educators. *Nurse Educator, 21*(6), 47–52; (erratum, 1997, 22(1), 49).
52. Curran, V., Solberg, S., LeFort, S., Fleet, L., & Hollett, A. (2008). A responsive evaluation of an Aboriginal nursing education access program. *Nurse Educator, 33*(1), 13–17.
53. Yearwood, E., Brown, D. I., & Karlik, E. C. (2002). Cultural diversity: Students' perspectives. *Journal of Transcultural Nursing, 13*(3), 237–240.
54. Padilla, R. V. (1999). College student retention: Focus on success. *Journal of College Student Retention: Research, Theory, and Practice, 1*(2), 131–146.
55. Knowles, M. (1984). *The adult learner: A neglected species.* Houston, TX: Gulf.
56. Roufs, A. (2007). In theory, advising matters. In: P. Fulson (Ed.), *The new advisor guidebook: Mastering the art of advising through the first year and beyond* (pp. 33–37). Kansas, MO: NACADA.
57. Braxton, J. M., & Mundy, M. E. (2001).Powerful institutional levers to reduce college student departure. *Journal of College Student Retention: Research, Theory, & Practice, 3*(1), 91–118.
58. Hammond, P. V., Davis, B. L., Hodges, G., & Warfield, M. (1997). Increasing retention rates of disadvantaged students through a faculty development program. *The Association of Black Nursing Faculty Journal, 8*(3), 51–53.
59. Hesser, A., Pond, E., Lewis, L., & Abbott, B. (1996).Evaluation of a supplementary retention program for African-American baccalaureate nursing students. *Journal of Nursing Education, 35*(7), 304–309.
60. Kirkpatrick, M. K., & Koldjeski, D. (1997). Career planning: The nurse educator as facilitator and career counselor. *Nurse Educator, 27*(3), 17–20.
61. Nora, A. (2001). The depiction of significant others in Tinto's "Rites of Passage": A reconceptualization of the influence of family and community in the persistence process. *Journal of College Student Retention: Research, Theory, & Practice, 3*(1), 41–56.

62. Rew, L. (1996). Affirming cultural diversity: A pathways model for nursing faculty. *Journal of Nursing Education, 35*(7), 310–314.
63. Sherrod, R. A., & Harrison, L. (1994). Evaluation of a comprehensive advisement program designed to enhance student retention. *Nurse Educator, 19*(6), 29–33.
64. Yoder, M. K. (2001). The bridging approach: Effective strategies for teaching ethically diverse nursing students. *Journal of Transcultural Nursing, 35*(7), 315–321.
65. Phinney, J. S. (1996). Understanding ethnic diversity. *American Behavioral Scientist, 40*(2), 143–152.
66. Andrews, M. (1995). Transcultural nursing: Transforming the curriculum. *Journal of Transcultural Nursing, 6*(2), 4–9.
67. Jeffreys, M. R. (2000). Development and psychometric evaluation of the Transcultural Self-Efficacy Tool: A synthesis of findings. *Journal of Transcultural Nursing, 11*(2), 127–136.
68. Jeffreys, M. R. (2010). *Teaching cultural competence in nursing and health care: Inquiry, action, and innovation* (2nd ed.). New York, NY: Springer Publishing.
69. Leininger, M. M. (1995). Teaching transcultural nursing in undergraduate and graduate programs. *Journal of Transcultural Nursing, 6*(2), 10–26.
70. Leininger, M. M. (2002). Essential transcultural nursing care concepts, principles, examples, and policy statements. In M. M. Leininger, & M. R. McFarland (eds.), *Transcultural nursing: concepts, theories, research, and practice* (3rd ed.) (pp. 45–69). New York, NY: McGraw-Hill.
71. Schon, D. (1987). *Educating the reflective practitioner*. San Francisco, CA: Jossey-Bass.

Expanding the Web of Inclusion Through Professional Events and Memberships

Participation in nursing conferences, workshops, events, meetings, and memberships exemplifies a professional commitment to lifelong learning that can be motivating and uplifting to students.

SNAPSHOT SCENARIO

Professor Bland arrives at the registration desk for a Nursing Alumni Association (NAA) annual conference and quickly nods a greeting to Jill and Richard, two of her undergraduate students enrolled in her nursing issues course. She thinks, "If I didn't have to obtain CEs [continuing education units] this year to renew my license, if my dean wasn't an alumnus here, and if I wasn't up for my annual evaluation, I certainly wouldn't be here. I only renewed my NAA membership because it gave me a discount at this conference. Hopefully, the awards luncheon has good food. Thank goodness, Jill and Richard are here together. Hopefully, they will just observe the conference and not bother me. It's just my luck that two of my students chose to complete the course requirement for attending a professional conference here. The last course coordinator added this requirement into the course with the approval of the curriculum committee so I have to comply."

Jill looks around thinking, "I better not take off my windbreaker. I don't see anyone else here wearing jeans and a T-shirt. I'll really stick out. At least Richard is with me; he's wearing a golf shirt, chinos, and high top sneakers."

Richard thinks, "I didn't expect to see so many people here of different ages. They can't all be undergraduates completing an assignment. I'm surprised to see many men here too. At school, there is only one other man in our class and he and I are so different, I'd been wondering if I really belonged in nursing."

Jill and Richard stay on the periphery of the conference activities, even during break time when others network. One of the speakers in front of Jill on the lunch buffet line introduces herself and says, "I see by your nametag that you are an undergraduate student. It's so nice to see undergraduate students here. How are you enjoying the conference so far?" Jill responds, "Fine" before turning quickly to Richard saying, "Why do you think the speaker's talking to me? What should I do? This is stressing me out." Richard says, "Forget about it. Some people are just chatty. Let's just get our lunch, sit at the back table, and cut out before the awards ceremony. We did our required 3 hours, got our 3.0 CE certificate, and Professor Bland already saw that we were here."

In contrast, Elle and Mario arrive at the registration desk dressed in neat business attire and are warmly greeted by Professor Bridges who says, "Elle and Mario, I'm so pleased to see you arrived early so we can network together. You both look very professional. You're already pre-registered, so this is where you check in to get your conference materials. Do you have any questions?"

Elle says, "Not right now, thanks. The chapter readings and class discussion about professional conferences, professional associations, memberships, nursing image, and networking makes me feel prepared."

Mario says, "Yes, I feel comfortable and have been looking forward to this day to experience my first of many professional conferences. The role-play activity we did in class helped me feel prepared too. But I especially liked the 20-minute video clips of a conference you attended last year. Reading conference proceedings just isn't the same as actually seeing a conference in action."

After check-in, Professor Bridges leads them to the coffee room and introduces them to several colleagues and speakers. Elle and Mario engage in conversation about professional topics, the conference, and share information about their future goals when asked. The students accept business cards from several of Professor Bridges's colleagues and one of the speakers. Elle and Mario are delighted when their business cards are graciously accepted too and they receive positive comments. Mario thinks, "I initially thought it was a waste of time to design and create a business card with 'RN student' after my name, but now I am glad we had this as a class assignment." Elle thinks, "Wow, we are being treated as if we are such important additions to the nursing profession. It feels good. Some of the stories Professor Bridges's colleagues shared are inspiring, especially the person who is receiving the most prestigious award. I couldn't believe all the struggles encountered along the journey toward becoming a nurse...and then to think what this person has accomplished now 30 years later! It's amazing! I feel more confident now about becoming a nurse despite all the struggles I might encounter along the way."

What thoughts and feelings do you have about the scenarios above?

Participation in professional events and memberships is viewed as an essential activity for professional growth and career mobility by providing unique opportunities for professional socialization, networking, skill enhancement, knowledge expansion, and professional attitude development (1). Professional events are nursing conferences, workshops, meetings, volunteer services, or social activities that have specific goals relevant for nursing education, practice, research, or theory. Memberships refer to affiliation or participation within nursing organizations or associations as a "member" prescribed by the respective bylaws (see Chapter 6).

Within the NURS model, participation in professional events and memberships is viewed as an essential component for enhancing professional integration and minimizing social isolation. Professional integration greatly enhances nursing student retention by promoting positive psychological outcomes and offering opportunities to enrich academic experiences and academic outcomes. It is proposed that positive experiences in professional event participation and memberships positively affect retention by enhancing self-efficacy and motivation, promoting professional integration, and facilitating positive psychological outcomes.

Although nursing students may feel a sense of cohesiveness or belonging within the classroom or clinical group, many still feel somewhat detached and disconnected from the nursing profession. This isolation is counterproductive and prevents students from achieving their optimal potential within nursing. Gaining entry and starting to feel part of the nursing professional is crucial. Nursing students must become "enculturated into nursing values, norms, and lifeways to survive, function, and become professional nurses"(2, p. 56).

Consequently, the nursing profession is challenged to include, embrace, and welcome nursing students as future valuable assets to the profession. Nurse educators are challenged to expand the web of student inclusion beyond the traditionally required educational curriculum and setting through professional events and memberships. In this book, the web of inclusion refers to an interwoven professional network that embraces students and strives to promote professional integration through participation in professional events and memberships.

Unfortunately, many nursing students (and nurse educators) undervalue and underestimate the significance of professional event participation and memberships. Visionary nurse educators are therefore challenged to develop innovative strategies and incentives to motivate students and encourage participation. Students often encounter numerous obstacles that discourage them from professional event participation and memberships. Nurse educators can first assist students by recognizing these obstacles, removing barriers, and offering acceptable solutions. Strategies that enhance student opportunities to participate in various professional integration factors will ultimately benefit students and the nursing profession. The purpose of this chapter is to discuss creative strategies for expanding the web of inclusion by enhancing student opportunities for participation in professional events and memberships. Barrier recognition, solutions, strategies, and incentives will be proposed.

> What are your views about the potential influence of students' participation in professional events and memberships on academic achievement, professional development, satisfaction, stress, and retention?

NURSE EDUCATORS AS ROLE MODELS

> To what degree are you an active promoter of student participation in professional events and memberships? What strategies do you actively implement consistently? What strategies can be enhanced or added?

Participation in nursing conferences, workshops, events, meetings, and memberships exemplifies a professional commitment to lifelong learning that can be motivating and uplifting to students. Professional nurses as role models can enhance self-efficacy and motivation, thereby enhancing student persistence and retention. Because students have most exposure to the nursing profession through faculty guidance, nurse educators exert powerful influence on them. If faculty do not value professional event participation and memberships for their own professional development, then it is hard to imagine that they would have a positive impact on encouraging student participation. Similarly, if nurse educators are actively involved in professional events and memberships, yet do not actively publicize their views, involvement, participation, and contribution to professional events and memberships, positive professional role modeling will not be evident to students.

Faculty self-assessment as active role model in promoting/facilitating student professional event participation and memberships is a necessary precursor for strategy development. Table 11.1 provides a guide for appraising values, beliefs, and actions and for determining whether one is an active role model. It is proposed that the actions taken to promote/facilitate participation make one an active role model. Table 11.1 can also provide a guide for organizational self-assessment to determine if organizations are "student friendly" (inclusive) or if there are obstacles obstructing student participation, thus creating "student unfriendly" (exclusive) environments (see Toolkit Item 18).

After self-assessment, nurse educators who have not optimally shared positive views, values, beliefs, and experiences with students should make a concerted effort to do so. However, it is not enough to profess

TABLE 11.1 Self-Assessment: Active Role Model in Promoting/Facilitating Student Professional Event Participation and Memberships

ROLE MODEL	VALUES, BELIEFS, AND ACTIONS	ROLE MODEL
Yes	Views professional event participation and membership as important in own life *and shares beliefs with students**	No
Yes	Views memberships in nursing organizations/associations as important in own life *and shares beliefs with students*	No
Yes	Views professional event participation as important in undergraduate students' education and/or professional development, and/or retention *and shares view with students*	No
Yes	Views student memberships in nursing organizations/associations as important in undergraduate students' education and/or professional development, and/or retention *and shares view with students*	No
Yes	Attends professional events *and shares positive and relevant experiences with students*	No
Yes	Maintains membership(s) in nursing organizations/associations *and shares positive and relevant experiences with students*	No
Yes	Recognizes actual and potential barriers hindering student's professional event participation *and initiates strategies to remove barriers*	No
Yes	Recognizes actual and potential barriers hindering student memberships *and initiates strategies to remove barriers*	No
Yes	*Offers incentives to encourage student participation in professional events*	No
Yes	*Offers incentives to encourage student participation in memberships*	No

*Active promoter/facilitator actions are indicated by italics.

values and beliefs to students; nurse educators must be sincerely committed and take positive actions in order to "make a difference" and enhance the "web of inclusion." In order to do this, they must recognize actual and potential barriers hindering students' participation, propose solutions, initiate strategies to remove barriers, and offer incentives to enhance participation.

Barriers may be practical or psychosocial. Practical barriers include financial cost, travel, and time (Table 11.2). Psychosocial barriers include perceived irrelevance to immediate educational goals, perceived irrelevance to future professional goals, multiple role stress, and fear of

TABLE 11.2 Student Participation in Professional Events and Memberships: Practical Barriers, Solutions, Strategies, and Incentives

BARRIERS	SOLUTIONS	STRATEGIES AND INCENTIVES
Financial cost	Waive fee Reduce fee	Sponsorship Award or scholarship Volunteer worker Service exchange Group discounts Student fee
Travel	Eliminate travel Enhance ease of travel	Host event Carpools Charter bus Public transportation group travel Clear directions
Time	Eliminate extra time needed Minimize time conflicts/ burden	Event corresponds with class time Sufficient advance notice Time exchange from class Schedule before or after class Readjust class assignment and test schedule Assistance with application related tasks

isolation (Table 11.3). Often, students are faced with a combination of practical and perceptual barriers.

What practical and psychosocial barriers are faced by your students?

PRACTICAL BARRIERS: RECOGNITION, SOLUTIONS, STRATEGIES, AND INCENTIVES

Financial Cost

For many students, the financial cost of a conference, workshop, or membership is a large deterrent. Although a reduced student fee or rate may be an incentive to some, it may not be enough to attract diverse student groups. For example, an economically disadvantaged student or a nontraditional student struggling with tuition, living expenses, and child-care costs may be unable to afford fees or may be unable to justify financial resource allocation to a "nonessential" expense. Even the "luxury" of a conference may not be justified for someone who is unsure of financial stability. As a strategy to increase membership participation, incorporating National Student Nurse Association (NSNA) membership as a mandatory

TABLE 11.3 Student Participation in Professional Events and Memberships: Psychosocial Barriers, Solutions, Strategies, and Incentives

BARRIERS	SOLUTIONS	STRATEGIES AND INCENTIVES
Perceived irrelevance to immediate educational goals	Demonstrate relevance to immediate educational goals	Link with course objectives Link with course assignments Link with test questions Provide background information Extra credit Mandatory participation Student certificates for participation
Perceived irrelevance to future professional goals	Demonstrate relevance to future professional goals	Faculty role models Student role models Professional role models Link with legal and ethical issues Link with criteria for a profession Professional portfolio and resume Educational mobility Career mobility
Multiple-role stress	Reduce role stress Demonstrate strategies to manage multiple roles effectively	Sufficient advance notice Case examples Letter to employer Written materials for significant others Extended college child-care services
Fear of isolation	Eliminate fear of isolation Minimize fear of isolation Promote feelings of inclusion	Link with faculty buddy or other RN Student role models Introduction to other students Introduction to presenters and/or members Networking during lunch and break times Encourage student involvement Publicize student involvement Student outreach and welcome

curricular requirement and instituting a student fee to cover this expense may assist financially challenged students to get this expense covered via financial aid, scholarships, and/or student loans.

Waiving of professional event fees may be a more productive option in yielding student participation; however, it may not always be feasible due to the need to meet overhead costs and expenses. An alternative to fee waivers may be soliciting sponsorship by nursing faculty, other nurses, alumni, deans, agencies, members of professional organizations, and organizations themselves. An incentive to individuals for sponsoring a student may be a reduction in conference or membership fees; for example, "sponsor a student, save 10%" or "sponsor one student, bring another student for free." Nurse educators can actively suggest options to sponsoring agencies or organizations such as offering an award or scholarship to student volunteers, students with the highest GPAs, or elected student nurse club (SNC) officers.

Another option may be to waive fees in exchange for volunteer services, such as assistance with workshop registration or stuffing membership renewal envelopes. Offering discounts for groups of students suggests that students are welcome and desired audience; group discounts encourage students to attend together while also sharing costs. Offering a 20% discount for every group of five students is one such example. Other expenses associated with attending a professional event may be travel, food, parking, lodging, or child care, which can impose severe restrictions for many students. Any effort to include these other expenses when approaching potential sponsors will enhance opportunities for many financially challenged students or financially unsure (insecure) students.

> What strategies and/or incentives do you implement to remove or reduce financial barriers for students' professional event participation and memberships? What else could you implement?

Travel

Travel costs and concerns can be minimized through the use of organized carpools, charter buses or vans, or group travel via public transportation. Ambiguous or unclear travel directions are a major deterrent. The nurse educator can facilitate the ease of travel by providing directions from the nursing school and/or organizing group car travel from the familiar location of the school. Assuring that directions are provided via the various modes of transportation available from the school will serve to include more students. By offering to host a professional event sponsored by a nursing organization, nurse educators can assure that students will have optimal opportunity to attend a professional event on campus in a nearby, familiar setting, thus easing travel concerns.

> What strategies and/or incentives do you implement to remove or reduce travel barriers for students' professional event participation? What else could you implement?

Time

Time demands from numerous responsibilities and roles may compete with participation in professional events and memberships. Sufficient advance notice of events is particularly important to allow for work schedule requests, child-care coverage, and other responsibilities that compete with the students' time in school, family, and work arenas. Nurse educators can minimize time demands by readjusting class schedules to accommodate participation in a professional event, such as shifting course topics and changing assignment due dates or test dates to avoid conflicts with the event.

Whenever possible, nurse educators should plan professional events into the class schedule in advance. This serves as a powerful incentive to students. Time exchange from class for events scheduled during the regular class meeting time accommodates students. For events scheduled outside the usual class session, time exchange minimizes burdens on time. Time exchange also demonstrates the nurse educator's commitment to the importance of professional event participation.

Complicated registration forms or membership application forms create additional time demands to complete them and may actually discourage students. Nurse educators can facilitate the ease of registration/application by distributing forms in class, providing clear instructions, allowing for in-class completion time, and assisting with other required tasks. For example, the nurse educator can coordinate group mailings, photocopying student identification cards, and collecting student fees.

What time incentive strategies do you implement to facilitate students' participation in professional events? What works? How have they been evaluated? What strategies could you implement?

PSYCHOSOCIAL BARRIERS: RECOGNITION, SOLUTIONS, STRATEGIES, AND INCENTIVES

What psychosocial solutions, strategies, and incentives for student's participation in professional events and memberships are implemented in your course? In your program?

Perceived Irrelevance to Immediate Education Goals

The perceived irrelevance to immediate educational goals is a major obstacle to student participation. Adult learners typically place importance on tasks directly and immediately related to the achievement of educational and/or career goals (3,4). Consequently, the nurse educator is challenged to change existing values and beliefs that negate or minimize the significance of professional events and memberships in achieving immediate goals. For the undergraduate student, immediate goals usually refer to successful achievement at the individual course level. Nurse educators can begin by tapping into the student's motivation at the immediate course level. By specifically addressing students' immediate desired educational goals, educators can link participation in professional events with course objectives, course assignments, and test questions. For example, the course outline can clearly delineate participation in professional events as a course objective that complements other course objectives and the course description. If a professional event will take place during the usual class time, the nurse educator can schedule the event as part of class. This is especially convenient if the event is held on campus or nearby. Time off from class can help accommodate students if the event is scheduled outside of the usual class meeting time.

Mandatory participation without a link to course objectives, assignments, test questions, or other incentives may not be sufficient to change students' attitudes toward valuing professional events and developing a commitment to lifelong learning. Course assignments connected to the professional event encourage students to become "active participants" rather than just attending. (See Chapter 4 concerning definitions of attendance.) Faculty requiring students to attend events to complete assignments or participate in class discussions means that students are involved with each other outside the classroom. This intentionally brings students in ongoing contact with one another and with other resources (5–7).

Engaging the student via written assignments, oral presentations, or class discussions should link some aspect of the professional event with course content and include a reflective component. Reflection encourages the transition from preprofessional education to professional education and is essential for affective learning (8). Affective learning refers to changes in attitudes, values, or beliefs. It is difficult to evaluate because it takes longer than psychomotor or cognitive learning and is difficult to measure; however it is critical for professional development (9,10). Multiple choice, short answer, and/or essay questions based on the professional event further validate professional event participation. A written assignment grade, test item points, or test grade that directly impacts upon the course grade validates professional event participation as significant enough to award a quantitative measure that will affect the immediate course grade and progression in the nursing curriculum.

Mandatory attendance (participation) assures that all students are exposed to a professional event; however, it does not assure that students will have a positive experience, develop a lifelong commitment to professional learning, or gain positive benefits associated with professional event participation. The nurse educator has the unique opportunity to provide necessary background information about the professional event that may enhance students' experiences. It may be necessary to focus students on a particular area or feature of the professional event. Preparing and reviewing expectations concerning assignments based on professional event participation may aid in focusing students on the most course-relevant features of the event. Assigned articles, chapters, movies, or other materials before the event serve as an advance organizer and provide essential background information to maximize the experience. Similarly, assigned reading or films after the event may support or expand upon the experience, rather than just complementing it.

Other incentives include offering extra credit for professional event participation. However, this will not affect all individuals. In fact, this strategy may really target the most self-directed, motivated individuals or, on the other end of the continuum, attract the most desperate, failing students who view professional event participation as a last resort for passing the course. Offering certificates for attendance, free books, or other items may not be sufficient enough to target students who are focused on immediate goals such as successfully achieving academic outcomes. Certificates, awards, and/or oral acknowledgment of students at the professional events may, however, assist in enhancing positive psychological outcomes for nursing.

Mandatory membership in the NSNA is a requirement in some nursing programs; the relevancy to immediate educational goals is evident. Writing a letter to the editor in response to an article in the NSNA journal, *Imprint*, can engage students more actively through participation rather than merely affiliation. Again, linking course objectives, assignments, course topics, and test questions with membership in NSNA will motivate students. Another incentive is to encourage active student participation in NSNA through NSNA Leadership U, where students can earn academic credit for their documented participation in NSNA leadership activities (11).

> How have activities for promoting students' participation in professional events and memberships been linked to immediate course goals in your course? What have other course instructors done in your program? What else can be done?

Perceived Irrelevance to Future Professional Goals

Frequently, students' myopic views fail to recognize the long-range benefits of professional event participation and memberships to future professional goals. This limited view is another barrier to participation.

First, nurse educators can provide personal testimonies about the numerous benefits attributed to professional event participation and memberships. For example, upon return from a nursing research conference sponsored by a nursing organization, the nurse educator can distribute or display materials relevant to the course and to possible future professional goals, such as a working nurse in a clinical specialty area. Second, soliciting advanced students to share their positive experiences in professional events and memberships and how these experiences enhanced and facilitated achievement of their educational goals and future professional goals further substantiates the nurse educators' perspective. Students are most influenced by peers with whom they most readily self-identify; therefore, the value of peer influence can be astounding. Third, professional role models such as clinical preceptors or invited guest speakers during class time can provide additional testimonies substantiating the significance of professional event participation and memberships in professional goal attainment. Fourth, faculty can mentor students at professional events, create an open and inclusive environment, transform the professional event into a reflective practicum, and pose probing questions to stimulate reflection-in-action thinking and dialogue. "A reflective practicum is an experience of high interpersonal intensity. The learning predicament, the students' vulnerability, and the behavioral worlds created by coaches and students critically influence learning outcomes" (8, p. 171).

Discussing legal and ethical issues in nursing (licensure, certification, competency, and standards of practice) within the context of the "criteria for a profession" has relevance to future professional goals. Exploration of individual future goals can personalize educational and career mobility options and the relevance of professional event participation and memberships beyond the broad topic of "professional issues." Professional events and memberships as part of professional portfolio and resume development can be introduced as a class topic and later evolve into an actual assignment to develop a professional portfolio, resume, and business card. Mock job interviews can also address professional event participation and membership.

> How have activities for promoting student participation in professional events and memberships been linked to future professional goals? What have other course instructors done in your program? What else can be done?

Multiple-Role Stress

> What are the multiple roles and responsibilities of your students outside the academic setting?

Stress related to multiple-role conflict is particularly relevant to nontraditional students with multiple-role responsibilities outside the academic setting. Eliminating, reducing, and managing multiple-role stress (MRS) effectively are all appropriate goals. To accomplish this, nurse educators must identify, introduce, and demonstrate strategies for decreasing stress and effectively balancing multiple roles. Anxiety may result when students perceive that professional event participation and membership adversely interfere with the management of multiple roles and responsibilities. They can perceive it to be "one more responsibility" that competes with precious time. Participation in this "extra" responsibility upsets the fragile balance between an overwhelming number of responsibilities. Stress and anxiety associated with school-related tasks adversely influence persistence and retention through negative psychological outcomes (see Chapter 7).

Therefore, it behooves nurse educators to develop and explore strategies to minimize stress and anxiety and assist students in managing multiple roles and responsibility. So what can nurse educators do? Sufficient advance notice is a primary strategy. Inadequate notice of a required or elective (extra credit) participation in an event or membership-related task increases stress and anxiety and decreases the probability that all students will be able to participate. Furthermore, the probability that students will associate positive psychological outcomes to the professional event participation is greatly reduced.

Acknowledging that students have multiple roles and busy lives, while also providing case examples of how other students have effectively balanced similar multiple roles is helpful. Asking nontraditional students with multiple roles who successfully managed professional events and memberships and multiple-role responsibilities to share experiences is a powerful incentive to students. Advance and ongoing collaboration with on-campus child-care facility to extend services beyond scheduled class sessions to allow for participation in professional events and memberships may be essential to students who rely solely on college child-care services.

Letters to employers and significant others may help obtain the necessary time off, reassigned time, or redelegated tasks to allow for student participation. For example, a letter that identifies the potential benefits to a hospital agency when a student working as a nursing assistant gets a requested day off to participate in a professional conference increases the likelihood that requested time off will be granted. A direct benefit may be that the knowledge learned at the conference will then be carried out in the workplace setting, potentially enhancing patient outcomes and satisfaction. Other indirect and direct benefits may include employee satisfaction, loyalty to the institution, employee retention, and the desire to continue working at the agency after licensure as a registered nurse. Similarly, written materials listing benefits can increase understanding among family members or essential support persons who may be asked to assume some additional household responsibilities or child-care tasks. For example, a spouse who reads that participation at a professional workshop is required and sees the listed benefits may be more willing to assume additional household or child-care tasks to permit attendance at this event. In contrast, an uninformed spouse may be opposed to what appears to be an unnecessary, optional event that he or she perceives will prevent the student from completing usually held household and/or child-care tasks.

What strategies have you implemented and evaluated to reduce possible stress associated with activities for professional event participation and memberships? What have other course instructors done in your program? What else can be done?

Fear of Isolation

Fear of isolation is an imposing barrier to many undergraduate nursing students. Ultimately, eliminating the fear of isolation and promoting feelings of inclusion are the desired goals. One effective strategy is to link student(s) with a buddy (faculty member, nursing alumni, or other RN). This may be done by assigning a buddy link at a professional event or within a nursing organization/association. It may be a one-time link for an event or may be more long term and evolve into a mentor–protégé relationship.

To enhance the web of inclusion at a professional event, nurse educators should make every effort to introduce students to professional colleagues and other students. If possible, introduction to key nursing leaders, presenters, or members can make an important impression on students through validation. Validation is especially important for nontraditional students (older, commuter, and/or minority) and has been positively linked with persistence behaviors and retention (12,13). Encouraging students to take part in picture-taking sessions, question–answer sessions, meetings, and evaluation questionnaire completion provides a realm of diverse opportunities for student inclusion. Informal and formal networking during lunch and break times also serves to include students. Seeking and innovatively shaping opportunities to mentor and connect students with each other and with diverse members of the nursing profession creates an open, inclusive environment (14,15).

The nurse educator who is actively involved in a professional event and/or nursing organization can enhance the web of inclusion more directly by means of a welcome address, closing address, editorial, newsletter, or letter that acknowledges and embraces students. Positive feelings associated with the professional event and/or organization will be promoted. Showcasing pictures of student participants via a webpage, website, poster display, slide show, newsletter, or bulletin board illustrates student-friendly (inclusive) environments. Other students as role models are a powerful influence on student motivation, self-efficacy, and persistence.

> What strategies have you implemented and evaluated to foster feelings of inclusion, equality, trust, and connection? What have other course instructors done in your program? What else can be done?

KEY POINT SUMMARY

- Professional events are nursing conferences, workshops, meetings, volunteer services, or social activities that have specific goals relevant for nursing education, practice, research, or theory.
- Memberships refer to affiliation or participation within nursing organizations or associations as a "member" prescribed by the respective bylaws.
- Positive experiences in professional event participation and memberships positively affect retention by enhancing self-efficacy and motivation, promoting professional integration, and facilitating positive psychological outcomes.
- The "web of inclusion" refers to an interwoven professional network that embraces students and strives to promote professional integration through participation in professional events and memberships.
- In order to "make a difference" and enhance the "web of inclusion," nurse educators must recognize actual and potential barriers hindering student's participation, propose solutions, initiate strategies to remove barriers, and offer incentives to enhance participation.

APPLICATION STRATEGIES

EDUCATOR-IN-ACTION VIGNETTE

Professor Webb teaches the first-semester nursing course and introduces the importance of professional organizations and memberships during the first class lesson. Background prerequisite reading assignments, an in-class video, and class discussion complement a brief lecture.

Heidi and several other students think, "This is nice, but it doesn't seem real."

Next, Professor Webb shares some lively yet relevant personal positive anecdotes concerning professional conferences, organizations, and networking. With student interest sparked, he invites students to attend a conference sponsored by a professional nursing specialty organization.

Heidi skeptically thinks, "It's a long way off before I'm a nurse. What does this have to do with me now?"

Professor Webb distributes a brochure to each student, pointing out that the intended audience listed in the brochure includes nursing students. The potential benefits of student attendance at the upcoming conference are highlighted and correlated with course objectives, course topics, and future professional development.

Heidi ponders, "Maybe this is relevant to me. But it is so expensive. I can't afford this. Besides, I might feel out of place."

As an added incentive, he announces that several faculty members and college administrators volunteered to sponsor students and pay for their conference fees. Arrangements for three clinical groups to attend the conference in lieu of clinical will permit three cohorts of students to attend together during regularly scheduled class time.

Tiffany feels elated that she is in one of the groups and thinks, "Faculty must really think it's important if they took all this effort and their own money to sponsor us."

Other students interested in attending are invited to enter a college "conference fee" raffle open to all undergraduate nursing students. Faculty colleagues publicize the conference and raffle in their respective courses; announcements are placed on bulletin boards and student e-mail listservs. The raffle will be held during a SNC meeting featuring an outside guest speaker from the conference planning committee.

Still somewhat skeptical and pessimistic, Heidi says to another student, "I never win at raffles, why should I bother?" Optimistically, Heidi's friend Petra says, "We have nothing to lose by going. Besides, the speaker might be interesting. If not, there's always the refreshment social to look forward to."

The enthusiastic and inspirational speaker networks with students during the SNC refreshment social. Student integration in nursing is enhanced and positive feelings about nursing are nurtured. The speaker stops to chat with Petra and Heidi about nursing. Heidi now thinks, "I really would like to go to the conference." When Petra wins the raffle, Heidi is happy for her friend but disappointed that she will not be able to attend.

Next week, Professor Webb coordinates the mailing of student registration forms and fees. Several students who are not selected via the raffle decide to pay for their own fees. Because the sponsoring organization offers one free student fee for every ten paid fees, additional students can attend. Heidi is thrilled that she is asked to attend but is concerned about traveling and feeling out of place.

Professor Webb organizes several carpools for students living in nearby neighborhoods. One instructor offers to meet other students at the bus stop for group travel via public transportation. Departure time, anticipated arrival time, professional dress code, and conference activity expectations are reviewed with students. Heidi and Petra join a carpool with three other students, confident that they know more about what to expect and what is expected of them.

Upon arrival, students are greeted by members of the sponsoring organization and by student volunteers from the sponsoring host site. Because students arrive early, they have the added opportunity to talk with other attendees, observe preconference networking in action, ask questions, become acclimated to the environment, and review conference packet materials. As a member of the nursing specialty organization, Professor Webb uses this opportunity to introduce featured speakers to students. Several of the speakers and organizational members engage in professional dialogue with students and provide encouragement for their educational and professional endeavors. Students comment that this made them feel "included," "welcome," "relaxed," and "excited about nursing." Heidi and Petra feel pleasantly surprised when the SNC guest speaker remembers them and comes over to talk with them.

Other opportunities for dialogue occur during coffee breaks, lunch, and the poster session. The welcome address, closing address, and keynote speakers direct several comments specifically to students, thus further promoting validation and professional integration. All attendees are invited to enter a raffle of select nursing items, including two memberships in the specialty nursing organization. One membership is specifically earmarked for an undergraduate nursing student and includes a subscription to the bimonthly specialty journal and quarterly newsletter. When Heidi wins the membership, she excitedly offers to share her journals and newsletters with other students in the class.

During the next class session, Professor Webb asks students to write what they most liked about attending the conference. A subsequent brief class discussion allows for the sharing of ideas between students. Overwhelmingly positive experiences and the desire for more opportunities to attend nursing conferences are voiced.

TOOLKIT RESOURCE BOX

Item 18—Active Promoter Assessment Tool: Student Professional Events and Memberships

Item 25—Professional Integration and Socialization

Items 3 and 4—Student Perception Appraisal—Revised Questionnaires Pretest and Posttest

DISCUSSION QUESTIONS

1. Professor Change proposes that faculty incorporate a professional event participation component in each undergraduate nursing course. She notes that only two of the six nursing courses currently include a required component in the course outline; one course lists professional event participation as an option for 5 extra points on the final exam. It is unclear if students are required to do anything besides produce a certificate or letter validating attendance at the event.

   Professor Clock says, "There is no time to add this in a busy course where I have to lecture fundamental content and skills. If students make it through my course and the high-tech course after mine, they can just have this requirement in the last semester's nursing issues course."

   Assume the role of Professor Change. How would you respond to Professor Clock?

2. Professor Uno says, "I once paid for the two sophomore class representatives to attend the conference sponsored by our nursing honor society chapter. One of them showed up 15 minutes late wearing sweaty workout clothes from a morning Latin dance aerobics class. The other student never showed up and told me she was home finishing a paper instead. I was very angry and vowed to never get involved with this again. I just stick with doing things in the classroom or clinical setting."

   Assume the role of Professor Change above. How would you respond to Professor Uno?

3. Professor Tech says, "Nowadays, there are more options for participating in professional conferences via independent or small group webinars and videoconferencing. Students don't even have to leave the campus or even their living rooms to get all they need to from professional events when using these media." How would you respond?

4. Professor Game proposes initiating an essay contest to enhance awareness of and participation in professional associations currently and for lifelong professional development. Three senior students would be chosen to receive paid memberships in the selected professional association. The ideas are outlined below:

   Students will
   (a) Select one professional association from a list of professional associations that permit student memberships
   (b) Review association's website, bylaws, journal or other publications, and event calendar
   (c) Write a 750–1000-word essay describing personal and professional rationale for desired membership with current role as a student and future nursing goals

   Professor Always says, "We always require our students to become members of the National Student Nurses Association. That should be sufficient. We don't need to change anything."

Professor Sloth says, "We have enough work to do already, especially with all these students dropping out or stopping out. I can't tell if they are serious or not about nursing. Organizing a contest and reading essays is just more work without any program results, especially if only three students get any benefits. It seems like three students win and the rest of us, especially overworked faculty, are losers."

How would you respond to each person? What additional suggestions would you propose?

5. How can the Educator-in-Action Vignette be adapted for use with students in your course?

REFERENCES

1. Joel, L. A., & Kelly, L. Y. (2002). *The nursing experience: Trends, challenges, and transitions*. New York, NY: McGraw-Hill.
2. Leininger, M. M., & McFarland, M. R. (2002). *Transcultural nursing: concepts, theories, research, and practice* (3rd ed.). New York, NY: McGraw-Hill.
3. Brookfield, S. D. (1990). *Understanding and facilitating adult learning*. San Francisco, CA: Jossey-Bass.
4. Knowles, M. S. (1984). *The adult learner: A neglected species* (3rd ed.). Houston, TX: Gulf.
5. Kuh, G. D. (2001). Organizational culture and student persistence: Prospects and puzzles. *Journal of College Student Retention: Research, Theory, and Practice, 3*(1), 23–40.
6. Tinto, V. (1997). Classrooms as communities. *Journal of Higher Education, 68*(6), 599–623.
7. Seidman, A. (2005). *College student retention: Formula for success*. Westport, CT: American Council on Education, Praeger.
8. Schon, D. (1987). *Educating the reflective practitioner*. San Francisco, CA: Jossey-Bass.
9. Bevis, E. O. (1989). *Curriculum building in nursing: A process* (2nd ed.). New York, NY: National League for Nursing.
10. Oermann, M. H., & Gaberson, K. B. (2009). *Evaluation and testing in nursing education*. New York: Springer.
11. National Student Nurses Association. (2012). *NSNA Leadership U*. Retrieved from http://www.nsnaleadershipu.org/nsnalu
12. Rendon, L. I. (1994). Validating culturally diverse students: Toward a new model of learning and student development. *Innovative Higher Education, 19*(1), 23–32.
13. Rendon, L. I., Jalomo, R. E., & Nora, A. (2000). Theoretical considerations in the study of minority student retention in higher education. In J. M. Braxton (Ed.), *Reworking the student departure puzzle* (pp. 127–156). Nashville, TN: Vanderbilt University Press.
14. Vance, C., & Olson, R. K. (1998). *The mentor connection in nursing*. New York, NY: Springer Publishing.
15. Vance, C. (2011). *Fast facts for career success in nursing: Making the most of mentoring in a nutshell*. New York, NY: Springer Publishing.

Promoting Positive and Productive Peer Partnerships

Creating caring communities of learners is essential for optimizing student success and retention.

After completing background reading, classroom, and nursing skills lab activity components on communication, infection control, and safety, beginning students meet for their first clinical preconference at the local hospital. After a brief welcome and introductions, Professor Light says, "I realize some of you may be anxious about your first day in the hospital and what the nursing unit may be like. Before you are assigned to interview or care for any patients, we will visit our assigned unit to get familiar with your new surroundings. Let's take a walk there and look around." After the group walks once around the busy medical unit, Professor Light pulls the group aside and says, "Now we will play a scavenger hunt game. I've assigned you a partner and have an index card listing several items. You will have 10 minutes to find each item and write down where it is located. You will not actually acquire the item or enter any patient rooms. You must remain with your partner at all times and work together. You cannot ask for or accept help from anyone else on the unit. We will then meet back in the conference room in 10 minutes. Let's see who will finish first."

Each card had a combination of similar and different eight items such as fire alarm, fire extinguisher, exit door, code cart, drug reference book, hospital policy and procedure book, telephone, staff bathroom, towel, pillow case, patient gown, scale, bandaid, clean (nonsterile) glove, toilet paper, garbage bag, bedpan, water pitcher, bath basin, blood pressure cuff, thermometer, and isolation cart. Students seemed surprised over the assignment; some pairs were hesitant to get started but after the first group got moving, the rest scattered across the unit more enthusiastically. Partners talked, walked, and smiled as they found items together.

When students returned to the conference room in 10 minutes, Professor Light asked each student to first reflect and then write down the following: (1) the most important thing they learned from the scavenger hunt (cognitive) and (2) what feelings they had during and after the learning activity (affective). Each student then shared his or her reflection, and a collaborative discussion ensued, with Professor Light modeling how to dialogue as colleagues, providing positive comments for insights shared, asking probing questions to prompt further dialogue when indicated, and openly valuing students' comments and questions. Here are some excerpts:

CHRIS: I discovered that I missed a lot when we first toured the unit. It made me realize I need to pay attention to details so I can function efficiently on the unit. It took a long time to find things because I didn't pay attention to important items like the fire alarm and the code cart. At first, I felt overwhelmed coming to the hospital. I felt less anxious working with a partner, especially after I discovered she also was feeling a lot of the same things I was feeling. I feel less alone now and feel like we can count on each other during the semester.

BRIDGET: I learned that it would be helpful to communicate with all staff members, even the housekeeping staff. Jamie and I were searching for toilet paper and it took forever. It would have been easier and quicker to just ask the housekeeper. That delayed us in finding other items on the list like the code cart—an item that a registered nurse needs to locate quickly. One of the nurses asked if we needed help so this made me feel relieved, welcome, and less anxious. I don't usually ask for help easily, but now I not only feel more comfortable asking friendly staff members but also realize that for the benefit of patient care and time management I must ask for help when needed.

RUTH: Well, I learned that I was overly confident in thinking that clinical would be easy because I am a nursing assistant. I work on a different unit in this hospital and things are organized differently here. I also learned that in my new goal to become a registered nurse, I would need to pay attention differently and look for different things. For example, I never needed to concern myself with knowing where the hospital policy and procedure book was, or the drug reference book. Initially, I felt scared and extremely anxious when my bubble of overconfidence burst, but working together with a kind partner who was more modest in her confidence put me at ease and showed me it's okay to not be totally confident about everything all of the time. At first, I felt angry being assigned a partner. I would have chosen Nancy as a partner because we work together, attend the same church, and live in the same neighborhood. Now I see the value of working with others of different backgrounds.

DEBBIE: I learned that there are two different types of bedpans that can be used for different patients and purposes. My partner works in a nursing home so she explained it to me. I always studied alone in the past but now I see the value of talking with my classmates. I felt angry initially about wasting valuable clinical time doing something so juvenile like a scavenger hunt game. My feelings changed once I realized that the activity was not a time waster but actually bringing together all the major points from this week's reading in a way I didn't understand before. I didn't value spending time learning about communication and professional collaboration but now I do.

> What are your views about the potential influence of class friends on academic achievement, professional development, satisfaction, stress, and retention? What are your views on student-centered activities? What peer partnerships do you encourage?

Interaction or "active engagement" is instrumental for effective learning (1). The educational literature profusely advocates multidimensional strategies that enhance opportunities for student-centered interactive learning experiences (1–37). Moreover, the quality of student interaction influences professional socialization, academic integration, psychological growth, self-efficacy, and motivation. In turn, such factors influence student persistence, academic outcomes, satisfaction, and levels of stress (38,39). Therefore, nurse educators have the responsibility to structure student-centered interactive experiences that enhance the potential for quality student interactions.

High-quality, rewarding, and positive student (peer) interactions may result in class friendships. Friends in class are mutually bonded in career goals, expectations, and stage of educational and professional development. The main focus of in-class friends is on the common academic goal of successfully completing course requirements and becoming a registered nurse. The NURS model proposes that encouragement by friends in class will actively promote positive psychological outcomes, self-efficacy, professional socialization, persistence, and retention (see Chapter 6). In contrast, lack of class friends will adversely affect retention through social isolation, dissatisfaction, stress, low self-efficacy, and decreased motivation.

Student interactions, however, do not automatically result in friendships; nurse educator intervention can be beneficial. While nurse educators cannot "make" classmates become friends, they can make a difference or assist in the process by creating opportunities and conditions that support and nurture peer interactions. Ultimately, a series of carefully patterned and interwoven student-centered interactive experiences throughout the nursing curriculum can be structured to promote positive and productive peer partnerships. In this book, positive and productive peer partnerships are those purposeful affiliations, alliances, and connections among peers that result in constructive, generative, creative, and desirable outcomes. Desirable outcomes include both the process and product of learning; quantitative (academic) and qualitative (psychological) outcomes are expected. One desirable outcome is that positive and productive peer partnerships are valuable precursors to initiating class friendships and to fostering encouragement by friends in class.

Desirable educational and professional outcomes can only be achieved through a faculty commitment to promoting positive and productive peer partnerships during all phases of the nursing educational process. Professional integration and partnerships must be seen as a priority and accepted as part of the mission, vision, and values of the school. Unfortunately, some nursing faculty may underestimate the potential influence of class friends in academic achievement, professional development, satisfaction, stress, and retention; student-centered activities may also be undervalued (18,40). Additionally, some nurse educators may lack prior experience with designing, implementing, and evaluating student-centered interactive learning experiences. Similarly, students may underestimate the influence of class friends and/or student-centered interactive learning activities. Student perceptions of friendships, learning, education, and peers can be influenced by student profile characteristics, affective factors, and environmental factors. Consequently, visionary nurse educators are challenged to structure quality student-centered experiences that are maximally valued, optimally utilized, and mutually desired. Nurse educators are also challenged to solicit support from colleagues and truly integrate student-centered interactive learning experiences throughout the curriculum with the specific aim of promoting positive and productive peer partnerships. The purpose of this chapter is to describe strategies for promoting positive and productive peer partnerships. Benefits, barriers, solutions, and strategies will be presented.

NURSE EDUCATOR AS ACTIVE PROMOTER

> To what degree are you an active promoter of positive and productive peer partnerships? What strategies do you actively implement consistently? What strategies can be enhanced or added?

Professional partnerships are a crucial part of future professional nursing roles (18,41–44). Students must not only be introduced to the concept of professional partnerships but also must acquire the necessary skills and learn to value partnerships throughout the educational process and a career as a professional nurse (14,44). This necessitates innovative strategies and sincere commitment on the part of nurse educators, who must be willing to become coparticipants and develop connections or partnerships with students. These connections can create communities of learners who are partners in the learning process whereby the nurse educator shifts the focus from teaching to learning (45,46). In this student-centered philosophy of learning, the role of the teacher is to guide, support, and coach learners throughout their educational journey and become active promoters of positive and productive peer partnerships.

As mentioned earlier, nurse educators exert powerful influence on students. If faculty do not value professional partnerships for their own professional development, then they are unlikely to encourage student interactions, partnerships, or friendships. Similarly, if nurse educators are actively involved in professional partnerships, yet are not vocal about their participation, students will be deprived of positive professional role modeling in this important area. For example, spending 2 minutes during class to tell students about positive experiences last week from work on a manuscript, research study, or college or clinical project with professional colleagues with periodic updates and other shared information strategically placed to correspond and tie with course or professional topics can do much to consistently and gradually shape students' perceived value of professional partnerships. In addition, a faculty member can share pertinent examples from his or her own undergraduate education in which positive and productive peer partnership enhanced learning, increased satisfaction, and decreased stress.

Comparable to faculty self-appraisal in the previous chapter, faculty self-assessment as active promoters of positive and productive peer partnerships is a necessary precursor for strategy development. Table 12.1 provides a guide for appraising values, beliefs, and actions and for determining whether one is an active promoter. It is proposed that the "actions taken" are what makes one an active promoter. Table 12.1 can also provide a guide for nursing curriculum self-assessment to determine if nursing programs actively promote positive and productive peer partnerships through their program philosophy, learner outcomes, and planned interventions or if there are obstacles present. Intentional planning in coordinated activities aimed at capturing the power of the peer group within the classroom should be a priority and is instrumental in developing a community of learners (47).

After self-assessment, nurse educators who have not optimally shared positive views, values, beliefs, and experiences with students should make a concerted effort to do so. However, it is not enough to profess values and beliefs to students; nurse educators must be sincerely committed and take positive actions. They need to recognize actual and potential barriers to students' development of positive and productive peer partnerships, propose solutions or goals, initiate strategies to remove barriers, and offer incentives.

TABLE 12.1   Self-Assessment: Active Promoter of Positive and Productive Peer Partnerships

PROMOTER	VALUES, BELIEFS, AND ACTIONS	PROMOTER
Yes	Views professional partnerships as important in own life *and shares beliefs with students**	No
Yes	Views positive and productive peer partnerships as important in undergraduate students' education, professional development, and retention *and shares view with students*	No
Yes	Views "encouragement by friends in class" as important in undergraduate students' education, professional development, and retention *and shares view with students*	No
Yes	Views own nurse educator role to include active involvement in promoting positive and productive peer partnerships among undergraduate students *and shares view with students*	No
Yes	Maintains professional partnerships *and shares positive and relevant experiences with students*	No
Yes	Updates own knowledge and skills about professional partnerships routinely *and shares relevant information with students*	No
Yes	Recognizes actual and potential barriers hindering student's development of peer partnerships *and initiates strategies to remove barriers*	No
Yes	*Implements strategies to encourage student development of positive and productive peer partnerships*	No
Yes	*Evaluates implemented strategies designed to encourage student development of positive and productive peer partnerships*	No

*Active promoter/facilitator actions are indicated by italics.

Although numerous barriers may exist, only the major ones will be highlighted here. Barriers may be categorized as practical or psychosocial. Practical barriers include (1) insufficient background information and/or skills, (2) insufficient in-class opportunities, (3) insufficient out-of-class opportunities, and (4) curricular inconsistency (see Table 12.2). Psychosocial barriers include perceived irrelevance to immediate educational goals, perceived irrelevance to future professional goals, stress, and fear of isolation (see Table 12.3). Students are often faced with a combination of practical and psychosocial barriers.

What practical and psychosocial barriers are faced by your students?

TABLE 12.2 Positive and Productive Peer Partnerships: Practical Barriers, Solutions, Strategies, and Incentives

BARRIERS	SOLUTIONS	STRATEGIES AND INCENTIVES
Insufficient background information and/or skills	Integrate adequate learning of the knowledge and skills necessary for developing positive and productive peer partnerships	Course outline Course objectives Course prerequisite assignments Course topics
Insufficient in-class opportunities	Integrate learner-centered student interactive teaching-learning strategies Maximize opportunities for positive and productive peer partnerships within class	Small group discussion Large group discussion Case study Gaming Group simulation Simulated role play Role play Debate Group presentation (oral, PowerPoint) Interview Storytelling Group film (video) production Group poster Paired writing draft critique Paired problem-based learning Paired computer-based learning Paired technical skills practice Paired technical skills testing Paired or group clinical assignment *For web-based courses*: Paired or group e-mails Paired or group course discussion boards Paired or group chat rooms
Insufficient out-of-class opportunities	Integrate learner-centered student interactive out-of-class activities Maximize opportunities for positive and productive peer partnerships outside of class	Assignments involving all of above Library literature review Paired or group computer-assisted instruction Professional event participation Professional memberships Enrichment programs Nursing student resource centers
Curricular inconsistency	Integrate learner-centered student interactive activities, opportunities, and incentives throughout the nursing curriculum	Systematic curriculum evaluation Concept-mapping Curricular threads Faculty development workshops

TABLE 12.3 Positive and Productive Peer Partnerships: Psychosocial Barriers, Solutions, Strategies, and Incentives

BARRIERS	SOLUTIONS	STRATEGIES AND INCENTIVES
Perceived irrelevance to immediate educational goals	Demonstrate relevance to immediate educational goals	Link with course objectives Link with course assignments Link with test questions Provide background information Pew Commission recommendations Low stakes writing assignments Reflection
Perceived irrelevance to future professional goals	Demonstrate relevance to future professional goals	Faculty role models Student role models Professional role models Link with legal and ethical issues Link with criteria for a profession Benefits to self and others Educational mobility Career mobility
Stress	Eliminate stress Reduce stress Manage stress	Stressor identification Realistic appraisal of strengths Realistic appraisal of weaknesses Strength enhancement Weakness remedies Student role models Judicious, positive feedback Realistic goals
Fear of isolation	Eliminate fear of isolation Minimize fear of isolation Promote feelings of inclusion	Acknowledge fears Open, caring, and trusting environment Value of all learners Initial student self-selection Appraisal of strengths and weaknesses Assigned partners or groups

PRACTICAL BARRIERS: RECOGNITION, SOLUTIONS, STRATEGIES, AND INCENTIVES

Insufficient Background Information and/or Skills

Students, especially beginning (novice) students, may lack sufficient background knowledge and/or skills necessary for developing positive and productive peer partnerships in nursing. Even more advanced students may need supplementary information to nurture, promote, foster, and expand the knowledge and skills needed to continue positive and productive peer partnerships throughout the formalized educational process and beyond. Nurse educators must aim to integrate the necessary background information and/or skills needed at various levels in the nursing curriculum.

Congruency between course objectives, prerequisite assignments, course topics, class activities, and methods of evaluation (with clear evidence of partnership development throughout) will help students integrate the necessary knowledge, skills, and attitudes needed to optimize positive and productive peer partnerships as an educational and professional outcome. For example, prerequisite readings related to group dynamics, communication, and group process, supplemented by an in-class video about professional collaboration and followed by an in-class discussion, can assist students in synthesizing information prior to initiating a small-group interactive teaching–learning strategy. Additionally, if students are to develop positive and productive peer partnerships, they must have sufficient background knowledge about a select topic to contribute equally as partners. Careful selection of prerequisite assignments that corresponds with intended interactive activities is a necessary precursor for success.

Insufficient In-Class Opportunities

What opportunities do you provide in class for promoting the development of positive and productive peer partnerships?

Perhaps one of the greatest barriers hindering students' development of positive and productive peer partnerships is insufficient in-class opportunity for quality student interaction. The most effective solution is to carefully integrate learner-centered student interactive teaching and learning strategies throughout the course, building upon previous interactive activities. Active learning is crucial for peer interaction. Because students have diverse learning needs, strengths, values, and beliefs, weaving multidimensional active learning activities throughout the course will be most beneficial. Student's cultural values and beliefs (CVB) will influence how various strategies are valued, interpreted, and used; therefore, nurse educators should take this into consideration while planning, implementing, and evaluating activities (48,49) (see Chapter 3).

Learner-centered student interactive strategies may involve students working in pairs, small groups, and/or large groups. Table 12.2 lists several examples. In general, strategies should involve collaborative or cooperative learning, in which all participating students are partners in the process. Collaborative learning experiences positively impact on learning outcomes, academic achievement, satisfaction, stress reduction, motivation, self-efficacy, and student retention, especially among diverse student populations (38,50,51). Additionally, problem-based collaborative

learning corresponds with Pew Commission competency recommendations (52), further impressing upon nurse educators to offer generous
in-class opportunities.

Specific strategies have advantages and disadvantages. Pairing students eliminates the potential for an audience and enhances the potential for in-depth quality student interactions that can foster cognitive and
affective growth (16). Groups, however, provide greater opportunities for
diverse thinking. Outcome benefits can be maximized with clear directions, group rules, well-matched group composition, effective leadership,
immediate feedback and guidance, reflection, and adequate time allocation (53). Storytelling with reflection is another effective strategy, especially
among culturally diverse learners (12,54–56). For many students, gaming, debate, and role play are effective mechanisms for active, enjoyable
learning that results in positive cognitive, psychomotor, and/or affective
outcomes (21,26,27,30,57–60); yet, individual competitiveness may be con-
trary to some students' CVB. Recently, the use of student response systems
or clickers in the classroom actively engage students simultaneously in a
nonthreatening way, provide immediate feedback to student and teacher,
foster climates of inclusiveness, thereby enhancing overall satisfaction for
learning (22–25). The Internet (web-based courses) provides opportunities
for interactive learning in pairs, small groups, and large groups via individual e-mails, group e-mails, course chat rooms, course discussion boards,
blogs, and wiki (61–67); however, awareness of potential online intercultural miscommunication partnered with proactive strategies to facilitate
intercultural communication is essential (68). Most recently, webcasting
permits audio and visual presentations via the Internet, including live class
participation via personal computers (63,69–71). Creatively integrating
YouTube within the classroom or online environment can stimulate active
learning, heighten relevance to actual real-life situations, and prompt lively
discussions (72). Other new technology, such as podcasting, permits various options that can enhance learning (but not replace in-classroom active
participation), especially among nontraditional learners with English as
a second language (ESL), dyslexia, and/or multiple-role responsibilities
(71,73,74). Virtual learning platforms offer students a unique opportunity to
transfer and apply knowledge and skills within a wide range of culturally
diverse and clinically diverse patients within a safe learning environment
(29,75,76). Students must be computer-literate, confident, and motivated if
computer-based strategies are to be effective. Conclusively, nurse educators have many learner-centered student interactive strategies from which
to choose; however, the educator must be adequately prepared, knowledgeable about student variables, committed, and caring.

In-class opportunities for positive and productive peer partnerships
critically depend upon a caring, safe, open environment that is intentionally shaped to embrace all students as unique, individual, and valuable contributors to the learning process. This is essential for optimizing

student success and retention, especially among nontraditional students (77). First, faculty attitudes and actions that demonstrate caring serve as a powerful role model to students. Next, faculty guidance, feedback, and intervention structure and nurture caring environments within the classroom, clinical, or laboratory setting. Subtle ways that certain students may become marginalized include unequal attention and respect to comments, method of calling on students, and type and amount of feedback and dialogue. Nurse educators should carefully observe small and large group dynamics noting hierarchical power distribution (who is the leader, who are delegates, who does what) in relation to gender, race, age, ethnicity, language (accent), religion, socioeconomic background, course grades, and so on, and encouraging equal opportunity for various group roles as needed. Both faculty and peers play a meaningful role in creating a caring, supportive environment (78).

> What strategies do you implement to create open, caring, classroom environments that facilitate the development of positive and productive peer partnerships? What works? How have they been evaluated? What strategies are implemented by your colleagues consistently throughout the program? What other strategies could be implemented?

Insufficient Out-of-Class Opportunities

> What out-of-class opportunities for peer partnerships do you encourage?

In-class opportunities are major factors in the initiation of positive and productive peer partnerships that can be overseen and guided by nurse educators. However, such partnerships can be enhanced greatly through ongoing out-of-class interactions as well. One benefit of out-of-class student interactions is that students may feel free to share ideas, thoughts, and opinions without the educator present. Partnerships, social networks, and friendships can develop, increasing academic and psychological benefits for all participants. One major drawback is that the potential for distraction may be greater.

Nurse educators have the opportunity and responsibility to provide incentives to enhance the quality of student interactions outside class. Extra-credit options provide an incentive for some, but not all, resulting in positive and productive peer partnerships developing between a more homogeneous group of self-selected students rather than a more diverse student group. A homogeneous group is self-limiting because diversity in learning ability, culture, age, and gender may not be present. Out-of-class required assignments have a greater potential for success. In the online environment, creating small subgroups within the discussion board or wiki and changing weekly or biweekly offer new opportunities for diverse thinking, dialogue, and roles.

Assignments involving the learner-centered student interactive strategies mentioned in the preceding section and listed in Table 12.2 provide a menu of strategies available to educators. For example, a literature review or survey of resources in the library may be one out-of-class paired or small-group activity. Paired or small group use of computer-assisted instructional programs can encourage critical thinking. Incentives for promoting student interaction via participation in professional events and memberships provide another aspect of professional socialization (see Chapter 11). Enrichment programs (EPs) and Nursing Student Resource Center (NSRC) services offer additional opportunities for high-quality peer interaction, positive and productive peer partnerships, and encouragement by friends (see Chapters 13 and 14). Active encouragement of student participation in EPs and NSRC services should be ongoing, especially during major transitional points in the educational process.

> What strategies do you implement to facilitate the development of positive and productive peer partnerships outside the classroom? What works? How have they been evaluated? What strategies are implemented by your colleagues consistently throughout the program? What other strategies could be implemented?

CURRICULAR INCONSISTENCY

Inconsistent and/or insufficient integration of activities, opportunities, and incentives throughout the nursing curriculum restricts professional development, confounds educational outcomes, and is confusing to students. Curricular inconsistency is incongruent with the creation of a true community of nursing learners, which is essential for professional socialization, development, and growth. It is also counterproductive to earlier partnership-promoting efforts. In contrast, consistent vertical and horizontal threads, critically woven throughout the curriculum, can support student success via positive academic and psychological outcomes.

Systematic curriculum evaluation via quantitative and qualitative methods helps identify program strengths, weaknesses, inconsistencies, and gaps (Toolkit Item 26).

Reflective self-appraisal on an individual and a program level is necessary for enhancing the scholarship of teaching (18,79,80). Concept mapping that focuses on partnership as a concept helps trace the concept throughout the curriculum. Strategy mapping that traces various student-centered learning approaches will assess another necessary dimension. Curricular vertical and horizontal threads should be complementary, consistent, and appropriate for each educational level. Finally, faculty development workshops targeting identified need areas assist faculty to integrate learner-centered student interactive activities, opportunities, and incentives throughout the nursing curriculum with the specific aim of promoting positive and productive peer partnerships and encouragement by friends in class.

> What activities, opportunities, and incentives are woven throughout your curriculum? What else can be done?

PSYCHOSOCIAL BARRIERS: RECOGNITION, SOLUTIONS, STRATEGIES, AND INCENTIVES

> What psychosocial solutions, strategies, and incentives for promoting positive and productive peer partnerships are implemented in your course? In your program?

Perceived Irrelevance to Immediate Education Goals

The perceived irrelevance to immediate educational goals serves as a major obstacle to student participation in positive and productive peer partnerships. Adult learners typically place importance on tasks directly and immediately related to the achievement of educational and/or career goals (15,17). Consequently, the nurse educator is challenged to change existing values and beliefs that negate or minimize the significance of peer partnerships and interactive student activities in achieving immediate goals. For the undergraduate student, immediate goals usually refer to successful achievement at the individual course level. Nurse educators can begin by sparking student's motivation at the immediate course level.

Communication can change the course of action (decisions and behaviors) and influence outcomes in the educational path toward professional socialization and development. Clearly identifying goals as student expected outcomes in a course outline clarifies any ambiguities and communicates the importance of positive and productive peer partnerships in nursing. The course outline can delineate participation in positive and productive peer partnerships as a course objective that complements other course objectives and the course description. Opportunities to develop positive and productive peer partnerships should take place as part of required class activities. For example, a topical outline may list the students' expected outcomes as follows:

At the completion of this class session, the student will be able to

1. Define positive and productive peer partnerships
2. Discuss examples of positive and productive peer partnerships in nursing
3. Identify desirable educational and professional outcomes (benefits)
4. Discuss the potential impact of desirable educational and professional outcomes on students, the academic institution, the nursing profession, the health care system, and society
5. Identify strategies for promoting positive and productive peer partnerships
6. Demonstrate skills for developing positive and productive peer partnerships in nursing

Multiple choice, short answer, and/or essay questions based on learning outcomes via student-interactive activities further validate the time engaged in quality student interaction and partnerships. A written assignment grade, test item points, or test grade that directly impacts upon the course grade validates interactive participation as significant enough to award a quantitative measure that will affect the immediate course grade and progression in the nursing curriculum. Assigning a portion of the course grade based on participation in student-interactive class activities and projects directly demonstrates relevance to immediate educational goals. Communicating consistency between the program's desired educational outcomes and Pew Commission (1995) recommendations concerning educational strategies, desired outcomes, and professional partnerships provides a broader view to students.

Communication may not be sufficient in changing students' attitudes toward valuing the potential of positive and productive peer partnerships and interactive student experiences. Students need to understand and appreciate the conditions under which specific learning strategies may be more or less effective rather than assuming that certain ones are best (81). Because reflection is essential for affective learning (82) and affective learning is most crucial for professional development (83), engaging the student through in-class or out-of-class learner-centered student interactive activities should include an individual reflective component. For example, students can be asked to write a "low-stakes" reflection of their in-class group experience. Low-stakes writing minimizes the pressure of "grading" associated with high-stakes writing (84) and optimizes affective learning outcomes. Reviewing and highlighting the immediate educational benefits obtained from positive and productive peer partnerships further confirms immediate relevance. Discussing the role of positive and productive peer partnerships and encouragement by friends in class in enriching learning, satisfaction, and stress management provides another important dimension to the achievement of immediate educational goals.

> How have activities for promoting positive and productive peer partnerships been linked to immediate course goals in your course? What have other course instructors done in your program? What else can be done?

Perceived Irrelevance to Future Professional Goals

Often, students' focus on short-term educational goals impedes their ability to recognize the long-range benefits of developing positive and productive peer partnerships. This limited perspective is another barrier to maximizing peer partnership possibilities. Discussions that appraise the relationship between professional standards, employer expectations, and professional partnerships illustrate relevance to future professional goals. Pew Commission (52) recommendations, Institute of Medicine (IOM) (43), and American Association of Colleges of Nursing (AACN) (44), the future of nursing recommendations, along with other international, national, and local nursing guidelines, document partnerships as a professional nursing practice expectation, exemplifying further justification.

Personal testimonies about the numerous benefits associated with positive and productive peer partnerships are a powerful incentive to students. For example, a nurse educator engaged in collaborative research can discuss both the personal and professional benefits of such a collaborative partnership. Sharing a story about patient-care benefits and staff satisfaction resulting from a collaborative partnership between two staff nurses provides a different, yet relevant perspective to students. Asking advanced students to share their positive experiences and how these experiences enhanced and facilitated achievement of their educational goals and future professional goals further substantiates the nurse educator's position. Professional role models such as clinical preceptors or invited guest speakers during class time can provide additional testimonies. Finally, asking students to explore their own individual goals can personalize educational and career mobility options and assist them in their understanding of professional relevance.

> How have activities for promoting positive and productive peer partnerships been linked to future professional goals? What have other course instructors done in your program? What else can be done?

Stress

Stress related to student interactive learning experiences threatens the development of positive and productive peer partnerships and adversely affects student academic outcomes, satisfaction, persistence, and retention (see Chapter 7). There may be several different underlying causes of stress associated with student interactive learning experiences; the major goal is stress reduction or elimination. Identifying the underlying cause of stress is an important precursor for stress reduction strategy development. For example, students may experience stress due to the need for self-disclosure or perceptions that group work is difficult (85), high responsibility for learning (86), and/or negative perspectives concerning active-learning strategies (86). Sources of stress are also interrelated with affective factors: CVB, self-efficacy, and motivation. CVB that do not comprehend and/or embrace student-centered interactive activities may cause stress. Inefficacious students may perceive their knowledge and skills as inadequate for successful student interactive experiences, positive and productive peer partnerships, and in-class friendships. Motivation will adversely be affected by stress (see Chapter 3).

Acknowledging that students have diverse learning styles, strengths, needs, values, and sources of stress should be followed by case examples of how other students have effectively reduced or eliminated stress associated with student interactive learning experiences. Hearing from diverse students who successfully managed stress, altered negative views, developed positive attitudes, built upon existing personal strengths, remedied personal weaknesses, enjoyed learning, and ultimately developed positive and productive peer partnerships is an inspiring incentive for students. Shared experiences, student interaction, and role modeling facilitate the development of effective coping strategies and positive self-efficacy appraisal (38). Offering a variety of teaching–learning strategies best accommodates the learning style preferences and needs within a diverse class. Sharing this evidence-based educational purpose with students can alleviate anxiety and help develop trust.

Judicious, immediate, and caring feedback for positive behaviors by educators and peers increases self-efficacy and motivation and reduces stress (38,87). Mutual assistance or reciprocation of academic and nonacademic (emotional) supports by peer partnerships can enhance confidence and independence and result in friendships. Friendships that encourage mutual reciprocation and individual independence rather than dependence can help with professional integration, growth, and development.

What strategies have you implemented and evaluated to reduce possible stress associated with activities for promoting positive and productive peer partnerships? What have other course instructors done in your program? What else can be done?

FEAR OF ISOLATION

Fear of isolation or actual feeling of disconnection, difference, detachment, or separateness from other students obstructs the development of quality student interactions, positive and productive peer partnerships, and friendships. Students who perceive themselves as "different" are less likely to engage in interactive behaviors that would promote a sense of belonging (88,89). Perceived differences may be based on academic ability and preparedness, motivational levels, age, gender, culture, economic status, neighborhood, and/or any other characteristics. Students who perceive themselves as similar frequently tend to congregate when faced with student interactive activities. This phenomenon has been referred to as in grouping (90), banding together syndrome (91), or classroom cliques (92). Although initially students may feel comfortable with the self-selected group, generally such homogeneous groups are counterproductive to the overall goals of interactive learning experiences, professional socialization, and positive and productive peer partnerships. In contrast, diverse, interactive groups have the greatest potential for maximizing outcomes (15).

Minority students with a sincere desire to engage with the larger, diverse college community will be more successful in meeting their personal, educational, and professional goals than minority students in predominantly White institutions who are hesitant or reluctant to do so (93,94). Nurse educators must be aware of the actual, potential, and perceived barriers stemming from past and present experiences with racism and discrimination that serve as barriers to inclusion. Good peer interaction with other students in an inclusive environment where students from all backgrounds experience equality and opportunity maximizes success through positive psychological outcomes, enhanced educational opportunities, and positive academic outcomes (93,94).

The literature abounds with techniques designed to maximize interpersonal group dynamics, learning outcomes, and psychological outcomes by offering suggested patterns of matching learners. Student self-selection of group members/partners has obvious advantages and disadvantages; however, premature nurse educator-determined groups/partners selection also has some limitations. Cravener (90) cautions against predicting student-learning behavior on an ethnic, racial, or cultural basis rather than individual evaluation. Antonio (95) points out that often "surface segregation" occurs in which outwardly a group may seem ethnically homogenous, but may actually represent diverse ethnic groups. For example, a non-Asian educator may label a group of "Asian" students as homogenous; however, the students within the group may perceive great diversity among group members. In another perspective, Pintrich and Garcia (81) propose that psychological mediators, such as self-efficacy and motivation, are more definitive than other student characteristics. Conclusively, nurse educators are challenged to select strategies that aim to replace the fear of isolation with feelings of inclusion and connection.

One strategy may be to allow students to self-select group members or partners during the first in-class student interactive activity. The nurse educator has the opportunity to observe individual student strengths and weaknesses in both the learning process and learning product. Additionally, opportunities to facilitate learning, group process, and satisfaction will assist students in developing positive and productive peer partnerships. During future student interactive activities, pairing or grouping students based on individual student strengths and weaknesses will enhance learning outcomes via positive and productive peer partnerships. Ongoing efforts to foster a caring, supportive, trusting, and open learning environment must be actively implemented throughout the nursing curriculum. Acknowledging that fears may occur yet can be effectively overcome accentuates the positive. Actions that sincerely strive to foster feelings of inclusion, equality, trust, and connection demonstrates a commitment to all learners.

> What strategies have you implemented and evaluated to foster feelings of inclusion, equality, trust, and connection? What have other course instructors done in your program? What else can be done?

FOSTERING OTHER PARTNERSHIPS

Creating networks of students who are socially connected to the academic community and have a commitment to learning, persistence, and success can make a marked difference in student retention (10,96). Nurse educators are in a key position to foster peer partnerships and class friendships. Friends in class have the ongoing opportunity to jointly discuss class expectations, course requirements, challenges, successes, difficulties, and career plans. They perceive a connection with each other because they are in the same stage of educational and professional development; struggles and joys of learning are mutually experienced.

One limitation, however, is that friends in class may be unable to comprehend the broader perspective, rationale for prerequisites or sequencing of courses, benefits of course assignments within the whole scope of the educational process, preparation for registered nurse licensing exam, next course, employment as a registered nurse, or continued education. Interconnectedness between courses and future professional role is frequently limited, skewed, or unknown. Partnership connections with peer mentor-tutors who are further advanced in the educational process can minimize this limitation. Nurse educators can "make a difference" in nursing student retention and success by fostering peer mentor-tutor partnerships. Chapter 13 will describe peer mentor-tutor partnerships as part of an enrichment program.

KEY POINT SUMMARY

- The NURS model proposes that encouragement by friends in class will actively promote positive psychological outcomes, self-efficacy, professional socialization, persistence, and retention.
- Nurse educators can make a difference by designing a series of carefully patterned and interwoven student-centered interactive experiences throughout the nursing curriculum structured to promote positive and productive peer partnerships.
- Positive and productive peer partnerships are those purposeful affiliations, alliances, and connections among peers that result in constructive, generative, creative, and desirable outcomes.
- Nurse educators must recognize actual and potential barriers to student's development of positive and productive peer partnerships, propose solutions or goals, initiate strategies to remove barriers, and offer incentives.
- In-class opportunities for positive and productive peer partnerships critically depend upon a caring, safe, open environment that is intentionally shaped to embrace all students as unique, individual, and valuable contributors in the learning process.

APPLICATION STRATEGIES

EDUCATOR-IN-ACTION VIGNETTE

Professor Webb has designed a series of carefully patterned and interwoven student-centered interactive experiences throughout the advanced medical–surgical nursing course. They are structured to encourage positive and productive peer partnerships, enhance critical thinking, maximize learning, promote satisfaction, minimize stress, and therefore promote retention. On the first day of the class, Professor Webb reviews the course outline, elaborates on the multidimensional teaching-learning strategies integrated throughout the course, and emphasizes their purposes and desired outcomes. First, he describes some lively, personal experiences in which professional partnerships enhanced his professional development, program of nursing research, teaching, and clinical practice. He briefly reminds students about the communication skills and interpersonal group dynamics essential to facilitate productive collaboration (learned last semester). A one-page handout summarizes major points. An overhead cartoon illustrates student behaviors that interfere with achieving positive learning outcomes and satisfaction. This serves as an icebreaker, and students laugh and comment on several of the cartoon scenarios (see Figure 12.1). Next, Professor Webb informs students that the next class will incorporate a small-group activity based on the assigned textbook reading *Nursing Care of the Client with AIDS* and the handout "Opportunistic Infections, Clinical Manifestations, Diagnostic Tests, and Drug Treatment."

On the second day of the class, Professor Webb allows students to self-select groups. Each five-member group is assigned a specific AIDS-related opportunistic infection and a specific drug used for treating the infection. Group tasks include determining (1) nursing interventions indicated for each clinical manifestation associated with the infection, (2) nursing implications indicated for each drug, and (3) relevant nursing diagnoses. Professor Webb moves throughout the room and guides students as needed, noting individual and group strengths and weaknesses. This information can guide future group activities and group assignments. After 20 minutes, each group briefly presents on their assigned topic while the remaining students take notes, ask questions, and provide additional suggestions. Professor Webb elaborates and comments as necessary, inviting further student comments and questions. During the two-hour class, all of the groups complete their presentations. However, five other unassigned opportunistic infections and ten drugs have not yet been discussed.

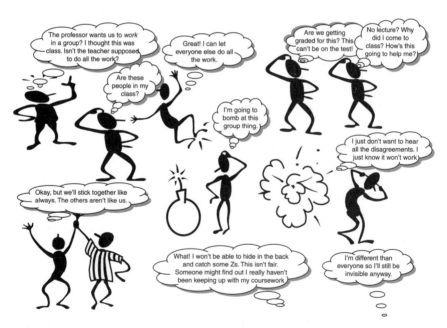

FIGURE 12.1 Group dynamics cartoon: Interfering behaviors.

Professor Webb proposes that a manageable option can be that groups meet outside of class and work together before next week. Students unanimously agree and volunteer to take specific topics.

At the beginning of the next class, students present their topics more quickly, accurately, and comprehensively than before. Next, Professor Webb asks students to individually reflect and write about their group activity experience. Select comments include:

SVETLANA: At first I didn't want to do a group activity because I didn't know anyone in my group. Because I had done the reading, I could contribute to the group and then everything was okay. As we discussed each clinical manifestation, everyone realized that it was nursing interventions and implications that were most important to know. I didn't focus my reading this way. Now I will read differently. Our group worked together after clinical to prepare for the next week. We finished up quicker than the first time so we decided to meet every week to prepare for class.

MINA: The group activity made the topics more fun and realistic. The book seems so abstract. Talking about nursing diagnoses and nursing interventions with my classmates will help me remember the information in clinic and on a test. Not everyone in our group met before class to work on the second assignment, but those of us who did meet got a lot accomplished. We even had time to review last week's class notes.

KEN: Working in the group in class made me feel like I wasn't alone in my questions, stress, or struggles. Dividing up the infections and drugs and sharing information about the nursing process made the content more manageable.

WILLA: Two people in my group were really smart. I thought I understood the material but after the group activity, I realized that I was trying to memorize instead of thinking critically like a nurse. Later, I asked one of those students how she studies. She was really nice and offered to help me if I need it.

Throughout the semester, Professor Webb implements and evaluates subsequent student-centered interactive activities that complement and build upon each other.

TOOLKIT RESOURCE BOX

Item 19—Active Promoter Assessment Tool: Positive and Productive Peer Partnerships

Item 26—Strategy Mapping Across the Curriculum

Item 24—Appraising Teaching Strategies: Potential Effect on Diverse Populations

Items 1–4—Student Perception Appraisal Questionnaires—Pretests and Posttests

---

DISCUSSION QUESTIONS

1. Professor Change proposes that faculty incorporate small-group interactive activities during the classroom component of "Nursing Fundamentals for Adult Health Nursing." She notes that currently the classroom component consists of lecture as a teaching strategy with few students asking questions. Recent test scores indicate that students have difficulty with critical thinking questions and application of theoretical material to actual patient scenarios. Student satisfaction surveys indicate moderate satisfaction with nursing as a career choice, the nursing program, and the college.

   Professor Clock says, "There is no time to do this in a busy course where I have to teach fundamental content and skills. I sometimes feel like I am talking nonstop to get everything in. A good lecture gives all the information students need to know to be successful in the course and as a nurse in the future.

   Assume the role of Professor Change. How would you respond to Professor Clock?

2. Professor Uno says, "I once tried to do a small group activity with first semester students. I gave them a case study and told them to work in groups on it. Students didn't know what to do. Many of the minority students and foreign-educated students just sat back and looked angry. They comprised about one-fourth of the class. My evaluations indicated that many students felt I wasted their class time and why didn't I just teach. I vowed never to try a group activity again."

   Assume the role of Professor Change above. How would you respond to Professor Uno?

3. A colleague says, "It is not the responsibility of nurse educators to manipulate peer partnerships by breaking up class cliques and forcing loners to participate in a classroom-based small group activity." How would you respond?

4. What part of the chapter captivated you the most? Why? How will this impact upon your future role?

5. How can the Educator-in-Action Vignette be adapted for use with students in your course?

REFERENCES

1. Kennerly, S. (2001). Fostering interaction through multimedia. *Nurse Educator,* 26(2), 90–94.
2. Conderman, G., Bresnahan, V., & Hedin, L. (2011). Promoting active involvement in today's classrooms. *Kappa Delta Pi Record, 47*(4), 174–180.
3. Brown, A. V. (2008). Effectively educating Latino/a students: A comparative study of participation patterns of Hispanic American and Anglo-American university students. *Journal of Hispanic Higher Education, 7*(2), 97–118.
4. Cejda, B. D., & Hoover, R. E. (2011). Strategies for faculty-student engagement: How community college faculty engage Latino students. *Journal of College Student Retention: Theory, Research, and Practice, 12*(2), 135–153.
5. Buch, K., & Spaulding, S. (2011). The impact of a psychology learning community on academic success, retention, and student learning outcomes. *Teaching of Psychology, 38*(2), 71–77.
6. Martin, A. J., & Dowson, M. (2009). Interpersonal relationships, motivation, engagement, and achievement: Yields for theory, current issues, and educational practice. *Review of Educational Research, 79*(1), 327–365.
7. Angelino, L. M., Williams, F. K., & Natvig, D. (2007). Strategies to engage online students and reduce attrition rates. *Journal of Educators Online, 4*(2), 1–14.
8. Callahan, K. M. (2009). Academic-centered peer interaction and retention in undergraduate mathematics programs. *Journal of College Student Retention: Research, Theory, and Practice, 10* (3), 361–389.
9. Oermann, M. H., & Gaberson, K. B. (2009). *Evaluation and testing in nursing education.* New York, NY: Springer Publishing.
10. Seidman, A. (2005). *College student retention: Formula for success.* Westport, CT: American Council on Education, Praeger.
11. Karp, M. M., Hughes, K. L., & O'Gara, L. (2011). An exploration of Tinto's integration framework for community college students. *Journal of College Student Retention: Research, Theory, and Practice, 12* (1), 69–86.
12. Bosher, S. D., & Pharris, M. D. (2009). *Transforming nursing education: The culturally inclusive environment.* New York, NY: Springer Publishing.
13. Wolf-Wendel, L., Ward, K., & Kinzie, J. (2009). A tangled web of terms: The overlap and unique contribution of involvement, engagement, and integration to understanding college student success. *Journal of College Student Development, 50*(4), 407–428.
14. American Association of Colleges of Nursing. (1998). *The essentials of baccalaureate education for professional nursing practice.* Washington, DC: Author.
15. Brookfield, S. D. (1986). *Understanding and facilitating adult learning.* San Francisco, CA: Jossey-Bass.
16. Christiaens, G., & Baldwin, J. H. (2002). Use of dyadic role-playing to increase student participation. *Nurse Educator, 27*(6), 251–254.
17. Knowles, M. (1984). *The adult learner: A neglected species.* Houston, TX: Gulf.
18. Young, P., & Diekelmann, N. (2002). Learning to lecture: Exploring the skills, strategies, and practices of new teachers in nursing education. *Journal of Nursing Education, 41*(9), 405–412.

19. Henry, P. R. (2006). Making groups work in the classroom. *Nurse Educator, 31*(1), 26–30.
20. Levey, J. (2010). Enhancing group interactions and reducing classroom cliques. *Nurse Educator, 35*(4), 144–145.
21. Alpers, R. R., Brown, G., Jarrell, K., & Wotring, R. (2007). That's edu-tainment! Using games to engage, excite, and educate. *Teaching and Learning in Nursing, 2*, 144–145.
22. Moredich, C., & Moore, E. (2007). Engaging students through the use of classroom response systems. *Nurse Educator, 32*(3), 113–116.
23. Smith, D. A., & Rosenkoetter, M. M. (2009). Effectiveness, challenges, and perceptions of classroom participation systems. *Nurse Educator, 34*(4), 156–161.
24. Jones, S., Henderson, D., & Sealover, P. (2009). "Clickers" in the classroom. *Teaching and Learning in Nursing, 4*, 2–5.
25. Patterson, B., Kilpatrick, J., & Woebkenber, E. (2010). Evidence for teaching practice: The impact of clickers in a large classroom environment. *Nurse Education Today, 30*, 603–607.
26. Raines, D. A. (2010). An innovation to facilitate student engagement and learning: Crossword puzzles in the classroom. *Teaching and Learning in Nursing, 5*, 85–90.
27. Royse, M. A., & Newton, S. E. (2007). How gaming is used as an innovative strategy for nursing education. *Nursing Education Perspectives, 28*(5), 263–267.
28. Stokes, L. G. (2003). Gatherings as a retention strategy. *Association of Black Nursing Faculty Journal, 14*(4), 80–82.
29. Schmidt, B., & Stewart, S. (2009). Implementing the virtual reality learning environment second life. *Nurse Educator, 34*(4), 152–155.
30. Jeffreys, M. R. (1991). Time out! Let's play charades. *Nurse Educator, 16*(5), 12, 34.
31. Ulrich, D. L., & Glendon, K. J. (1999). *Interactive group learning: Strategies for nurse educators.* New York, NY: Springer Publishing.
32. Jeffreys, M. R. (2010). *Teaching cultural competence in nursing and health care: Inquiry, action, and innovation.* New York, NY: Springer Publishing.
33. Lowenstein, A. J., & Bradshaw, M. J. (2004). *Fuszard's innovative teaching strategies in nursing* (2nd ed.). Boston, MA: Jones & Bartlett.
34. Svanum, S., & Bigatti, S. M. (2009). Academic course engagement during one semester forecasts college success: Engaged students are more likely to earn a degree, do it faster, and do it better. *Journal of College Student Development, 50*(1), 120–132.
35. Chaves, C. (2006). Involvement, development, and retention: Theoretical foundations and potential extensions for adult community college students. *Community College Review, 34*(2), 139–152.
36. Callahan, K. M. (2009). Academic-centered peer interaction and retention in undergraduate mathematics programs. *Journal of College Student Retention: Research, Theory, and Practice, 10* (3), 361–389.
37. Goguen, L. M. S., Hiester, M. A., & Nordstrom, A. H. (2011). Associations among peer relationships, academic achievement, and persistence in college. *Journal of College Student Retention: Research, Theory, and Practice, 12*(3), 319–337.
38. Bean, J. P., & Eaton, S. B. (2001). The psychology underlying successful retention practices. *Journal of College Student Retention: Research, Theory, & Practice, 3*(1), 73–90.
39. Bean, J. P. (2005). Nine themes of college student retention. In A. Seidman (Ed.), *College student retention: Formula for success* (pp. 215–244). Westport, CT: Praeger.

40. Braxton, J. M., & McClendon, S. A. (2001). The fostering of social integration and retention through institutional practice. *Journal of College Student Retention: Research, Theory, & Practice, 3*(1), 57–72.
41. Vance, C., & Olson, R. K. (1998). *The mentor connection in nursing.* New York, NY: Springer Publishing.
42. Vance, C. (2011). *Fast facts for career success in nursing: Making the most of mentoring in a nutshell.* New York, NY: Springer Publishing.
43. Institute of Medicine. (2010). *The future of nursing: Leading change, advancing health.* Washington, DC: Author.
44. American Association of Colleges of Nursing. (2010). *The future of higher education in nursing: 2010 annual report.* Washington, DC: Author.
45. Bevis, E. O. (1989). *Curriculum building in nursing: A process* (2nd ed.). New York, NY: National League for Nursing.
46. Diekelmann, N., Swenson, M. M., & Sims, S. L. (2003). Reforming the lecture: Avoiding what students already know. *Journal of Nursing Education, 42*(3), 103–105.
47. Kuh, G. D. (2001). Organizational culture and student persistence: Prospects and puzzles. *Journal of College Student Retention: Research, Theory, & Practice, 3*(1), 23–40.
48. Bastable, S. B. (2003). *Nurse as educator: Principles of teaching and learning for nursing practice* (3rd ed.). Boston, MA: Jones & Bartlett.
49. Campbell, E. T. (2009). Teaching Korean RN-BSN students. *Nurse Educator, 34*(3), 122–125.
50. Cabrera, A. F., Crissman, J. L., Bernal, E. M., Nora, A., Terenzini, P. T., & Pascarella, E. T. (2002). Collaborative learning: Its impact on college students' development and diversity. *Journal of College Student Development, 43*(1), 20–34.
51. Gumbs, J. (2001). The effects of cooperative learning on students enrolled in a level 1 medical-surgical nursing course. *Journal of Cultural Diversity, 8*(2), 45–48.
52. Pew Health Professions Commission. (1995). *Health professions education and managed care: Challenges and necessary responses.* San Francisco, CA: Center for the Health Professions.
53. Huff, C. (1997). Cooperative learning: A model for teaching. *Journal of Nursing Education, 36*(9), 434–436.
54. Davidhizar, R., & Lonser, G. (2003). Storytelling as a teaching technique. *Nurse Educator, 21*(5), 217–221.
55. Koenig, J. M., & Zorn, C. R. (2002). Using storytelling as an approach to teaching and learning with diverse students. *Journal of Nursing Education, 41*(9), 393–399.
56. Curran, V., Solberg, S., LeFort, S., Fleet, L., & Hollett, A. (2008). A responsive evaluation of an Aboriginal nursing education access program. *Nurse Educator, 33*(1), 13–17.
57. Candela, L., Michael, S. R., & Mitchell, S. (2003). Ethical debates: Enhancing critical thinking in nursing students. *Nurse Educator, 28*(1), 37–39.
58. Cowan, D. T., & Tesh, A. S. (2002). Effects of gaming on nursing students' knowledge of pediatric cardiovascular dysfunction. *Journal of Nursing Education, 41*(11), 507–509.
59. Kramer, N. (1995). Using games for learning. *Journal of Continuing Education in Nursing, 26*, 40–42.

60. Pimple, C., Schmidt, L., & Tidwell, S. (2003). Achieving excellence in end-of-life care. *Nurse Educator, 28*(1), 40–43.
61. Ciesielka, D. (2008). Using a wiki to meet graduate nursing education competencies in collaboration and community health. *Journal of Nursing Education, 27*(6), 276–282.
62. Dorrian, J., & Wache, D. (2008). Introduction of an online approach to flexible learning for on-campus and distance education students: Lessons learning and ways forward. *Nurse Education Today, 29*, 157–167.
63. O'Neill, C. A., Fisher, C. A., & Newbold, S. K. (2009). *Developing online learning environments in nursing education.* New York, NY: Springer Publishing.
64. Rash, E. M. (2008). A problem-based learning hybrid in a women's health course. *Journal of Nursing Education, 47*(10), 477–479.
65. Wink, D. (2009). Teaching with technology: Finding information on the Internet. *Nurse Educator, 34*(2), 51–53.
66. Grassley, J. S., & Bartoletti, R. (2009). Wikis and blogs: Tools for online interaction. *Nurse Educator, 34*(5), 209–213.
67. Merrill, E. B., Reinckens, T., Yarborough, M., & Robinson, V. I. (2006). Retaining and assisting nontraditional nursing students in a baccalaureate nursing program utilizing Blackboard and Tegrity technologies. *Association of Black Nursing Faculty Journal, 17*(3), 107–110.
68. Russell, C. K., Gregory, D. M., Care, W. D., & Hultin, D. (2007). Recognizing and avoiding intercultural miscommunication in distance education: A study of the lived experiences of Canadian faculty and Aboriginal nursing students. *Journal of Professional Nursing, 23*, 351–361.
69. Ostrow, L., & DiMaria-Ghalili, R. A. (2005). Distance education for graduate nursing: One state school's experience. *Journal of Nursing Education, 44*(1), 5–10.
70. DiMaria-Ghalili, R. A., Ostrow, L., & Rodney, K. (2005). Webcasting: A new instructional technology in distance graduate nursing education. *Journal of Nursing Education, 44*(1), 11–18.
71. Pressler, J. L., & Kenner, C. (2009). Embracing new directions in curricula and teaching. *Nurse Educator, 34*(2), 49–50.
72. Agazio, J., & Buckley, K.M. (2009). An untapped resource: Using YouTube in nursing education. *Nurse Educator, 34*(1), 23–28.
73. Kemp, P. K., Myers, C. E., Campbell, M. R., & Pratt, A. P. (2010). Student perceptions and the effectiveness of podcasting in an associate degree nursing program. *Teaching and Learning in Nursing, 5*,111–114.
74. Forbes, M. O., & Hickey, M. T. (2008). Podcasting: Implementation and evaluation in an undergraduate nursing program. *Nurse Educator, 33*(5), 224–227.
75. Edwards, H., Nash, R., Sacre, S., Courtney, M., & Abbey, J. (2007). Development of a virtual learning environment to enhance undergraduate nursing students' effectiveness and interest in working with older people. *Nurse Education Today, 28*, 672–679.
76. Giddens, J. F. (2007). The Neighborhood: A web-based platform to support conceptual teaching and learning. *Nursing Education Perspectives, 28*(5), 251–256.
77. Tinto, V. (1997). Classrooms as Communities. *Journal of Higher Education, 68*(6), 599–623.
78. Nora, A. (2001). The depiction of significant others in Tinto's "Rites of Passage": A reconceptualization of the influence of family and community in

the persistence process. *Journal of College Student Retention: Research, Theory, & Practice, 3*(1), 41–56.

79. Drevdahl, D. J., Stackman, R. W., Purdy, J. M., & Louie, B. Y. (2002). Merging reflective inquiry and self-study as a framework for enhancing the scholarship of teaching. *Journal of Nursing Education, 41*(9), 413–418.

80. Diana, T. J. (2011). Becoming a teacher leader through action research. *Kappa Delta Pi Record, 47*(4), 170–173.

81. Pintrich, P. R., & Garcia, T. (1994). Self-regulated learning in college students: Knowledge, strategies, and motivation. In: P. R. Pintrich, D. R. Brown, & C. E. Weinstein, (eds.), *Student motivation, cognition, and learning: Essays in honor of Wilbert J. McKeachie* (pp. 113–133). Hillsdale, NJ: Lawrence Erlbaum Associates.

82. Schon, D. (1987). *Educating the reflective practitioner.* San Franscisco, CA: Jossey-Bass.

83. Bevis, E. O., & Watson, J. (1989). *Toward a caring curriculum: A new pedagogy for nursing.* New York, NY: National League for Nursing.

84. Elbow, P. (1997). High stakes and low stakes in assigning and responding to writing. *New Directions for Teaching and Learning, 69,* 5–13.

85. Drevdahl, D. J., & Dorcy, K. S. (2002). Using journals for community health students engaged in group work. *Nurse Educator, 27*(6), 255–259.

86. Martens, K. H., & Stangvik-Urban, L. (2002). Views on teaching-learning: Lessons learned from nursing education in Sweden. *Nurse Educator, 27*(3), 141–146.

87. Bandura, A. (1986). *Social foundations of thought and action: A social cognitive theory.* Englewood Cliffs, NJ: Prentice-Hall.

88. Astin, A. W. (1975). *Preventing students from dropping out.* San Francisco, CA: Jossey-Bass.

89. Chaney, B., Muraskin, L. D., Cahalan, M. W., & Goodwin, D. (1998). Helping the progress of disadvantaged students in higher education: The federal student support services program. *Educational Evaluation and Policy Analysis, 20*(3), 197–215.

90. Cravener, P. (1996). Multicultural education: A second look. *Nurse Educator, 21*(4), 6–7.

91. Hummel, M., & Steele, C. (1996). The learning community: A program to address issues of academic achievement and retention. *Journal of Intergroup Relations, 23*(2), 28–33.

92. Levey, J. (2010). Enhancing group interactions and reducing classroom cliques. *Nurse Educator, 35*(4), 144–145.

93. Bessent, H. (1997). *Strategies for recruitment, retention, and graduation of minority nurses in colleges of nursing.* Washington, DC: American Nurses Publishing.

94. Tidwell, R., & Berry, G. (1997). Higher education and the African American experience: Barriers to success and remedies for failure. In H. Bessent (Ed.), *Strategies for recruitment, retention, and graduation of minority nurses in colleges of nursing* (pp. 55–62). Washington, DC: American Nurses Foundation.

95. Antonio, A. L. (2001). Diversity and the influence of friendship groups in college. *Review of Higher Education, 25*(1), 63–89.

96. Skahill, M. P. (2002). The role of social support network in college persistence among freshman students. *Journal of College Student Retention: Research, Theory, & Practice, 4*(1), 39–52.

Enrichment Program Design, Implementation, and Evaluation

The enrichment experience expedites enhanced excellence for everyone.

SNAPSHOT SCENARIO

PROFESSOR BLAZE: At the conference last week, I was most impressed with one school's presentation about a special, comprehensive program designed to help nursing students succeed. We should have something like that here for our students.

PROFESSOR ALWAYS: Well, I always invite questions during my class, and I always stay 5 minutes after class to answer extra questions. The weak students always fail out or drop out anyway, so why waste our efforts in trying to remediate students?

PROFESSOR NUMBERS: I've heard of remedial programs to help at-risk students succeed. Urban University reported an increased retention and graduation rate from 65% to 80% and a below-state-average, registered nurse (RN) licensing, first-time pass rate that increased to state average in 1 year after implementing the program. We can identify the weakest nursing students by the lowest grade point averages (GPAs) and put them all in a remediation group and track them until they graduate, fail, or drop out.

PROFESSOR BLAZE: Well, I was really suggesting the development of a program focused on enrichment rather than remediation. The presenters coined several phrases that really resonated with me—"The enrichment experience expedites enhanced excellence for everyone," or a short version, "Enrichment is for everyone," meaning that everyone's potential can be enhanced. The presenters also shared that the initiation of the enrichment program also enriched their own teaching, revitalized their career, and generated professional rewards beyond just improved retention, progression, graduation, and licensure rates. The enrichment also resulted in more satisfaction among students and faculty, results they quantified by using a psychometrically tested satisfaction questionnaire.

PROFESSOR PONDER: This all sounds interesting, but I don't really know what you mean by a comprehensive enrichment program.

PROFESSOR BLAZE: The presenters discussed a multidimensional program that was actively encouraged for all students. It consisted of an orientation program, mentoring and tutoring by paid peer mentor-tutors, online newsletters with discussion board, career advisement and guidance, test-prep workshops, and study groups. A faculty member with some released time from teaching coordinated the proactive, ongoing, and transitional components of the program; however, she shared that some schools have a full-time position allocated for this role.

PROFESSOR ALWAYS: We have always separated our nursing faculty role from the student support services in the college. Students can just go over to the general college tutoring services over in the large library complex across campus.

PROFESSOR PONDER: That place is so big, and I imagine it could be very scary and intimidating for a nursing student to go over there. Are any staff members there to answer nursing type questions? Can general staff members or student tutors be the best role models for our nursing students if they aren't nurses and may not even know about or respect the nursing profession?

PROFESSOR NUMBERS: I think we should start with something small first. Let's identify the weak students by lowest GPA and then offer them some remedial services to get them equal to the other students.

PROFESSOR PONDER: Couldn't labeling students as weak, less than other students, and in need of remediation do the opposite of what we want to do, by decreasing their confidence and further isolating them from their peers and the nursing profession? Aren't there other factors besides GPA that influence students' persistence and success?

PROFESSOR BLAZE: The presenters shared that a multidimensional enrichment program should be inclusive for everyone and about everything that potentially influences students' success, rather than exclusive to some students and about some select things. Especially for many nontraditional students and students in accelerated nursing programs, environmental factors outweigh academic factors in influencing their progress and success.

PROFESSOR PONDER: How does one start an enrichment program? Where should we begin?

An enrichment program (EP) is a formally designed multiservice program that aims to enrich the total nursing student experience by maximizing strengths, remedying weaknesses, promoting positive psychological outcomes, facilitating positive academic outcomes, and nurturing professional growth and development. Services may include several of the following: orientation, mentoring, tutoring, newsletters, career advisement and guidance, workshops, study groups, networking, transitional support, financial stipends, and referral. Services are best facilitated through a collaborative partnership in learning and professional development among nursing faculty, other professional nurses, and students. The ongoing opportunities for professional integration and socialization offer tremendous possibilities for optimizing academic and psychological outcomes. Nurse educators can make a difference in nursing student retention and success through a carefully designed EP.

The main purpose of this chapter is to describe the process of designing, implementing, and evaluating an EP. An illustrative case exemplar using the prenursing enrichment program (PEP) will complement each step of the process. The PEP consisted of free services for students; orientation, mentoring, tutoring, career advisement and guidance, workshops, networking, and transitional support services facilitated through a collaborative partnership in learning and professional development. Evaluation of EP components, including academic outcomes, psychological outcomes, and variables influencing retention, will conclude the chapter.

ENRICHMENT PROGRAM DESIGN, IMPLEMENTATION, AND EVALUATION

EP design, implementation, and evaluation should be a well-planned process. This involves time, energy, money, commitment, collaborative partnerships, and a systematic plan. Figure 13.1 presents the 11-step process that can guide EP development. Each step will be described followed by a case exemplar. The PEP case exemplar illustrates how this process can be adapted by other nurse educators interested in developing diagnostic-prescriptive enrichment programs for undergraduate nursing students. Although the PEP was designed for nontraditional undergraduate nursing students, the case exemplar has applicability for traditional students as well as those in accelerated undergraduate programs.

The first phase of the process might appear to be "design," but there is really a predesign phase. This involves five steps: assessing the current situation, reviewing the literature, searching for grants, drafting a plan, and soliciting support. Each step will be described individually and within the context of the PEP case exemplar.

Step 1: Assess Current Situation

What is the profile of your program's student retention and success pathways? What departmental and administrative supports exist and/or are needed for EP design, implementation, and evaluation? What college resources currently exist?

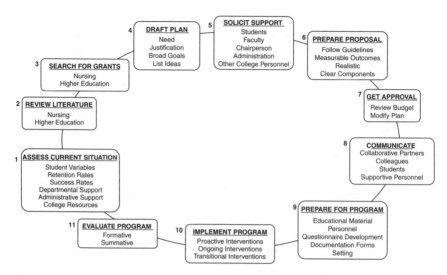

FIGURE 13.1   Enrichment program design, implementation, and evaluation process.

A retention strategy or EP should be designed for a specific situation and have empirical support (1). The first step is to systematically assess the current situation, including student profile variables, retention rates, success rates, departmental support, administrative support, and the existing college resources.

A systematic assessment of the targeted student population can be initiated using the NURS model. The realization that there are multi-dimensional variables influencing retention and success is often overwhelming; yet, it is essential to evaluate them before designing the EP. The assessment of student profile variables can give a general description of the student population or can help the nurse educator target a specific student group. For example, a nursing program with many ESL (English as a second language) students may need to incorporate language enhancement strategies into an EP.

In the PEP case example, student perceptions had been assessed in a previously funded study. Descriptive results from the study of first semester nontraditional associate degree nursing students found that environmental variables were perceived as more influential for academic achievement and retention than academic variables (2–4). Students felt that family, faculty, and friends greatly influenced retention; however, family responsibilities were thought to be severely restrictive. Overly confident students who rated their academic factors as greatly supportive had significantly lower nursing course grades. Students with a more conservative self-appraisal of academic and environmental factors had higher nursing course grades. This suggested that some students did not have realistic self-appraisals of strengths and weaknesses, or accurate comprehension of the skills needed for professional nursing education. Because inaccurate perceptions could be detrimental to student retention and success, it was believed that an EP consisting of proactive, ongoing, and transitional interventions would be most effective.

Assessment of current retention rates should differentiate between course retention, ideal program retention, program retention, and interim program retention (see Chapter 1, Exhibit 1.1, and Figure 1.1). Course retention is the easiest to assess. Comparison of course retention rates across various semesters and between courses can help identify trends within the overall program. However, tracking nontraditional students throughout the program is difficult for a variety of reasons. First, nontraditional students often attend college part-time, and therefore, a cohort group for analysis is difficult to identify. Second, nontraditional students often must "stop out" for nonacademic reasons such as pregnancy, child care, care of a sick family member, financial strain, employment constraints, and other examples. Full-time students including traditional students and those enrolled in accelerated programs may also stop out for nonacademic reasons. Third, the institution's computer capability for tracking such nontraditional students who frequently attend college part-time and stop out one or more times may be limited. Fourth, the individual tracking of students who stop out and attend part-time is labor-intensive, costly, at increased risk for human error, and results in a small number of students in many different cohorts. A small sample cohort becomes problematic when trying to use inferential statistical analyses.

One recommendation would be to calculate three different program retention rates: ideal program retention, program retention, and interim program retention. After several semesters, a trend and student profile would emerge. This assessment could guide EP design to specific groups. For the purposes of the PEP, course retention rates across various semesters and for each of the clinical nursing courses was the primary focus.

Assessment of current success rates should differentiate between program success and ideal program success (see Chapter 1, Exhibit 1.1, and Figure 1.1). Additionally, the various components of "success" should be operationalized, measured, and compared for several semesters to look for common trends and/or gross disparities in trends. This means measuring graduation rates, RN licensing exam pass rates, employment rates, and enrollment rates in more advanced nursing program. A problem in one area could have an impact on other areas. For example, failing the RN licensing exam will affect employment and enrollment in a more advanced nursing program because an RN license is usually required for both options. Inclusion of program success was beyond the scope of the PEP; however, with future expansion of student support strategies and ongoing measurement strategies, it could be possible to evaluate the entire process of retention and success.

Determining departmental support should address both conceptual and instrumental support. Conceptual support refers to the support of the idea of an EP and can range from passive (listening without offering opinions and suggestions) to active (advocacy, suggestions, and verbal commitment). It is valuable to have conceptual support from the chairperson, deputy chairperson, faculty, and staff. Instrumental support refers to allocation of resources such as expertise, money, released time, secretarial services, supplies, space, and teaching load distribution.

After appraising departmental support, administrative support should be assessed. Determining administrative support first requires a comprehensive understanding of the institution's administrative structure, organizational culture, politics, policy, and procedures. Formal meetings with key administrators can provide a valuable guide for EP development. Careful review of current and proposed college resources available to all college students and the adequacy or inadequacy of such services for nontraditional undergraduate nursing students is important to avoid duplication of existing services, substantiate the need for absent or insufficient services, and explore partnership possibilities and pooling of resources.

After assessing each of these areas individually, the overall strengths and weaknesses in the already existing college resources can be evaluated. This overall assessment should reveal areas that need development and provide some basis to determine costs and feasibility. Without the conceptual support of the department and administration, there are too many obstacles that would impair feasibility and implementation. Conceptual support without some commitment to instrumental support also would pose obstacles, although with generous grant funding this could be overcome.

Before designing the PEP, collaboration with the department chairperson resulted in both conceptual and instrumental support. The chairperson readily gave active support by offering encouragement for the idea and advocating the pursuit of the project. Instrumental support ranged from the chairperson sharing her expertise to acknowledging the future access to secretarial services and supplies. Administrative support was assessed during formal meetings with the divisional dean and vice president of the college. College resource assessment revealed the absence of college tutoring services for nursing courses and the presence of several support services for student referral, such as personal counseling. College resources for the project director such as services by the institution's office of grants and research were identified. Collaborative partnerships with measurement experts and the director of institutional research were discussed in anticipation of the evaluation phase of the PEP. Conclusively, the overall assessment revealed that the institutional climate was favorable toward PEP development.

Step 2: Review Literature

Next, a review of the nursing and higher education literature should be conducted. Materials should be reviewed for gathering background information about student retention, nontraditional students, retention strategies, evaluation methods, and funding sources. Choice of a relevant conceptual framework can be instrumental to the organization. When reviewing literature concerning other student support strategies, educators should determine strategy strengths, limitations, and appropriateness of fit to the targeted population. One must be aware, however, that there is no panacea; EPs will not solve all problems, nor will they help every student succeed. Realistically weighing the possible benefits against the risk of doing nothing can help in the decision-making process. The quote "we cannot do everything at once, but we can do something at once" (5) captures the importance of taking action and making a difference, rather than waiting for the perfect or idealistic situation. But planning ahead for the future is crucial for the longevity and improvement of situation. Actually, slight imperfections and less than ideal situations may reap more benefits long term. For example, limited funds for a pilot peer mentor-tutoring EP may initially limit services to 45 minutes weekly per six-member study group; however, documented use of services, quantifiable positive academic outcomes, and student and faculty requests for expanded services may result in getting more than originally desired. In addition, students receiving modest services are gaining benefits even if not the ideal, so a positive difference is being achieved. Keeping a list of future desired areas for expansion and enhanced services and resources is an efficient way to always keep something on hand when organizational climate and funds become available. In addition, if the literature documents successful outcomes, the probability for support is increased because proposed EP initiatives are evidence-based and not haphazard.

In the PEP, a previous compilation of literature on retention necessitated an updated review of the nursing and higher education literature. Published journal articles and books were reviewed and organized into specific categories, expanding the current literature files and making future retrieval and updates easy.

When was the last time you conducted a review of the literature concerning nursing student retention and success? What books, book chapters, websites, journal articles, dissertations, and other scholarly resources can help you plan the EP?

Step 3: Search for Grants

The search for grant resources can be conducted via computer by the nurse educator or by requesting assistance from the institution's office of grants and research. For the PEP, one specific funding source was selected. The funding was specifically allocated for public institutions, associate degree programs, and vocational education. Additionally, specific populations of students were targeted. Prior assessment of student variables in step 1 supported that many students fell into the targeted categories; therefore, it was appropriate to pursue this grant opportunity.

> What small institutional seed grants are available in your institution? What professional, local, state, and national grants are available? Which one(s) would be most feasible to get your initial EP started? Which one(s) might be easier attainable after an initial EP pilot?

Step 4: Draft Plan

Next, a written draft is developed. Familiarity with the grant's terminology, goals, format, funding capabilities, and guidelines is important prior to drafting a plan. Grant specifications must guide the draft development. Relevant issues reported in the literature and assessment findings (step 1) also should be incorporated throughout the plan. Clear identification of the need and justification based on the literature and assessment findings is a necessary precursor to establishing goals. At this point, goals should be broad and relate directly to the identified need. The draft should include an "idea" list, leaving details for later consideration (see Toolkit Item 27).

In the case example, data from the preliminary study of nontraditional associate degree nursing students strongly supported the need for the PEP. The use of a conceptual model as a proposed organizing framework for designing a retention strategy was an added strength. This suggested that the strategy would not haphazardly use a trial and error approach but, based on available conceptual and empirical literature, would use a systematic and detailed approach. The broad goal was to improve student retention. Brainstorming resulted in a list of possible retention strategy components. Reviewing the list for feasibility eliminated some strategies. Finally, prioritizing the remaining components provided an outline of ideas that could be a starting point for soliciting support.

Step 5: Solicit Support

Although soliciting support can be time consuming, the benefits of conceptual and instrumental support commitments are invaluable and help build alliances and partnerships. Although both are important here, soliciting significant number of instrumental support commitments is an essential precursor to preparing a proposal.

Although this step may seem similar to the assessment of support in step 1, it has many important differences. First, it builds on the collaborative relationship initiated in step 1 that should then evolve or be nurtured into a collaborative partnership. A collaborative partnership can have varying degrees of direct or indirect supportive involvement but all could be potentially critical to the funding of an EP and ultimately its success.

At this point of more formalized commitment to specific tasks, the anticipated time line for the tasks should be mentioned. This gives more structure and organization. If the timeline is not realistic, it can be adjusted now before writing it in the proposal and setting the plan up for failure. Before preparing a proposal, it is important to tease out what strategies are feasible and realistic and which would be problematic. In this way, the presence or absence of support will result in a modified list of possible strategy components. Instrumental support cannot occur without conceptual support; however, conceptual support without instrumental support greatly limits the possibilities of EP success. Evaluating student support for various components is crucial before entering the design phase (proposal preparation and approval).

The following examples were applicable to the PEP:

- Students agree to use PEP services and/or encourage their use.
- Faculty members agree to make announcements in class to encourage students to use PEP services.
- Chairperson agrees to reserve an empty adjunct office to be used for possible peer mentor-tutoring.
- Administrators commit to support release time for project director.
- Director of Institutional Research agrees to actively assist with transcript data retrieval and data analysis.
- Colleagues agree to review questionnaire drafts and serve as expert reviewers for content validity.

> What specific supportive tasks have your departmental and college colleagues, students, and administrators agreed to perform? How have these expected tasks and time frames been communicated, agreed upon, and documented?

Step 6: Prepare Proposal

In the PEP, the broad goals listed in the draft plan (step 4) needed to be rewritten to fit with the terminology used in the grant proposal guidelines. The initial draft was decreased to pilot several of the strategy components first, followed by an evaluation. This was done for three main reasons. First, there would not be enough time for the project director to carry out all interventions, along with teaching and other faculty responsibilities, even with released time. Second, students would be overwhelmed with so many choices that it would be confusing and would encourage fragmented use of many services rather than promote a concentrated effort and consistency in one or two services. Third, financial constraints limited what could be done.

PEP strategy components were organized to include proactive, ongoing, and transitional interventions. Theoretical and empirical support for this approach and its components were documented in the proposal. Using grant specific guidelines and terminology, the evaluation plan included formative and summative evaluation measures. Although the grant's guidelines focused primarily on quantitative results documenting improved academic outcomes, the measurement of students' psychological outcomes (satisfaction) and perceived variables influencing retention were written into the evaluation plan. The justification for their inclusion was based on prior research and the underlying conceptual model. Instrument development and evaluation (reliability and validity studies) were accordingly incorporated into the proposal. Several revisions resulted in a final proposal that was submitted on time according to the procedure at the educational institution.

> Have you customized your grant proposal to meet the specific requirements of the agency while also customizing it to meet your program's needs? Are your plans realistic, feasible, and sustainable given the specifics of the grant and program, time, money, and resources available and desired? What components should be deferred to a later date and time? Why?

Step 7: Get Approval

When a project or grant proposal is approved, it is important to review the budgetary allocations for specific categories and check if there are any restrictions or added guidelines. Budgetary constraints may require some modifications from the original proposal plan. These modifications should be finalized before entering the next phase of preimplementation. The preimplementation phase acknowledges that there are two essential steps that need to be done before program implementation: communication and preparation. For the PEP, no major changes from the original proposal were noted.

> What are the budgetary allocations for specific categories? Are there any changes from the original proposal? Are there any restrictions or added guidelines? How will this affect the overall EP?

Step 8: Communicate

Once grant funding is awarded and the budgetary plan modifications are finalized, the project director should communicate that funding has been received. The important questions to consider are with whom to communicate, what needs to be communicated, and how to communicate. Essentially, what must be communicated is the fact that a grant was received and how this will involve the other collaborative partner(s).

Collaborative partners or those individuals who committed time, expertise, service, or some other instrumental support toward the proposed project should be contacted personally. A telephone contact followed by a written memo or copy of the grant award and proposal may be indicated, depending on the type of partnership required and level of involvement. Memos that communicate the necessary details serve as reinforcement to the verbal communication.

A copy of the grant award may be forwarded to the administration as part of the grant notification process. If not, a copy should be forwarded to all administrators. Announcements made at faculty, curriculum, and other pertinent meetings can be made both verbally and in the form of a written memo or information sheet. Students can be notified about the upcoming services via classroom announcements, memos, and student club meetings.

In the PEP, announcement of the grant award was automatically forwarded to administrators by the institution's office of grants and research. A scheduled meeting with the department chairperson tried to build on the communication, commitments, and partnerships established previously in steps 1 and 5. Because the grant was awarded after classes had ended, chairperson support for communicating with students via a mailed letter was greatly welcomed. A letter outlining the main features of the PEP was mailed to all students listed as prenursing or associate degree nursing students, along with an application for an orientation session and study group sessions. A letter explaining the funded project also was mailed to all full-time nursing faculty members.

Students already enrolled in the associate degree or RN to BS program received an invitation to apply for a peer mentor-tutor (PMT) position. Job qualifications and responsibilities were included along with a blank application form. PMT qualifications included (1) current enrollment in an upper-level, associate-degree nursing course or in the baccalaureate program after completion of the college's associate degree program, (2) above-average grades in prenursing and nursing courses and in clinical evaluations, and (3) excellent communication skills. Responsibilities included assistance with orientation sessions, tutoring for prenursing and/or nursing courses, individual and small group mentoring sessions, and collaborating with the project director. Hours were advertised as flexible and negotiable with wages set at a rate competitive with other college assistants, work-study, and unlicensed hospital personnel wages. Copies of all letters were posted on bulletin boards.

> With whom do you need to communicate? What, where, when, how, and why do you need to communicate initially? What type of follow-up communication would be beneficial?

Step 9: Prepare for Program

Allocating a sufficient amount of time for program preparation is important. Making a list of what needs to be done, by whom, and the needed date of completion can help prioritize program preparation components. Preparation may include creating or obtaining educational materials and documentation forms, selection and orientation of personnel, questionnaire development and evaluation, and arranging the physical setting.

In the PEP, a timeline was originally submitted with the project proposal and served as a valuable guide. Two tasks that had the highest priority, because they involved a series of steps, were time-consuming, and involved several people, were questionnaire development and the selection and orientation of personnel (project assistants and PMTs).

Questionnaire Development

Several instruments were developed as proposed in the grant proposal. A cover letter explaining some background information and purpose of the instruments, the requested due date, a self-addressed stamped envelope, and an instruction sheet for rating content validity accompanied the instruments. The ratings and comments of the content reviewers provided the basis for minor revisions. Review by a psychometric expert confirmed that the instruments were in a format that could easily be scanned, interpreted, and analyzed, using the statistical package for the social sciences (SPSS) statistical program. The instrument drafts were then given to a project assistant who had computer expertise in creating optical scanning instruments, scanning, and conversion into SPSS. All instruments needed a trial run for scanning to assure ease with future data processing.

Selection and Orientation of PMTs

The selection of PMTs first involved a review of completed applications by the requested due date. The next step involved a review of student transcripts and clinical evaluations for each course completed so far. The review of clinical evaluations was quite time consuming but provided insightful information, such as a record of the student's verbal communication and interaction with others, attendance, tardiness, and other important qualities and skills.

The highest-ranking applicants were then invited for an interview. Scheduling and arranging the interviews as well as conducting the interviews were time consuming, yet essential to the selection process. During interviews, it was emphasized that a collaborative partnership among PMTs, students, and the project director was an important goal.

The next priority was to organize and prepare the educational and documentation materials needed for the PMT orientation. A 90-minute orientation session was held with the PMTs. The overall purposes and goals of the EP, particularly detailing the significance of mentoring in nursing and the role of PMT and student as partners in learning, were described (Figure 13.2). The expected benefits of specific PMT roles and interventions were discussed. This discussion clarified the scope of the PMT role and emphasized the importance of conveying this information during the first contact meeting with students.

Documentation forms for recording the study group's activities and for recording anticipated plans for the next meeting were reviewed with PMTs. The documentation forms would serve as a weekly communication between the PMT and project director. Strategies for enhancing student survival skills addressed issues such as academic support strategies, time management, stress reduction techniques, assisting students throughout the educational process, promoting professional growth, and balancing multiple role responsibilities. Handouts and lists of referral resources within the college complemented this discussion.

Next, the simulated situations and group discussion provided an opportunity for PMTs to use problem-solving strategies for academic and nonacademic problems that could potentially arise. Decision-making dilemmas and varying opinions identified areas that required further clarification and guidance. It was emphasized that the PMT would have an ongoing collaborative relationship with the project director throughout the semester.

Finally, PMT study group schedules were confirmed. Because several study groups would occur at the same time, finding sufficient space necessitated organizing room arrangements and reservations via the college's protocol. A written evaluation of the PMT orientation concluded the meeting.

What are your three highest priority tasks? Why? What is the best way for you to successfully complete tasks?

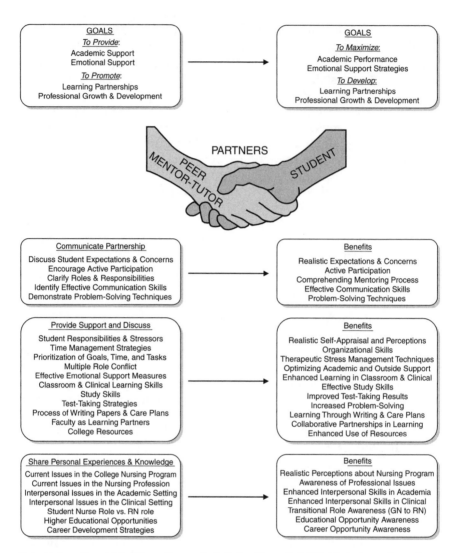

Select information obtained from Alvarez, A., & Abriam-Yago, K. (1993). Mentoring undergraduate ethnic-minority students: A strategy for retention. *Journal of Nursing Education*, 32(5), 230–232.

FIGURE 13.2   Peer mentor-tutor and student as partners in learning and professional development.

Step 10: Implement Program

A well-developed and detailed proposal, accompanied by an itemized timeline, can be the guide for program implementation. To facilitate implementation, the program should be divided into various intervention categories: proactive, ongoing, and transitional. Each category should complement the others and easily flow among them. There may be some eventual overlap in categories as students participate in an EP throughout several semesters.

Proactive interventions are interventions implemented before the beginning of the semester and aim to prepare students academically, psychologically, and practically, and to enhance performance, satisfaction, and success. Preparation may allow for opportunities to review previously learned skills, ask questions, review pertinent information, assist with time management strategies specific to the new nursing course, interact with students who previously completed the course, and informally meet the new course instructors.

Ongoing interventions aim to maximize student success by the early identification of student strengths and weaknesses before academic difficulties, role conflicts, or stress onset. Early identification of the at-risk student can prevent failure or withdrawal. Often students do not seek help until difficulty arises, and then it is often too late to improve an academically precarious situation.

Another benefit of ongoing interventions is that collaborative and productive partnerships can flourish. For example, the PMT–student partnership can only develop with consistent and frequent contacts. Students also can feel more at ease with study group peers, offering both emotional and academic support strategies. This peer interaction helps develop professional socialization, integration, and acculturation into the nursing student role and future RN role (6–33). The opportunity to share experiences and watch role models and peers struggle with similar academic and nonacademic challenges can help increase self-efficacy and motivation to persist (34,35).

As students move from one phase of the educational process to the next, *transitional interventions* should be implemented (36). Transition from preprofessional to professional education (first nursing course) and one nursing course to the next level challenges students to embark on a new, unknown path in their journey toward becoming an RN. Guidance at these transitional stages is crucial to encourage retention, enhance achievement, promote satisfaction, and minimize stress.

The PEP encompassed the various stages of the educational process and included proactive, ongoing, and transitional interventions. Activities will be described in the sections that follow.

Orientation

The piloted program included a 2½-hour orientation program before the start of the semester. Although the orientation targeted prenursing students not yet enrolled in a clinical nursing course, several students already in the first nursing course attended. All students were invited to bring a family member, friend, or support person. Each student was personally greeted by a PMT. Everyone received an orientation folder, calendar, and study skill handouts. Several of the participants had just enrolled at the college for the first time; other prenursing students had completed all prenursing required courses.

The agenda included: (1) purposes and goals of the PEP, (2) nursing program requirements, (3) student information, (4) family, friend, and faculty support network, (5) time management strategies, (6) enhancing textbook reading comprehension, (7) enhancing learning skills in the classroom, including taking notes effectively, and (8) collaborating with the PMT. Prenursing students then met with their PMT. Following a brief introduction, a follow-up meeting date or phone call was set up based on the individual needs of the student.

Next, students completed a satisfaction questionnaire. All students found the orientation session to be "very helpful and informative." Written and verbal comments by students provided additional information. For example, one student commented that the mentor encouraged her to keep trying. Many students commented that it was helpful to have someone to talk to who had already been through the nursing courses. A few students realized the need to resolve personal and/or family issues before trying to take a full-time course schedule. Most students commented that the handouts and orientation session provided them with new study skills and time management strategies. One student commented that she would share the handouts on family–student–faculty partnerships with her family so that her requests for assistance with household responsibilities would be respected and honored. In subsequent years, all nursing students enrolled in the first clinical nursing course were invited to attend a presemester 2-hour orientation session that incorporated the above components, specific information about course requirements, resources specifically available to assist students in meeting specific course requirements, plus an interactive component with clinical group members to enhance professional integration and socialization and decrease social isolation. Although attendance was not mandatory, participation was approximately 95% or higher over several semesters. Student feedback was consistently positive for all orientation components.

Newsletter

The newsletter was created to enrich the prenursing and nursing program experience by broadening information access to students. The biannual newsletter addressed relevant issues such as requirements of the nursing program, student responsibilities, strategies for enhancing academic success, career advisement and guidance, management of work and family responsibilities, and services available to assist students. Announcements concerning workshops, tutoring, and nursing application dates, and notices about the EP were included.

Feature article sections were presented. Questions frequently asked by students or questions submitted by students were selected for answers in the featured section "What Enquiring Students Want to Know." The "Stories From the Field" feature provided some clinical case scenarios and attempted to showcase how nursing students can make a positive difference in the clinical setting. Tear-off application forms for PMT study groups comprised the last two pages of the newsletter.

Study Groups

The study groups, led by PMTs, were in great demand. Application forms submitted by the deadline exceeded available openings. Registration was done on a first-come, first-serve basis on the assigned registration date and time before the beginning of the semester. Students who submitted applications by the deadline had first choice in selecting study group sessions and were required to commit to regularly scheduled group meetings (usually weekly) starting at the beginning of the semester. The study group registration session also allowed for informal meeting among peers, PMTs, and the project director. Marketing the EP and study group spots in the best way possible to increase perceived value, usage, and satisfaction should be carefully considered. Free services are often unvalued and taken for granted; however, sharing with students the concept that what is offered free is often desired but not available in other programs suddenly puts a higher value on it. This enhances usage and satisfaction that something unavailable somewhere else is available here and now. Published articles in the nursing magazine showcasing the EP, especially if student testimonies to its positive academic and professional development outcomes are featured, increased the perceived value among doubtful faculty and students. Publicized success via publications and personal testimonies and can do much to validate the allocation of resources in economically challenging times.

Students in the study groups developed a working partnership with the PMT and other group members. Study groups usually consisted of five students per one PMT. Additional in-person meetings, telephone meetings, and/or referrals were individualized as needed. Frequently, the project director met with referred students about academic and nonacademic problems. The project director was informed about group activities weekly through personal visits and/or study group documentation forms. These forms focused the group on the day's tasks or topics, identified specific areas for the following week's session, and documented attendance. Additionally, a PMT comment section informed the project director about individual and group concerns, strengths, weaknesses, and other pertinent academic and nonacademic issues. The documentation forms also helped maintain consistency and structure between groups and within groups on a regular basis while keeping the project director informed. Updated information technology innovations (such as e-mail, documentation forms via attachments, and text messages) offer newer, efficient methods for ongoing communication.

Transitional Workshop

All nursing students were invited to attend a brief transitional workshop prior to the beginning of the next semester. Although there was some overlap between proactive and transitional interventions, the main difference was that transitional interventions targeted students who had already participated in the PEP. The agenda included the purposes and goals of the PEP, nursing student transitional process, strategies for successful transition, collaborating with a PMT, and study group selection. The workshop addressed the transitional process and issues that nursing students often face when moving from one phase of their professional nursing education to another. Each phase offered different challenges and required students to modify previous successful study strategies to accommodate these new challenges.

For example, study time allocation for a six-credit, 15-week course would have to be adjusted to meet the demands of a nine-credit course or a five-credit half semester course. Sometimes students needed assistance in changing the focus from an adult client with medical or surgical problems to pregnant women, children, or mentally ill clients. Although many of the essential underlying professional skills had been learned previously, guidance through the transition from one phase (course) to another could be eased by acknowledging that a transitional process existed and by learning effective strategies to meet transitional challenges. Nursing students stated that working with a PMT has assisted them through this transitional process. Spontaneous testimony by more advanced students as role models assisted novice students to develop resilient self-efficacy and adapt previous skills to new circumstances and motivated them to further develop skills.

Other transitional support measures included the PEP nursing skills lab practice sessions prior to the beginning of the new semester. Nursing students were encouraged to practice any previously learned and evaluated technical skills during the supervised PEP practice session in preparation for clinical. New students accepted into the first clinical course were invited to participate in a nursing skills lab and educational resources tour led by a PMT guide. The tour familiarized students with their new environment and showed students what resources were available to assist them throughout their educational experience.

> What proactive, ongoing, and transitional strategies are consistently implemented for your course, other courses, and throughout your program?

Step 11: Evaluate Program

A carefully orchestrated evaluation should be tied explicitly to the proposal's measurement plan and should include both formative and summative components. Formative evaluations assess the process of a program rather than outcomes. They can be monitored as the program is implemented and can document specific activities, identify difficulties, and allow for diagnostic and prescriptive modifications based on participants' feedback, using both quantitative and qualitative data.

Summative evaluations should be monitored every semester and compared globally at the completion of the program to assess the achievement of desired program outcomes. Because student retention is a dynamic and multidimensional phenomenon, the success of any teaching, support, or enrichment strategy requires a multidimensional evaluation strategy.

The NURS model may be used to identify desired program outcomes as academic, psychological, and affective. Academic outcomes may include course retention, course success, course withdrawal, continuous program retention, interim program retention, ideal program retention, total program retention, total program success, and ideal program success. Psychological outcomes may include measures of satisfaction or stress; affective outcomes may include self-efficacy (confidence) perceptions.

Following the preestablished plan for data collection and analysis consistently and rigorously will help make the evaluation results more valid and reliable. This includes working diligently with previously established partners in the evaluation process such as the data collectors, director of institutional research, project assistant, and psychometric expert. Once the results are obtained and reviewed for statistical and practical significance, inferences from the data can guide future EP activities, outcome measures, and desired outcomes.

The process of evaluation naturally leads into the beginning of the enrichment design process (step 1) again, in which the nurse educator would assess the new current situation and compare with the EP evaluation just completed. Assessment would include the appropriateness of generalizing findings to the new situation. The ultimate goal of the EP design, implementation, and evaluation process is that empirical and conceptually based EPs will address the holistic needs of students.

A study was undertaken to evaluate select aspects of the PEP among students who participated in PMT-led study groups throughout the semester. The evaluation addressed academic outcomes, psychological outcomes (satisfaction), and perceived variables influencing retention. Academic outcomes targeted course retention by measuring course success rates, course failure rates, and course withdrawal rates for the intervention group and a control group. Comparisons were done between the clinical nursing courses, within courses, and throughout several semesters.

Overall, the intervention (PEP) group had lower failure rates, lower withdrawal rates, higher course success rates, and positive psychological outcomes (satisfaction). Students also perceived that environmental variables were more influential than academic variables in influencing retention. Social integration variables such as faculty advisement and helpfulness, tutoring, and the EP were perceived as highly supportive. Details concerning the PEP evaluation, including instrumentation, are described in two published articles (37,38).

High student satisfaction with the PEP and perceptions that the PEP supported retention emphasize the continued need for strategies that enrich the nursing student experience. Formative evaluations of EP interventions and comments on the Satisfaction Questionnaire (Toolkit Item 6) also provided valuable information to guide future enrichment strategies. For example, students' written request for extended study group hours, especially in the beginning nursing courses, substantiated the need for greater allocation of resources to the beginning students. Additionally, request for longer study group sessions increased the sessions from an average of 45 to 90 minutes.

> What formative and summative evaluations are consistently conducted for proactive, ongoing, and transitional strategies implemented in your course, other courses, and throughout your program? How have the results guided subsequent design, implementation, and evaluation strategies?

KEY POINT SUMMARY

- An EP is a formally designed multiservice program that aims to enrich the total nursing student experience by maximizing strengths, remedying weaknesses, promoting positive psychological outcomes, facilitating positive academic outcomes, and nurturing professional growth and development.
- The 11-step EP design process includes: assess current situation, review literature, search for grants, draft plan, solicit support, prepare proposal, get approval, communicate, prepare for program, implement program, and evaluate program.
- The PEP case exemplar illustrates each step individually, describes PEP activity components, and highlights the main benefits of PMT partnerships and other essential partnerships.
- The PEP consisted of free services for students: orientation, mentoring, tutoring, career advisement and guidance, workshops, networking, and transitional support services facilitated through a collaborative partnership in learning and professional development.

- Evaluation included the assessment of academic outcomes, psychological outcomes, and variables influencing retention.

APPLICATION STRATEGIES

EASY APPLICATION ACTION STEPS

Assessing the Current Situation Before EP Design

1. Apply easy application action steps from Chapter 2.
2. List details of conceptual and instrumental support currently available, unavailable, essential, and desired.
3. List existing college resources aimed at enhancing college student retention and success.

Touring the 11-Step EP Design, Implementation, and Evaluation Process

1. Contemplate the big picture of the 11-step process depicted in Figure 13.1 (panoramic view).
2. Beginning with step 1, consider the interaction between all steps and possible obstacles along the way.
3. Propose strategies for eliminating obstacles or adapting to challenges.

EDUCATOR-IN-ACTION VIGNETTE

Professor Bridges is the project director of an EP that includes weekly study groups led by PMTs. Although the PMT orientation addressed roles and responsibilities of study group participants as well as PMT roles and responsibilities, PMTs expressed concern that study group participant expectations were often different and sometimes inappropriate. To address this issue, Professor Bridges prepared a handout on "Study Group Etiquette: Dos and Don'ts to Maximize Success" (see Exhibit 13.1). After reviewing the handout with PMTs, she distributed it to first semester nursing students, briefly reviewed it, and invited students to sign up for study groups. PMTs reviewed the handout again with students on the first study group meeting day and clarified any ambiguities. PMTs reported positive results from this approach:

MAURA: Because I did this on the first day, students knew more what to expect from the study group. When one student asked me about what might be included on an exam, another student was quick to say that this was inappropriate. Besides, I could just refer to the handout if it came up again. I felt more comfortable with setting limits.

LYNN: Overall, students seemed to come to the study group on time and be more prepared than last semester. They didn't expect me to summarize

---

EXHIBIT 13.1   Study Group Etiquettes: Dos and Don'ts to Maximize Success

DOs:

1. Join a study group at the beginning of the semester.
2. Attend group meetings regularly.
3. Complete prerequisite class readings.
4. Expect to contribute to the group discussion.
5. Plan to study individually in addition to the group study.
6. Respect each individual group member.
7. Ask questions related to group focus topic.
8. Bring notes and other necessary materials to group session.
9. Tell group facilitator if study session is meeting your needs.
10. Set a target plan for the next meeting.

DON'Ts:

1. Wait until after the first exam to join a study group. Your success can be enhanced by group study.
2. Attend groups intermittently. This disrupts group effectiveness and cohesiveness.
3. Expect that others will read the chapters for you. Actively reading chapters *before* enhances classroom learning and group interaction.
4. Expect everyone else to do all the discussion. Actively discussing material identifies your strengths and weaknesses. Everyone has strengths and weaknesses. Remedying weaknesses *before* an exam maximizes your chances for success. *The group facilitator is a RESOURCE person available to ASSIST you. The group facilitator is not a lecturer.*
5. Substitute group study sessions for individual reading, writing, and studying. Study groups should **supplement, complement, and enhance** your individual study time. Study groups are not a substitute for meeting with your course instructor when you have difficulty or class-specific questions.
6. Make biased assumptions about individual group members or treat some members with less respect. Mutual respect enhances group interpersonal dynamics and interaction effectiveness.
7. Ask questions just to show off, change the topic, challenge the group facilitator, or obstruct the group process. Questions asked for the right reasons should always be asked; questions asked for the wrong reasons should be avoided.
8. Leave notes, study guides, care plan information, etc., at home. It is an unnecessary disadvantage to you and other group members when essential materials are not available.

(continued)

9. Expect the group facilitator to read your mind. Your input is not only valuable, it is essential.
10. Leave the group session without having an idea about what will occur at the next meeting. This will save time at the beginning of the next meeting. Additionally, everyone should be focused on what needs to be done before the next meeting (reading) and what essential materials should be brought.

DON'T ASK THE GROUP FACILITATOR — (PEER MENTOR-TUTOR):

1. "What's going to be on the exam?" This is unethical. Besides, it is unknown. Remember, you are studying to become a qualified, safe, registered professional nurse who will care for human lives. Therefore, you are not simply studying for an exam but for a life-long career.
2. "Can I see the paper/care plans you did when you were in nursing class?" Again, this is unethical. The most valuable learning occurs from the **PROCESS** of learning to write a paper, rather than simply the finished product.
3. "Can I copy your notes when you took the nursing class?" You will learn more by active note-taking and immediate review of notes after class.

---

their readings, but came prepared to ask me specific questions about the readings.

TONY: Last semester a student kept asking me for my old care plans. Although I knew I was doing the right thing by refusing, I still felt uncomfortable. With these written guidelines, I'm more comfortable about this issue. This semester students showed me parts of their care plan as they were working on it and asked me for guidance when they got stuck. They didn't expect the answer but rather were satisfied when I asked them a series of questions to help them come up with the answer.

Student study group participants also reported positive responses:

TAMIKA: I always studied on my own before so I didn't really know what to expect about a study group. The handout and explanation set everything straight at the beginning.

TOMAS: Last semester I was in the enrichment program study group. Some of the people just listened and never contributed anything. After awhile three of us just dropped out and formed our own study group without the PMT, but we missed her guidance and mentoring. This semester everyone is contributing in some way. Everyone has learned a lot, and we enjoy studying together.

DOMINIQUE: I am a person who needs structure so the guidelines of do's and don'ts really helped me.

Professor Bridges continually evaluates the multidimensional aspects of the EP using student feedback and academic outcome measures to guide future interventions.

TOOLKIT RESOURCE BOX

Item 27—Enrichment Program
Item 6—Enrichment Program Satisfaction Survey
Item 22—Peer Mentoring and Tutoring
Items 1–4—Student Perception Appraisal Questionnaires—Pretests and Posttests

---

DISCUSSION QUESTIONS

1. Which two steps do you view as most challenging? Why? What are some strategies to assist you in meeting these challenges?
2. How can the Educator-in-Action vignette be adapted for use with students in your course, other courses, and PMTs?
3. A faculty member says, "It's a waste to have any study groups at the beginning of the semester because students won't want to use them until they're failing. I don't want to label students as weak, so I wait to suggest meeting with a PMT until after the first exam. If students are weak and lack confidence in clinical, PMTs are no help at all. They're not in clinical to help them." How would you respond?
4. Professor Always says, "Before the EP proposal that included PMTs tutoring students, we always had a problem with the integrity of exams, and students sharing test questions and papers with newer students. I have a set of validated questions that I always use on my exams and a paper format that I always use. PMTs are going to jeopardize the integrity of our exams, papers, and adversely affect our program. It is like we will be promoting academic dishonesty and creating more work for us in the long-run." How would you respond?
5. A colleague says, "We could create a very tight research study design by creating an experimental group and a control group using matched sampling based on GPA, ethnicity/race, enrollment status (full-time or part-time) and number of college credits. The experimental group would be assigned to a PMT-led study group that would meet weekly. Both groups would receive other EP services such as the online monthly newsletter, and the one-hour presemester orientation session. All students would receive usual instruction, advisement, and opportunities to use college-wide resources such as the library. We can then track students

and compare withdrawal rates and course grades in the matched sub-groups." What ethical, legal, conceptual, and empirical/methodological issues make this a poor suggestion? How would you respond?

REFERENCES

1. National League for Nursing Accrediting Commission. (1999).*Criteria and guidelines for the evaluation of associate degree programs in nursing 1999.* New York, NY: National League for Nursing.
2. Jeffreys, M. R. (1993). *The relationship of self-efficacy and select academic and environmental variables on academic achievement and retention.* Unpublished doctoral dissertation, Teachers College, Columbia University, New York.
3. Jeffreys, M. R. (1995). Joining together family, faculty, and friends: New ideas for enhancing nontraditional student success. *Nurse Educator, 20*(3), 11.
4. Jeffreys, M. R. (1998). Predicting nontraditional student retention and academic achievement. *Nurse Educator, 23*(1), 42–48.
5. Coolidge, C. (n.d.) Great-quotes.com. Retrieved May 30 2011, from http://www.great-quotes.com/quote/437692
6. Alvarez, A., & Abriam-Yago, K. (1993). Mentoring undergraduate ethnic-minority students: A strategy for retention. *Journal of Nursing Education, 32,* 230–232.
7. Baldwin, D., & Wold, J. Students from disadvantaged backgrounds: Satisfaction with a mentor-protégé relationship. *Journal of Nursing Education, 32,* 225–226.
8. Bessent, H. (Ed.). (1997). *Strategies for recruitment, retention, and graduation of minority nurses in colleges of nursing.* Washington, DC: American Nurses Publishing.
9. Perry, L. (1997). The bridge program: An overview. *Association of Black Nursing Faculty Journal, 8*(1), 4–7.
10. Ramsey, P., Blowers, S., Merriman, C., Glenn, L. L., & Terry, L. (2002). The NURSE Center: A peer mentor-tutor project for disadvantaged students in Appalachia. *Nurse Educator, 25*(6), 277–281.
11. Tucker-Allen, S., & Long, E. (1999). *Recruitment and retention of minority nursing students: Stories of success.* Lisle, IL: Tucker Publications.
12. Vance, C., & Olson, R. (1998). *The mentor connection in nursing.* New York, NY: Springer Publishing.
13. Vance, C. (2011). *Fast facts for career success in nursing: Making the most of mentoring in a nutshell.* New York, NY: Springer Publishing.
14. Bosher, S. D., & Pharris, M. D. (2009). *Transforming nursing education: The culturally inclusive environment.* New York, NY: Springer Publishing.
15. Stokes, L. G. (2003). Gatherings as a retention strategy. *Association of Black Nursing Faculty Journal, 14*(4), 80–82.
16. Giordana, S., & Wedin, B. (2010). Peer mentoring for multiple levels of nursing students. *Nursing Education Perspectives, 31*(6), 394–396.
17. Colalillo, G. (2007). Mentoring as a retention strategy in a diverse, multi-cultural, urban associate degree nursing program. *Teaching and Learning in Nursing, 2,* 28–33.
18. Campinha-Bacote, J. (2010). A culturally conscious model of mentoring. *Nurse Educator, 35*(3), 130–135.

19. Dennison, S. (2010). Peer mentoring: Untapped potential. *Journal of Nursing Education, 49*(6), 340–342.
20. Dorsey, L. E., & Baker, C. M. (2004). Mentoring undergraduate nursing students: Assessing the state of the science. *Nurse Educator, 29*(6), 260–265.
21. Dunham-Taylor, J., Lynn, C. W., Moore, P., McDaniel, S., & Walker, J. K. (2008). What goes around comes around: Improving retention through more effective mentoring. *Journal of Professional Nursing, 24*, 337–346.
22. Bulut, H., Hisar, F., & GulerDemir, S. (2010). Evaluation of mentorship programme in nursing education: A pilot study in Turkey. *Nurse Education Today, 30*, 756–762.
23. Bensfield, L., Solari-Twadell, P. A., & Sommer, S. (2008). The use of peer leadership to teach fundamental nursing skills. *Nurse Educator, 33*(4), 155–158.
24. Robinson, E., & Niemer, L. (2010). A peer mentor tutor program for academic success in nursing. *Nursing Education Perspectives, 31*(5), 286–289.
25. Sprengel, A. D., & Job, L. (2004). Reducing student anxiety by using clinical peer mentoring with beginning nursing students. *Nurse Educator, 29*(6), 246–250.
26. Scott, E. S. (2005). Peer-to-peer mentoring: Teaching collegiality. *Nurse Educator, 30*(2), 52–56.
27. Sweet, S., & Fusner, S. (2008). Social integration of the advanced placement LPN: A peer mentoring program. *Nurse Educator, 33*(5), 202–205.
28. Rudel, R. J. (2006). Nontraditional nursing students: The social influences on retention. *Teaching and Learning in Nursing, 1*, 47–54.
29. Higgins, B. (2004). Relationship between retention and peer tutoring for at-risk students. *Journal of Nursing Education, 43*(7), 319–321.
30. Sutherland, J. A., & Goodman, N. (2007). Affirming at-risk minorities for success (ARMS): Retention, graduation, and success on the NCLEX-RN. *Journal of Nursing Education, 46*(8), 347–353.
31. Rees, B. B. (2006). Can you have both retention and increased pass rates on the NCLEX-RN? *Teaching and Learning in Nursing, 1*, 18–21.
32. Valencia-Go, G. (2005). Growth and access increase for nursing students: A retention and progression project. *Journal of Cultural Diversity, 12*(1), 18–25.
33. Watts, T. E. (2011). Supporting undergraduate nursing students through structured personal tutoring: Some reflections. *Nurse Education Today, 31*, 214–218.
34. Bandura, A. (1986). *Social foundations of thought and action: A social cognitive theory.* Englewood Cliffs, NJ: Prentice-Hall.
35. Zimmerman, B. J. (1995).Self-efficacy and educational development. In A. Bandura (Ed.), *Self-efficacy in changing societies* (pp. 202–231). New York, NY: Cambridge University Press.
36. Schon, D. (1987). *Educating the reflective practitioner.* San Francisco, CA: Jossey-Bass.
37. Jeffreys, M. R. (2001). Evaluating enrichment program study groups: Academic outcomes, psychological outcomes, and variables influencing retention. *Nurse Educator, 26*(3), 142–149.
38. Jeffreys, M. R. (2002). Students' perceptions of variables influencing retention: A pretest and post-test approach. *Nurse Educator, 27*(1), 16–19 [Erratum, 2002, 27*(2), 64].

The Nursing Student Resource Center: A Place for Linking Strategies Together

The Nursing Student Resource Center (NSRC) is a place that creates a caring, local nursing neighborhood of learners that holistically fosters professional growth, development, and socialization through the careful integration of various strategies, thereby enhancing student persistence and retention through the attainment of positive academic and psychological outcomes.

SNAPSHOT SCENARIO

As part of the new nursing student orientation program, Bianca, a second year peer mentor-tutor (PMT) begins the Educational Resources Tour by leading newly admitted students through the nursing building. Bianca says, "Last year, I was in your place, a new student who felt overjoyed at being accepted to the nursing program yet overwhelmed at all the requirements, clinical, and new places and faces. The faculty here have so many resources for students. My PMT helped me a lot during the Educational Resources Tour and the weekly study groups she facilitated. My study group partners provided a good support system. I did not have to journey alone in this foreign place. I felt like an outsider at first, but after this tour, I hope you feel more part of the nursing neighborhood. The philosophy is that everyone is part of the neighborhood. Here is the NSRC, one part of the nursing neighborhood where study groups meet and students practice computerized National Council Licensure Examination (NCLEX) questions individually or in small groups. The listening center was especially helpful for me because I am only speaking English for 4 years. I could listen to the narrator read English words on the screen in the computer-assisted instructional programs, videos, and videoclips. My friend who has dyslexia also found the listening center programs to be extremely helpful. Actually, everyone can benefit from these types of programs because the audio and visual interactive components really make everything come alive and help you learn better that way."

Here are some of the thoughts of several students on the tour:

RAVI: Wow, look at that study group actually having fun and helping each other as they review class notes with their PMT. I usually study alone because I have always done this and I'm not sure I would fit in with a group; I'm one of the few guys in class and I am self-conscious about my accent. But now, I see men and women of different ages and backgrounds together in a group. Our tour guide and the other students don't seem to mind that she has an accent. Maybe I'll have to give this study group thing a try.

LOURDES: I really like that poster on the wall with the Black nurse, White nurse, and Latina nurse working together in the ER. I also like that picture of the young Latina nurse with the newborn infant and mother. They all look so happy. I've been having a lot of doubts about whether I as a Mexican American would fit in nursing. These posters are motivating and so is the NSRC. It seems warm and friendly.

SUNHEE: My family expects me to excel, so it's great that there are extra resources available to enhance my learning. They will be happy to hear about these opportunities.

LASHAUN: Can't wait to use the computers. Those two students over there with the headphones who are watching the program and taking notes don't seem too stressed. They live in my neighborhood and graduated a year before I did in high school. Guess I can see myself part of this nursing neighborhood too. If they could get through the first year, I can too. And, I don't have to do it alone. What a relief.

KYLE: I've made it through college this far. What can be so difficult about nursing that I need to come here? Hmm . . . That sign says food or drinks permitted in designated areas and now I see those two students in the big lounge chairs eating a bagel and drinking coffee. It looks so comfortable and clean here. And now, I hear them talking about a surgery they watched in the OR. A circulating nurse and a nurse anesthetist? Interesting. . . . Maybe there's more to nursing than I thought. Well, I guess it's a good place to hang out for a few minutes between nursing classes.

GRACE: The faculty really must want us all to succeed if they have a place just for nursing students with lots of services and supports. Look, that professor is stopping in to wave at her students and offers them encouragement. Now one student is thanking her for a test prep workshop that increased her confidence and skills in nursing type questions. That makes me feel good. My cousin goes to a different nursing school and they don't have any of this. She almost dropped out a few times because she feels so lost, overwhelmed, and often says the faculty just don't seem to care. I was almost ready to drop out of nursing and college because of the horror stories she told me. Now I see something different.

LEONIA: Hey, that bulletin board has a photo of some PMTs featured on the cover of the regional nursing magazine. That's impressive. Oh…our tour guide is in the photo too. She said she was scared and struggled last year but got through it by using the many resources here. I felt really scared this morning about what to expect in nursing, but now I feel better. If she can do it, and all these other students here can do it, I can do it too. If I get scared again, I'll just know I am part of the nursing neighborhood and can come here for support.

All students, regardless of background, age, academic preparedness, or other influencing factors will benefit from coordinated, interactive, and multimedia student support services and resources. Support services and resources may encompass a variety of strategies based on students' diverse needs. According to Tinto (1) effective strategies must demonstrate commitment to the welfare and education of all students above other institutional goals and aim to integrate all students as full members into a cohesive learning community. In professional programs, students benefit from disciplinary-specific strategies for easing the transition from preprofessional educational into professional education and then into the profession (2).

Unfortunately, nursing student services that are fragmented rather than complementary and centrally located may discourage student use. For example, services that are scattered throughout the campus isolate users by physically distancing students and preventing the development of nursing discipline-specific group solidarity. Absent or inconsistent faculty commitment towards the promotion of resources and services available confuses students and discourages ongoing enrichment strategies throughout the curriculum. Unused or underused student services are tragic; their untapped potential in enhancing student academic and psychological outcomes could have a significant positive impact on nursing student retention and professional development. Some services still need to be referred to such as writing center, disability center, personal counseling, and so on. The NSRC is not a substitute for these services but is meant to enhance overall services with its discipline-specific focus and nurturing atmosphere that welcomes all nursing students to the neighborhood of learners and begins socialization for lifelong professional learning.

There is no single solution or strategy for improving student retention; therefore, an approach that links multiple strategies is most effective. The well-designed NSRC offers a place for effectively linking multiple strategies together. Nurse educators are in the key position to develop and coordinate complementary nursing student support strategies via the design of a NSRC. The main purpose of this chapter is to describe the process of designing, operating, and evaluating a NSRC. Key definitions, concepts, decisions, and considerations will be discussed.

NSRC DEFINED

A center is a "place of concentrated activity, influence, or importance" (3). The word "place" indicates that the center is a space designated for a specific purpose. A NSRC is the heart or focus for specifically designed and coordinated resources and activities that are important in influencing student outcomes. The NSRC is a central place where learning, resources, support, peer interaction, professional socialization, and other activities enrich other learning experiences and settings separate from the classroom, clinical, and nursing skills laboratory. It is a place where students can seek help, support, and guidance through a coordinated effort between several activities and multimedia resources to enhance success, enrich learning, and promote positive academic and psychological outcomes. The positive benefits of organized student support interventions within a central location or NSRC has been discussed in the literature (4–6).

The philosophy behind designing a "center" is that creating a niche for nursing students will promote professional socialization, satisfaction, positive academic outcomes, persistence, and stress reduction. The word "room" is avoided as more passive, suggesting a storage facility of resources rather than a learning philosophy that promotes active learning and ongoing interaction. A center promotes active engagement of learners in various levels of the educational and professional development process that actively and purposely coordinates multidimensional and multimedia efforts and strategies to maximize learning and satisfaction and minimize stress. The center is where all points come together, that is, all phases and components of nursing education become integrated appropriately and in a complementary fashion that seeks to elevate learning to a higher level (synthesis) between all components. This is enhanced by the positive influences of peers and students in more advanced levels in the educational and professional development process.

> Reflect back on the snapshot scenarios at the beginning of the chapter. What multidimensional strategies are evident? What are the potential effects on student learning, satisfaction, stress, self-efficacy (confidence), persistence, retention, and success?

ANTICIPATING STUDENT NEEDS: INTEGRATING COMPUTER TECHNOLOGY

In a seamless student retention system, student needs and student profile characteristics are anticipated well in advance (7). Preparing graduates of nursing programs who are computer-literate and who exercise critical thinking, clinical decision making, and reflection is an absolute necessity (8). Empirical evidence shows that computer-assisted instruction (CAI) can enhance self-efficacy in clinical decision making and create a link between theoretical and clinical learning without the fear of jeopardizing client safety (9–13). Students may have guided practice without the instructor present (14). Especially for adult learners who are self-directed and desire immediate feedback for performance, CAI offers a forum for independent learning, immediate feedback, clinical decision making, and critical thinking in a nonthreatening environment. Additionally, computer-based learning tools can influence life-long learning (15).

Previous computer experience and faculty promotion of software programs has a direct impact on student use (16). Previous computer experience may include degree of comfort and familiarity with computer use, satisfaction with software programs, correlation of CAI material with course content and immediate goals, self-efficacy about computer skills, easy access to CAI, satisfaction, and support services associated with CAI use. For example, the quality of the software program can influence student learning, interest, and motivation. A high-quality program is one that is interactive, stimulating, uses multimedia format, permits user control, and provides immediate and descriptive feedback in questioning (17). If software programs are to be perceived as user friendly, programs must be promoted consistently by faculty throughout the curriculum, beginning students must be introduced to CAI early in the curriculum, and software programs must complement and enhance learning via other educational media (e.g., film, video, reading, and lecture). Using a standardized, reliable, and valid evaluation tool for appraising instructional software can enhance the probability that programs will meet overall curricular objectives (14).

Unfortunately, the growing numbers of minority students and new immigrants in higher education have limited resources. Furthermore, limited access to computer technology will be characteristic of many minority and lower income students (7). Shared computers within households and costly Internet charges may be a major barrier for economically challenged students. Integrating computer technology throughout the nursing curriculum must be accompanied by strategies to enhance nursing students' computer technology access, skills, use, and values (18).

The nontraditional student is older, with multiple role responsibilities competing with academic demands. For such students, the opportunity for social integration, professional socialization, professional development, and exploration of new educational technology resources is usually limited. These students mainly attend classes, with little interaction outside the classroom. Furthermore, their organized study time and opportunities to use educational resources are often limited. Some students are inefficacious in their ability to use computers and other educational resources; interaction with student peers and more advanced students who use nursing resources and equipment effectively will assist them to achieve academic success and positive psychological outcomes (satisfaction).

Additionally, minority students in predominantly White institutions may experience social isolation and therefore require extra measures to encourage interaction with nonminority students and among culturally different minority peers, explore new technologically enriched learning strategies, and feel integrated within the college and nursing profession. Socialization and interaction across racial and ethnic groups can have a strong positive impact on retention by increasing satisfaction and self-confidence (19–20).

Traditional students may feel isolated from older students or other nontraditional students. Although traditional students may not have multiple role responsibilities or other barriers typically faced by minority students, they often require assistance with college adjustment, time management, developmental issues related to adolescence and young adulthood, and transition into professional responsibilities and expectations. Such issues may detract from the traditional students' integrated use of CAI and/or their perceived value of CAI. Interaction and coordinated support strategies can have a positive impact on CAI use and overall traditional student retention.

> What are your students' values, skills, knowledge, self-efficacy, strengths, and weakness concerning computer technology, learning, and persistence? What challenges do your students face concerning computer and Internet access? What strategies can be implemented to enhance students in your course and other courses in the nursing program?

LINKING STRATEGIES TOGETHER: A HOLISTIC APPROACH

The literature supports interaction or "active engagement" as the key to effective learning (21–33). Students, especially adult learners, demand student-centered learning and environments that are multidimensional, flexible, nurturing, and holistic. Holistic factors address academic and nonacademic needs. Student-centered learning encourages interaction. Interaction implies that the student is in contact with information, resources, or people so that opportunities for information exchange and new experiences are accessible (21). Nurse educators have the responsibility to structure student-centered experiences that enhance the potential for interaction (21).

The NSRC can enhance student interactions with peers, resources, and information. Developing a social environment that engages students and enhances student interaction is crucial, especially for commuter students (30,31,34). The NSRC offers such an environment of opportunities.

Additionally, the presence of a NSRC demonstrates to students that the institution cares and is committed to nursing student success by providing them with a special place of their own. Institutional commitment to student success and student needs and concerns helps foster positive attitudes toward the institution. The organizational environment impacts greatly on student persistence and retention through student perceptions (30,35).

Linking strategies together in a flexible yet complementary fashion will not only enhance learning opportunities but can influence student choice, use, persistence, satisfaction, and outcomes. Choices that respond to the multidimensional nature of learning, learning styles, time constraints, multiple role responsibilities, and other factors influencing student persistence and retention will enhance student use (36). For example, offering workshops on days and times that complement students' class schedule and without requiring an additional trip to campus may increase opportunities for many nontraditional commuter students.

Meeting the needs of learners in various stages of the educational process necessitates a NSRC that holistically accommodates students' changing academic and nonacademic needs. The mentoring needs and types of partnerships developed change over time, necessitating flexibility and anticipatory planning (37,38), and attention to the quality of student interaction (39). The quality of interaction influences (professional) socialization, academic integration, psychological growth, self-efficacy, and motivation. Such factors influence student persistence, academic outcomes, satisfaction, and levels of stress (40).

Creative means of bringing together students in ongoing contact with one another and with various educational resources, working with students in cohorts, and creatively linking beginning and advanced students not only captures the power of peer group interaction and develops a supportive environment outside of the classroom but provides the foundation for initial and ongoing (lifelong) professional socialization, mentoring, and commitment. The literature repeatedly states that peer interaction and a supportive environment outside the classroom are vital (41–43). Kuh (41), for example, speaks about "academic neighborhoods" while Tinto (44,45) talks about "learning communities." Successful learning communities strategically link faculty, students, staff, and other resources into a cohesive network; students take the responsibility for peers (46). The concept of creating an environment conducive to learning and socialization outside the classroom is what underlies these and other similar terms. It is proposed that the NSRC is a place that creates a caring, local nursing neighborhood of learners that holistically fosters professional growth, development, and socialization, through the careful integration of various strategies, thereby enhancing student persistence and retention through the attainment of positive academic and psychological outcomes (satisfaction and decreased stress). Creating such an environment requires strategic planning, careful decision making, flexibility, and ongoing commitment.

DESIGN DECISIONS AND PLAN

What is the profile of your program's student retention and success pathways? What departmental and administrative supports exist and/or are needed for NSRC design, implementation, and evaluation? What college resources currently exist?

Similar to the design of an enrichment program (Chapter 13), the predesign phase involves five steps: assessing the current situation, reviewing the literature, searching for grants, drafting a plan, and soliciting support. Readers are encouraged to review Chapter 13 for details and rationale about these steps as overlapping areas will not be repeated here.

Together, literature support and student survey responses can justify the need for designing a NSRC. For example, among several student sample populations, survey responses indicated great interest and need for student support services, including study assistance, workshops, career advisement, computer resources, educational resources, and peer support (47–49). Easy access to current nursing resources and assistance with educational resources and equipment (books, computers, etc.) was also identified needs. Furthermore, grant opportunities existed towards the development of nursing student retention strategies. This vital information strengthens justification for a NSRC when soliciting support and preparing a proposal.

Conceptual and instrumental support by the nursing faculty and administrators is essential. Although conceptual support is fundamental to promoting success of a NSRC, accurately appraising the amount of instrumental (monetary and service) support is crucial. Inaccurate estimates of needed services or funds will obstruct or prevent the eventual development and operation of a NSRC. Consequently, systematic decision making sets the framework for a realistic and feasible plan. Suggestions for systematic decision making will follow.

First, a checklist approach offers a quick appraisal of desired resources, activities, and services that can later be revised and/or refined when the overall checklist results are reviewed. After deciding upon desired educational resources, educators need to consider the necessary equipment and furniture (see Figure 14.1). For example, computer-assisted instructional programs with videos require earphones. A listening center composed of earphones, jack box with individual volume controls, rack, and plastic cover will allow groups of students up to four to view CAI video together

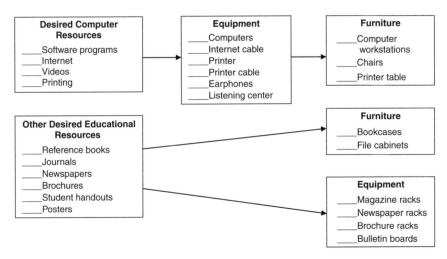

FIGURE 14.1   Planning the nursing student resource center: Checklist of desired educational resources, equipment, and furniture.

or individually and to keep equipment clean and well organized. An adequate size workstation for the computer, large monitor, listening center, and adequate seats will therefore be needed.

Consideration of desired student support activities precedes the decisions on needed personnel, required furniture and equipment, and miscellaneous materials for enhancing these activities (see Figure 14.2). For example, a telephone link to a peer mentor or tutor may provide opportunities for easy and quick access to social and academic support that does not necessitate lengthy intervention. Often, the knowledge that a caring peer mentor or tutor is available by telephone to answer a quick question, verify a study group meeting, offer positive encouragement for continued study behaviors, offer a suggestion on prioritizing assignments, and suggest ways of balancing multiple role responsibilities is valuable in minimizing stress, enhancing satisfaction, and promoting positive academic outcomes. Especially for commuter students and nontraditional students with multiple role responsibilities, quick access to support without commuting is comforting. Obviously, a peer mentor, telephone, telephone-jack box, and telephone service are necessary.

If a nursing skills practice laboratory or simulation center does not already exist within a school of nursing, nurse educators may wish to allocate a separate section of the NSRC for technical skills practice. A separate, sufficiently large area is recommended to accommodate equipment and minimize the noise associated with technical skills practice. Many schools of nursing have a separate classroom and laboratory for teaching and practicing technical skills; therefore, the NSRC design in this chapter will exclude the details necessary in planning nursing skills practice laboratory

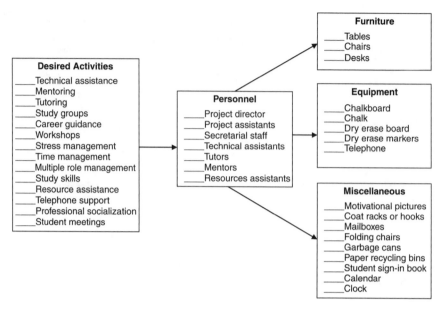

FIGURE 14.2 Planning the nursing student resource center: Checklist of desired student support activities, needed personnel, equipment, furniture, and miscellaneous items.

or a simulation center. The philosophy behind a NSRC is to complement, enrich, and coordinate learning in various course components (classroom, clinical, nursing skills laboratory, or simulation center); thus the assumption is that a nursing skills practice laboratory and/or simulation center already exists. Interested readers are referred to sources in the literature discussing the teaching and learning involved with technical nursing skills, simulation, and design.

It is especially important to evaluate the actual, potential, and hidden costs and services sometimes overlooked in design planning that underlie the desired resources and activities. For example, the need to rewire a room that is going to be converted into a NSRC to accommodate computer stations will require electricians and possibly contractors and painters, if walls and ceilings need to be opened. An architect and campus-planning expert will need to evaluate fire and building safety issues and prepare a floor plan. Installation of computer software programs requires institutional and technical support. Special security measures may be required. Construction of a new building or an addition to an already existing building will require more time, consultation, services, and money.

Once the checklists are completed, revisions and refinement will be required. Deleting unrealistic resources or activities based on insufficient conceptual and instrumental support or available space may be necessary. Detailing the amount, type, and cost of desired resources, equipment, furniture, activities, and personnel may necessitate arriving at more feasible and realistic cost estimates. Soliciting support via formal commitment to specific tasks, time allocation for specific tasks, and ongoing availability to assist/consult with specific tasks should be finalized in written follow-up letters or memos.

Willingness to further refine details and make additional revisions is important. However, a sparse selection of resources, services, and activities without the potential opportunity for future expansion will probably not make a significant impact on nursing student retention. With a large one-time grant or benefactor, a NSRC may need to be clearly delineated with a final plan. However, allocation of funds for the ongoing operation of the NSRC needs to be realistically appraised. With the distribution of funds over several years, it may be important to delineate several phases in the overall development of the NSRC. For example, purchase of five computers each year over a 4-year period will lead to 20 computers. Advanced planning concerning sufficient space, electrical requirements, and technical support is therefore important. Modifications based on grant proposal guidelines and/or institutional guidelines should be strictly followed to optimize funding opportunities and approval.

Once the NSRC project or grant is approved, it is important to review the budgetary allocations for specific categories and check if there are any restrictions or added guidelines. Budgetary constraints may require some modifications from the original proposal. Once modifications are finalized, the project director should communicate to faculty, administrators, students, support personnel, and collaborative partners that funding has been received. Collaborative partners (those individuals who committed time, expertise, service, or some other instrumental support toward the proposed project) should be contacted personally. A telephone contact followed by a written memo or copy of the grant award and proposal may be indicated, depending on the type of partnership or services required and level of involvement. Memos that communicate the necessary details reinforce the verbal communication. Publicizing available job openings for positions associated with the NSRC should be done early to permit a larger pool of applicants for best selection. Written and verbal announcements should describe roles and responsibilities, qualifications, hours, wages, and any other important information.

When was the last time you conducted a review of the literature concerning nursing student retention and success? What books, book chapters, websites, journal articles, dissertations, and other scholarly resources can help you plan the NSRC?

What small institutional seed grants are available in your institution? What professional, local, state, and national grants are available? Which one(s) would be most feasible to get the NSRC started?

What specific supportive tasks have your departmental and college colleagues, students, and administrators agreed to perform? How have these expected tasks and time frames been communicated, agreed upon, and documented?

PREPARATION

Coordination of all tasks, services, and activities associated with developing, operating, and evaluating the NSRC is a complex responsibility of the project director. Allocating a sufficient amount of time for program preparation is essential. Adequate released time for the project director is integral to the overall success of the NSRC. Making a list of what needs to be done, by whom, and the needed date of completion can help prioritize program preparation components. If a timeline was originally submitted with the NSRC proposal, it can be a valuable guide for organization. Preparation may include ordering furniture and equipment, creating or obtaining educational materials and documentation forms, selection and orientation of personnel, questionnaire development and evaluation, and arranging the physical setting. Dividing tasks between NSRC development, operation, and evaluation can help prioritize them.

Tasks associated with the NSRC setting and development take first priority. Minor remodeling, reconstruction, electrical work, painting, floor waxing, security measures, and cleaning need to be completed before furniture and equipment can be set up. Therefore, early initial contact and ongoing contact and collaboration with associated services will be necessary. Anticipating that work schedules may fall behind due to unexpected complications will ease frustration and stress. For example, a leak discovered during remodeling may delay further action until plumbers are contacted and subsequently complete their work.

After contacting appropriate personnel for remodeling/reconstruction or construction, the project direct should order equipment, furniture, and educational resources. Sometimes, delays in processing purchase order requests may occur; early submission enhances the probability that ordered items will arrive well before the anticipated NSRC opening date. Previewing and reviewing educational resources before proposal preparation decreases preparation time now; however, if previews and reviews were not done previously, the project director will need sufficient preview and review time for self and/or other faculty members. Prearranging for a safe and secure storage area for equipment and furniture is advisable in the event that the NSRC remodeling is delayed.

While waiting for the NSRC setting to be completed, the project director can move to the high priority tasks involved with NSRC operation and evaluation. Two tasks that usually have the highest priority because they involve a series of steps, are time consuming, and concern several people are the selection and orientation of personnel who will work in the NSRC (operation) and questionnaire development (evaluation).

Selection and Orientation of NSRC Personnel

The desired activities checklist (Figure 14.2) provides a guide for the selection of NSRC personnel. Criteria for selection may include (1) current enrollment in an upper-level nursing course, (2) above-average grades in prenursing and nursing courses, (3) above-average clinical evaluations, (4) excellent communication skills, (5) basic computer skills, and/or (6) recommendation from a previous course instructor. For the purposes of this chapter, a student personnel worker employed in the NSRC will be referred to as a Nursing Student Resource Assistant (NSRA). The application form, the applicant's written statement of reason for interest, college transcripts, clinical evaluations, written recommendations, prior work history, and experience provide baseline information about the applicant prior to an invited interview. The interview process should allow for dialogue concerning expected responsibilities and necessary skills.

If assistance with CAI is an expected responsibility, noting applicants' technical finesse with computers as well as their attitude concerning the value of CAI is important. Willingness, motivation, and eagerness to build upon existing computer skills to accommodate new software programs are helpful assets. The applicant's sensitivity to students inefficacious in their learning abilities and/or computers is an important quality to note. Scheduling, arranging, and conducting interviews are time consuming yet essential to the selection process. During the interview, it should be emphasized that a collaborative partnership among NSRC personnel and the project director is an important goal.

The next priority is to organize and prepare the educational and documentation materials needed for the NSRA orientation and the operation of the NSRC. A NSRC brochure detailing hours of operation, services, equipment, NSRA role, and CAI programs succinctly conveys the main features of the NSRC and can easily be distributed to students. A separate CAI brochure or NSRC brochure insert listing alphabetized topics, names of corresponding computer software programs, icons, method for accessing, and suggestions for use becomes another valuable tool for guiding students through the use of various software programs throughout the educational process. Noting the recommended user level assists users in avoiding programs that are too advanced while minimizing the risk that available and appropriate programs are inadvertently overlooked. Maximizing CAI use appropriate to the target learner audience will minimize stress and dissatisfaction. Other necessary educational support materials may include handouts on time management, stress reduction, balancing multiple roles, test-taking strategies, study skills, college adjustment, and other college

resources. Documentation forms or ID card scanners for recording attendance, CAI use, study group topics, and other proposed NSRC activities
and resources should be well designed to enhance the efficiency of record
keeping, data management, and data analysis.

Orientation offers structure and direction for NSRAs; it assists in organizing and coordinating NSRC activities, services, and resources via the
NSRA role. An orientation session should review the overall purposes
and goals of the NSRC, particularly detailing the significance of mentoring in nursing and the role of NSRA and student as partners in learning.
The expected benefits of specific NSRA roles and interventions should be
highlighted, clarifying the scope of the NSRA role, and emphasizing the
importance of sharing this information with students. Documentation
forms for recording the study group's activities and anticipated plans
for the next meeting and other activities must be clearly reviewed with
NSRAs. Some documentation forms can serve as a weekly communication between the NSRA and project director. Strategies for enhancing
student survival skills may address such issues as academic support
strategies, time management, stress reduction techniques, assisting
students throughout the educational process, promoting professional
growth, and balancing multiple role responsibilities. Handouts and lists
of referral resources within the college should complement this discussion, along with detailed procedures for contacting technological support personnel (for computers, software, e-mail, telephones) and security
personnel. Hands-on practice with various CAI software programs and
other educational media helps develop NSRA confidence and familiarity
with new equipment.

Simulated situations and NSRA group discussion allow NSRAs to
use problem-solving strategies for academic, nonacademic, and computer technology–related problems that can arise. Simulated situations
related to computer technology include dealing with students who
(1) misuse the Internet for nonacademic purposes, (2) misuse the
Internet to obtain papers via online papermills, (3) misuse the Internet
for other unethical and/or illegal purposes, (4) are afraid to use the
computer, (5) are reluctant to do RN licensing practice questions for
fear of being wrong, and (6) see little value in CAI. Decision-making
dilemmas and varying opinions identify areas that require further clarification and guidance. Continued emphasis that the NSRA will have an
ongoing collaborative relationship with the project director throughout
the semester offers reassurance. The NSRA's written evaluation of the
orientation also gives information to guide future orientations.

Questionnaire Development

Evaluation measures should include academic and nonacademic components. Measures of satisfaction, stress, student perceptions concerning

strategy components on retention, or self-efficacy may all be appropriate; however, evaluation measures should be carefully selected based on predetermined desired outcomes. The review of existing instruments for use and/or adaptation as part of the initial review of the literature in the pre-design, decision, and planning phase can save time when deciding upon evaluation measures. If existing instruments are selected, collaboration with content and psychometric experts will further determine the appropriateness of the selection. Obtaining formal permission for instrument use from its author and/or a publisher should be initiated early, combined with a request to possibly collaborate on its intended use. Sometimes, existing questionnaires may require minor or major adaptations, requiring permission for use. Determining collaboration or negotiation with the author concerning intended changes, method of administration, scoring, data collection, data analysis, and/or final adapted questionnaire revision also should be done early to avoid delays. Development and evaluation of a new questionnaire is time consuming and requires a systematic plan (50). Review by a psychometric expert should affirm that the paper format will be easily scanned, interpreted, and analyzed, using statistical software programs. A project assistant with computer expertise in creating optical scanning instruments, scanning, and conversion into statistical packages for the social sciences can format the instrument. However, all instruments need a trial run for scanning to assure ease with future data processing. Another option is creating online survey instruments, which also require trial runs for use, interpretation, and analysis. As reliability and validity tests must be routinely done with each sample—whether old, new, or adapted questionnaires are used—plan for additional time for data collection and analysis.

> What are your three highest priority tasks in the preparation phase? Why? What is the best way for you to successfully complete tasks?

OPERATION

Operation of the NSRC consists of proactive, ongoing, and transitional interventions. A smoothly running NSRC begins with good publicity and reliable, conscientious, and caring NSRAs. Proactive announcements of NSRC services, resources, and hours also offer assurance that student support services are available and should be used throughout the semester before academic difficulties arise. Before the beginning of the semester, information can be distributed via the nursing Webpage, listserv, group e-mail, postal mail, presemester orientation meetings, registration, and bulletin boards. At the beginning of the semester, distribution of NSRC brochures accompanied by an in-class personal greeting and invitation from the project director and/or NSRA will serve as a reminder to use services proactively throughout the semester. Highlighting the main features and benefits of select services, resources, and activities particularly pertinent to each course will help optimize use of coordinated resources and activities within the NSRC and throughout the curriculum. An orientation or introduction to the NSRC can be scheduled for new students.

Early formation of weekly study groups, practice test question groups, CAI user groups, care plan groups, student peer support groups, and other student groups will maximize student success by identifying student strengths and weaknesses before academic difficulties, stress, or role conflicts arise. Early identification of the at-risk student also can prevent failure or withdrawal. Often students do not seek help until difficulty arises, and then it is often too late to improve an academically precarious situation. (See Chapter 13 for details concerning enrichment programs and study group strategies.) Early planned scheduling for weekly individual tutoring, self-CAI study, and other self-directed study strategies can also promote success, and facilitate weekly contact with NSRAs and other students at various stages of the educational and professional development process.

NSRA-student partnerships cannot truly develop without consistent and frequent contacts. Ongoing contact can evolve into interactions that flourish into collaborative and productive partnerships. Students also can feel more at ease with group peers, offering emotional, academic, and technological support strategies. This peer interaction helps develop professional socialization, integration, and acculturation into the nursing student role and future RN role. The opportunity to share experiences and watch role models and peers struggle with similar academic, technological, and nonacademic challenges can help increase self-efficacy and motivation to persist (51,52).

By linking various strategies, the NSRC offers the unique opportunity for students at various stages of their educational and professional development to share experiences while observing role models and peers use multimedia approaches to learning with varying levels of ease, difficulty, and satisfaction. More advanced students can be role models to guide students through transitional stages and encourage persistence through personal, academic, and professional challenges typically associated with transitional points. Here, guidance is crucial to encourage retention, enhance achievement, and promote satisfaction and minimize stress. As students move from one level of the educational process to the next, publicizing activities, resources, and services particularly important for this new level (course) helps spark ongoing energy to persist and build upon previously used NSRC services.

Certainly, a brief orientation session can complement an announcement. Activities, services, and resources should be woven into a pattern that has easily identifiable vertical and horizontal curricular threads that create a strong and durable fabric to ensure positive academic and psychological outcomes. By requiring CAI programs and/or study group participation within the first 2 weeks, beginning students get accustomed to the multidimensional learning environment and become socialized with peers and more advanced learners.

Ongoing collaboration between NSRAs and the project director is crucial to the smooth operation of the NSRC. Collaboration may occur during regularly scheduled intervals and/or as needed via in-person meetings, telephone calls, e-mail, documentation forms, or other written communication. It may not be feasible for the project director to be on-site during all NSRC hours; however, open channels of communication are necessary to facilitate success and create an atmosphere of the "nursing learning neighborhood." Anticipating problems, facing existing problems immediately, suggesting solutions, and verbally praising positive actions will enhance the function of the NSRC and maximize efficient use of the project director's time.

> What are your three highest priority tasks for the operation phase? What are your three hardest challenges? Why? What is the best way for you to successfully complete tasks?

EVALUATION

A carefully orchestrated evaluation should be tied explicitly to the NSRC's plan, with formative and summative components. Formative evaluations, which assess the functioning or operation of the NSRC (rather than outcomes), can be monitored as the program is implemented—documenting specific activities, identifying difficulties, and allowing for diagnostic-prescriptive modifications based on participants' feedback via quantitative and qualitative data. Formative evaluations can provide immediate feedback for initiating needed changes at any point in the semester. (Toolkit Item 7 may be adapted for formative evaluation and should include open-ended questions.)

Summative evaluations should be monitored and compared globally at the completion of each semester to assess the achievement of desired outcomes over a period of time. The NURS model may be used to identify academic, psychological, and affective outcomes. Academic outcomes may include course retention, course success, course withdrawal, continuous program retention, interim program retention, ideal program retention, total program retention, total program success, and ideal program success. Psychological outcomes may include measures of satisfaction or stress; affective outcomes may include self-efficacy (confidence) perceptions.

Because student retention is a dynamic and multidimensional phenomenon, the NSRC evaluation should include academic and nonacademic (psychological and/or affective) outcomes. In one evaluation study, academic outcomes (nursing course grade and withdrawal) were measured by the student transcript record and compared with the previous year's retention rates (53). During the second year of NSRC operation, student NSRC use, course pass rates, and course retention rates increased; failure rates and course withdrawal rates decreased. Results demonstrated a 6% increase in course retention from one spring semester group to the next spring semester group. For the fall semester groups, an 8% increase in course retention was noted. Course retention greatly impacted upon program retention as greater number of students successfully completed courses and could therefore progress in the program.

In the same study, student psychological outcomes (satisfaction) were measured by a satisfaction questionnaire (see Toolkit Item 7). To maintain consistency in data collection, the project director administered the satisfaction questionnaire at the end of the semester during lecture class sessions. Overall, students were satisfied with nursing and/or prenursing courses, nursing discipline as a career choice, college, and NSRC services. Qualitative comments on student questionnaires further attested to their general satisfaction with the NSRC. Requests for continued and expanded NSRC services and hours were noted.

Following the preestablished plan for data collection and data analysis consistently and rigorously will help make the evaluation results more valid and reliable. This includes working diligently with previously established partners in the evaluation process such as the data collectors, director of institutional research, project assistant, and psychometric expert. Once the results are obtained and reviewed for statistical and practical significance, inferences from the data can guide future NSRC activities, resources, services, outcome measures, and desired outcomes. The ultimate goal of the NSRC is for empirical and conceptually based retention strategies to continue to address the holistic needs of changing student populations.

> What formative and summative evaluations are consistently conducted for proactive, ongoing, and transitional strategies implemented in the NSRC? For equipment and resources in NSRC? How have the results guided subsequent design, operation, and evaluation strategies?

KEY POINT SUMMARY

- The NSRC is a central place where learning, resources, support, peer interaction, professional socialization, and other activities enrich other learning experiences and settings separate from the classroom, clinical, nursing skills laboratory, and simulation lab.

- The philosophy behind designing a "center" or "nursing neighborhood" is that creating a niche for nursing students will promote professional socialization, satisfaction, positive academic outcomes, persistence, and stress reduction.
- The predesign phase involves five steps: assessing the current situation, reviewing the literature, searching for grants, drafting a plan, and soliciting support.
- Preparation may include ordering furniture and equipment, creating or obtaining educational materials and documentation forms, selecting and orienting personnel, developing and evaluating questionnaires, and arranging the physical setting.
- Operation of the NSRC consists of proactive, ongoing, and transitional interventions; evaluation should include academic and nonacademic (psychological and/or affective) outcomes.

APPLICATION STRATEGIES

EDUCATOR-IN-ACTION VIGNETTE

Professor Booke is the project director of a newly funded NSRC. Furniture and equipment include: eight small study tables, 16 computers with nursing interactive and multimedia programs, two printers, two bookcases with resource books, two small sofas, a file cabinet, a large chalkboard, motivational pictures, a bulletin board, a telephone, and a small desk. Student services include enrichment program study group sessions, individual peer tutoring, peer mentoring, career guidance, CAI and practice test questions, and workshops. The new project is publicized to students via in-person announcements in class and flyers.

As part of the evaluation plan, Professor Booke prepares to evaluate the functioning of the NSRC after 6 weeks of operation. Her formative evaluation targets both the student users and the student workers and includes both qualitative and quantitative assessments. For example, all students using the NSRC during the sixth week are asked to complete an anonymous ten-item satisfaction questionnaire and write additional comments in the comment section. Student workers are asked to complete a similar survey concerning the NSRC equipment, facilities, and overall functioning. A quick scan of survey responses and written comments indicate overall satisfaction; however, several emerging themes are apparent. To gain further insight, Professor Booke invites ten students in the NSRC to a brief, 30-minute open roundtable discussion about the NSRC services and facilities. Several student comments and subsequent educator actions follow below:

NORI: The NSRC is a great place. I can come and practice NCLEX questions and discuss them with my classmates and mentor. We can look up information in the resource book if we get stuck. Everything is right here.

JEAN-PAUL: The NSRC is a place to stop in before class or after class, study, talk about our stress, or practice questions. You always see someone you know. It helps us nursing students feel like one big family. That doesn't happen in the library—it is too big. There is always someone here in the NSRC to answer a nursing question.

SUSANNA: Sometimes it gets really crowded and noisy so I can't really concentrate to do reading or answer practice test questions. Sometimes I have to wait to use a computer. There are no other computers on campus with the nursing computer programs.

MARTINE: I wish the NSRC were open on weekends, especially before test days. The PMT and the study groups really help me a lot.

EBONY: Samantha, one of the PMTs, is the best. She offered to help me outside of the study group during the NSRC morning hours. It's quiet at the NSRC in the mornings. My grades have really improved with the extra tutoring. I even enjoy learning!

NANCY: I live far away so I can't come in extra to use the NSRC. A few times I got stuck at home and called the NSRC. Samantha was able to guide me through by asking me a series of questions until I figured out the answer myself. That's what is good about the PMTs—they help you through the process; they don't give you the answer. I was able to continue studying at home without any problems.

Discussions with the student PMTs indicated that the NSRC was noisy and crowded on certain days and times. During these times, PMTs felt that resources and services could not be used optimally and individual attention to students was impossible. Based on the formative evaluation findings, Professor Booke implements the following actions:

- Gathers detailed data on student use of different types of services, time, and day
- Schedules open NSRC hours on alternating weekend days
- Schedules additional open hours closely before midterms and final exams
- Schedules two PMTs during busy hours
- Explores the possibilities for expanding the facility, equipment, and services

Summative evaluation (academic outcomes, retention rates, and student satisfaction) will provide valuable outcome data that can substantiate ongoing and/or expanded student services via the NSRC.

TOOLKIT RESOURCE BOX

Item 28—Nursing Student Resource Center (Nursing Neighborhood)
Item 7—Nursing Student Resource Center Satisfaction Survey
Items 3 and 4—Student Perception Appraisal Questionnaires—Revised, Pretest and Posttest

DISCUSSION QUESTIONS

1. Professor Bridges proposes to write a grant proposal to support the conversion of a classroom into a multiservice NSRC along with purchase of educational programs, wages for PMTs, and released time coverage or salary for a nursing retention coordinator. Professor Hurdles verbalizes opposition, saying, "This will just confuse students and they won't know how to go to the library and use learning resources there. Why do we want to compete with the library and other college resources such as counseling and tutoring located in the campus center? Why do we have to pay PMTs to facilitate study groups? Many students already study with their classmates or friends. There is already a nursing faculty shortage in this department and nationwide. Why do we want to take teaching time away from a faculty member to coordinate a nursing retention program? We can just let the college retention center do its job. With the 10,000 students on campus, I'm sure they're way more experienced about dropout prevention than nurses are." Assume the role of Professor Bridges. How would you respond to Professor Hurdles?
2. Which character in the snapshot scenario could you relate to most? Why? How will this influence your future role when teaching, advising, and interacting with students?
3. Several students in the first semester nursing course express various academic and/or nonacademic issues causing them to contemplate dropout or stopout. The course instructor tells the students, "go and see the nursing student retention coordinator. It's not part of my job to help you about dropout or stopout decisions." As the nursing student retention coordinator, how would you handle this situation with the students, course instructor, and other program faculty?
4. Which part of NSRC/nursing neighborhood design process do you find the most challenging? Why? What strategies and resources could you employ to meet these challenges effectively?

5. How can the snapshot scenario and Educator-in-Action Vignette be adapted for use with new nursing students, new PMTs, nursing faculty, and college administrators?

REFERENCES

1. Tinto, V. (1993). *Leaving college: Rethinking the cause and cures of student attrition.* Chicago, IL: University of Chicago Press.
2. Schon, D. (1987). *Educating the reflective practitioner.* San Franscisco, CA: Jossey-Bass.
3. *Roget's II: The new thesaurus* (3rd ed.). (1995). Boston, MA: Houghton Miflin.
4. Ankele, R., Lohner, L., & Masiulaniec, B. A. S. (2001). Innovative teaching within the nursing resource center: A blueprint for student success. *Journal of Multicultural Nursing & Health, 7*(3), 6–9.
5. Ramsey, P., Blowers, S., Merriman, C., Glenn, L. L., & Terry, L. (2000). The NURSE Center: A peer mentor-tutor project for disadvantaged nursing students in Appalachia. *Nurse Educator, 25*(6), 277–281.
6. Dennison, S. (2010). Peer mentoring: Untapped potential. *Journal of Nursing Education, 49*(6), 340–342.
7. Burr, P. L., Burr, R. M., & Novak, L. F. (1999). Student retention is more complicated than merely keeping the students you have today: Toward a "seamless retention theory." *Journal of College Student Retention: Theory, Research, and Practice 1*(3), 239–253.
8. Mueller, S. S., Pullen, R. L., & McGee, K. S. (2002). A model nursing computer resource center. *Nurse Educator, 27*(3), 115–117.
9. Madorin, S., & Iwasiw, C. (1999). The effects of computer-assisted instruction on the self-efficacy of baccalaureate nursing students. *Journal of Nursing Education, 38*(6), 282–285.
10. Weis, P. A., & Guyton-Simmons. (1998). A computer simulation for teaching critical thinking. *Nurse Educator, 23*(2), 30–33.
11. Edwards, H., Nash, R., Sacre, S., Courtney, M., & Abbey, J. (2007). Development of a virtual learning environment to enhance undergraduate nursing students' effectiveness and interest in working with older people. *Nurse Education Today, 28,* 672–679.
12. Mertig, R. G. (2003). *Teaching nursing in an associate degree program.* New York, NY: Springer Publishing.
13. Rouse, D. P. (2007). Computer-assisted instruction: An effective instructional method. *Teaching and Learning in Nursing, 2,* 138–143.
14. Boyce, B. A. B., & Winne, M. D. (2000). Developing an evaluation tool for instructional software programs. *Nurse Educator, 25*(3), 145–148.
15. Zinatelli, M., Dube, M. A., & Jovanovic, R. (2002). Computer-based study skills training: The role of technology in improving performance and retention. *Journal of College Student Retention: Research, Theory, & Practice, 4*(1), 67–78.
16. Thede, L. Q., Taft, S., & Coeling, H. (1994). Computer-assisted instruction: A learner's viewpoint. *Journal of Nursing Education, 33*(7), 299–305.
17. Khoiny, F. E. (1995). Factors that contribute to computer-assisted instruction effectiveness. *Computers in Nursing, 13*(4), 165–168.

18. Pressler, J. L., & Kenner, C. (2009). Embracing new directions in curricula and teaching. *Nurse Educator, 34*(2), 49–50.
19. Astin, A. (1993). Diversity and multiculturalism on campus: How are students affected? *Change, 25*(2), 44–49.
20. Luo, J., & Jamieson-Drake, D. (2009). A retrospective assessment of the educational benefits of interaction across racial boundaries. *Journal of College Student Development, 50*(2), 115–134.
21. Kennerly, S. (2001). Fostering interaction through multimedia. *Nurse Educator, 26*(2), 90–94.
22. Conderman, G., Bresnahan, V., & Hedin, L. (2011). Promoting active involvement in today's classrooms. *Kappa Delta Pi Record, 47*(4), 174–180.
23. Brown, A. V. (2008). Effectively educating Latino/a students: A comparative study of participation patterns of Hispanic American and Anglo-American university students. *Journal of Hispanic Higher Education, 7*(2), 97–118.
24. Cejda, B. D., & Hoover, R. E. (2011). Strategies for faculty-student engagement: How community college faculty engage Latino students. *Journal of College Student Retention: Theory, Research, and Practice, 12*(2), 135–153.
25. Buch, K., & Spaulding, S. (2011). The impact of a psychology learning community on academic success, retention, and student learning outcomes. *Teaching of Psychology, 38*(2), 71–77.
26. Martin, A. J.; & Dowson, M. (2009). Interpersonal relationships, motivation, engagement, and achievement: Yields for theory, current issues, and educational practice. *Review of Educational Research,m 79*(1), 327–365.
27. Angelino, L. M., Williams, F. K., & Natvig, D. (2007). Strategies to engage online students and reduce attrition rates. *Journal of Educators Online, 4*(2), 1–14.
28. Callahan, K. M. (2009). Academic-centered peer interaction and retention in undergraduate mathematics programs. *Journal of College Student Retention: Research, Theory, and Practice, 10* (3), 361–389.
29. Oermann, M. H., & Gaberson, K. B. (2009). *Evaluation and testing in nursing education.* New York, NY: Springer Publishing.
30. Seidman, A. (2005). *College student retention: Formula for success.* Westport, CT: American Council on Education, Praeger.
31. Karp, M. M., Hughes, K. L., & O'Gara, L. (2011). An exploration of Tinto's integration framework for community college students. *Journal of College Student Retention: Research, Theory, and Practice, 12* (1), 69–86.
32. Bosher, S. D., & Pharris, M. D. (2009). *Transforming nursing education: The culturally inclusive environment.* New York, NY: Springer Publishing.
33. Wolf-Wendel, L., Ward, K., & Kinzie, J. (2009). A tangled web of terms: The overlap and unique contribution of involvement, engagement, and integration to understanding college student success. *Journal of College Student Development, 50*(4), 407–428.
34. Braxton, J. M., & Mundy, M. E. (2001). Powerful institutional levers to reduce college student departure. *Journal of College Student Retention: Research, Theory, & Practice, 3*(1), 91–118.
35. Berger, J. B. (2001). Understanding the organizational nature of student persistence: Empirically-based recommendations for practice. *Journal of College Student Retention: Research, Theory, & Practice, 3*(1), 3–22.

36. Bork, A. (2000). Futurespective. *Technological Horizons in Education, 27*(6), 49.
37. Vance, C., & Olson, R. K. (1998). *The mentor connection in nursing.* New York, NY: Springer Publishing.
38. Vance, C. (2011). *Fast facts for career success in nursing: Making the most of mentoring in a nutshell.* New York, NY: Springer Publishing.
39. Ishitani, T. T.,.& DesJardins, S. L. (2002). A longitudinal investigation of dropout from college in the United States. *Journal of College Student Retention: Research, Theory, & Practice, 4*(2), 173–202.
40. Bean, J. P., & Eaton, S. B. (2001). The psychology underlying successful retention practices. *Journal of College Student Retention: Research, Theory, & Practice, 3*(1), 73–90.
41. Kuh, G. D. (2001). Organizational culture and student persistence: Prospects and puzzles. *Journal of College Student Retention: Research, Theory, & Practice, 3*(1), 23–40.
42. Nora, A. (2001). The depiction of significant others in Tinto's "Rites of Passage": A reconceptualization of the influence of family and community in the persistence process. *Journal of College Student Retention: Research, Theory, & Practice, 3*(1), 41–56.
43. Stokes, L. G. (2003). Gatherings as a retention strategy. *Association of Black Nursing Faculty Journal, 14*(4), 80–82.
44. Tinto, V. (1997). Classrooms as communities. *Journal of Higher Education, 68*(6), 599–623.
45. Tinto, V. (2000). Linking learning and leaving: Exploring the role of the college classroom in student departure. In J. M. Braxton (Ed.), *Reworking the student departure puzzle* (pp. 81–94). Nashville, TN: Vanderbilt University Press.
46. Soldner, L., Lee, Y., & Duby, P. (1999). Welcome to the block: Developing freshman learning communities that work. *Journal of College Student Retention: Research, Theory, & Practice, 1*(2), 115–130.
47. Jeffreys, M. R. (1998). Predicting nontraditional student retention and academic achievement. *Nurse Educator, 23*(1), 42–48.
48. Jeffreys, M. R. (2001). Evaluating enrichment program study groups: Academic outcomes, psychological outcomes, and variables influencing retention. *Nurse Educator, 26*(3), 142–149.
49. Jeffreys, M. R. (2002). Students' perceptions of variables influencing retention: A pretest and post-test approach. *Nurse Educator, 27*(1), 16–19 [Erratum, 2002, 27(2), 64].
50. Jeffreys, M. R., & Smodlaka, I. (1996). Steps of the instrument-design process: An illustrative approach for nurse educators. *Nurse Educator, 21*(6), 47–52 [Erratum, 1997, 22(1), 49].
51. Bandura, A. (1986). *Social foundations of thought and action: A social cognitive theory.* Englewood Cliffs, NJ: Prentice-Hall.
52. Zimmerman, B. J. (1995). Self-efficacy and educational development. In A. Bandura (Ed.), *Self-efficacy in changing societies* (pp. 202–231). New York, NY: Cambridge University Press.
53. Jeffreys, M. R. (2002). *Evaluation of the nursing student resource center.* Unpublished report.

Future Directions: A Vision for Tomorrow

Whatever is done (or not done) today will influence what happens tomorrow and beyond. Every nurse educator or future nurse educator is empowered to make a positive difference in the world of nursing education and in the lives of students.

SNAPSHOT SCENARIO

During a faculty discussion about improving student retention and success, Professor Uno thinks, "I'm only one person. I'm struggling to keep up with all my teaching responsibilities. We're so short on nursing faculty that I'm teaching an extra course this semester. What could I ever do to make a difference in student retention? It takes more than one person."

Professor Frank says, "We can't do everything at once, or solve all the problems interfering with nursing student retention and success, but we can do something now to make it better."

Professor Ponder shares, "I was wondering so much about what factors restricted or supported student success and retention that I decided to give one day a month to reading new journal articles in higher education and nursing concerning this topic. Each article gave me new insight into the complexities surrounding individual nursing student success. I realized that faculty actions and inactions might unintentionally ignore students' needs and contribute to stress and dissatisfaction. I've been thinking about how I might make a more positive difference with students in the future, and I've been thinking about how I might prevent other new faculty from making mistakes without making them feel patronized or inadequate."

PROFESSOR WEBB: Well, some universities have formalized mentoring programs for new faculty. Every new faculty member is paired with an experienced, tenured nursing faculty member. The roles of mentor and mentee are delineated in writing to clarify purposes, goals, expectations, boundaries, limits, anticipated outcomes, and duration. Sometimes there are also combined small group meetings with several new mentees and mentors. This enhances dialogue, mutual bonding from shared experiences, and role modeling. Of course, once the formalized mentoring period is over, it usually evolves into an informal mentor–mentee relationship with mutual exchange of information and shared expertise. Like all good professional mentor–mentee relationships, change is expected and desired. One benefit of a formal mentoring program is that everyone is interconnected and empowered within the web of inclusion rather than feeling alone, lost, tangled up, and trapped within a web of confusion.

PROFESSOR ELLIS: Before I moved here to be closer to my aging parents, another university hired me for my first tenure-track teaching position. I was paired with a tenured, full professor in the nursing department's yearlong faculty mentoring program. I had been a nurse administrator in a large hospital for 6 years so it was quite a change to be mentored. At first, I was resentful because my mentor was much younger than me but then I began to appreciate her years of experience in academia, impressive program of research that focused on educational strategies to enhance National Council Licensure Examination (NCLEX) success rates for ESL (English as a second language) students, willingness to share personal stories to enhance my understanding about new student and academic situations, and commitment to assisting me to create my own way in academia where I could make a difference. After the year, our informal mentor–mentee relationship changed in ways that were mutually rewarding. We wrote an article together; she was first author and guided me along the way. Later, I wanted to write about a teaching strategy that I designed, implemented, and evaluated in the classroom that improved test scores among all students, but especially among new immigrant students. She then reviewed my article outline and several drafts before I submitted the manuscript as sole author. She was tough on me … but caring … and refused to coauthor the article or do any of the writing. She kept sending me back to do drafts saying I wasn't ready …. until the 13th draft … but it paid off. The article was published in a good peer-reviewed journal. Now, I would like to do the same for someone else, mentor a new faculty member, but we don't have a formalized program here.

PROFESSOR FRANK: We can all do something individually and collectively to make a positive difference in nursing student retention and success. Let's start developing an action plan.

Clearly, nursing student attrition persists. Current and future enrollment trends predict a more academically and culturally diverse nursing student population, suggesting that nursing student persistence, retention, and success will be even more complicated in the future. Furthermore, the escalating nursing shortage and the rising health care needs of the future urgently demand immediate and future attention toward promoting nursing student retention and success. Every nurse educator has the potential to make a positive impact on nursing student retention. Nurse educators will always be in the most strategic position to influence retention positively. Unfortunately, the rising nursing faculty shortage; the declining number of nurses who will be adequately prepared for the educator role; the disturbing, ongoing need to defend, define, and redefine the "scholarship of teaching;" compounded by the substantial gaps in high quality, comprehensive nursing student retention research impose grave obstacles for the future. The purpose of this chapter is to propose future directions and create a positive vision for tomorrow, including recommendations for nurse educators.

FUTURE DIRECTIONS

Stimulate Interest and Commitment

Without deep commitment and sincere interest in nursing student retention, the future of nursing education, nursing, and health care will be bleak. Nurse educators are challenged to look beyond their immediate daily educator responsibilities, beyond tomorrow, and toward the vast future ahead for nursing education and nursing. This requires a broader worldview in which all nurse educators must consider how to promote nursing student retention. Visionary nurse educators are further challenged to spark interest in others by sharing insights, disseminating information, questioning, and mentoring. Nurturing beginning levels of commitment, invigorating ongoing interest, and clarifying conflicting values will present future challenges as well.

In what ways do you demonstrate and stimulate interest and commitment to nursing education and retention research? What else can be done?

Value Retention Research

Nursing student retention research must be valued especially by nurse educators, nurse researchers, nurses in clinical agencies, undergraduate nursing students, graduate nursing students, college administrators, members of tenure and promotion committees, funding agencies, and legislators. The value of educational research, including retention research, must become equitable with other areas of research. Unfortunately, not everyone believes that student retention or other educational research is a serious priority or legitimate area for scholarly research (1–5).

One controversy surrounds the association of research value with the amount of funding received. The expenses of retention research may be significantly less than those of clinical research; therefore, comparison based on financial cost is invalid. The amount of funding available for educational research is also significantly less. The value of the research must not be equated with the amount of grant funding received. If college administrators or members of tenure and promotion committees view retention research as less important than clinical research, despite evidence of a well-designed, rigorous research study, then nurse educators/researchers may be discouraged from pursuing a program of research in nursing education and retention. In the future, the active valuing of retention research through the publicized, tangible benefits of career advancement, grant funding, tenure, and promotion must complement the intangible benefits of positive morale, satisfaction, and self-actualization. This visionary future must begin with all members of the nursing profession valuing its rich diversity, including nursing educational research and scholarship.

> To what extent do you value retention research for yourself, your colleagues, and in comparison to other topics of research? To what extent is retention research valued in your institution? What should be done in the future?

Expand Specialized Knowledge Base

Expanded knowledge of the complex process of undergraduate nursing student retention should be systematically organized so that concepts, constructs, and variables are linked in a comprehensive fashion and are specific to undergraduate nursing student retention. Both conceptual and empirical literature must be routinely reviewed and synthesized so that increasing quality of knowledge will sufficiently complement the increasing quantity. Specialized knowledge must build on previous nursing knowledge, as well as interdisciplinary conceptual and empirical knowledge. In this book, the Nursing Undergraduate Retention and Success (NURS) model presented an organizing framework for examining the multidimensional factors that affect undergraduate nursing student retention and success that can be used to guide further knowledge expansion and literature reviews. Following well-established protocols for a systematic literature review will further assure that a comprehensive literature synthesis includes valid worldwide resources (books, journal articles, online materials, video, etc.).

> What have you done to expand the specialized retention literature knowledge base for yourself, colleagues in your institution, and the broader nursing community? What else can be done?

Test Conceptual and Theoretical Directions

Theory testing and new theory development will add richness to the current paucity of retention theory and research. The NURS model was proposed as an organizing framework that will need modification and repatterning as more data become available. The model is flexible enough to allow for the introduction and testing of new variables. Researchers may wish to test select components of the model and validate existing directional propositions or propose alternative patterns of indirect and direct relationships. Future research on indirect relationships will enrich the comprehension of the retention process (6).

Testing components of the model, or the model in entirety with different student populations, is also needed. At first, local studies are advocated to control for extraneous variables. Multi-institutional studies should be disaggregated based on program type or other pertinent differing characteristics (7). Past retention studies in higher education and nursing frequently lacked the guidance by an underlying conceptual framework, thus confounding comparison between studies. In the future, it will become increasingly crucial for nurse educators to develop a program of nursing student retention research using the same conceptual framework. The benefit of using the same model to guide research is the ability to compare results between various student groups over time, thus adding depth to retention research.

What conceptual model(s) guide your nurse educator role now? In the future?

Adopt Consistent Definitions

Adopting consistent, conceptual, and operational definitions within and between nursing student retention studies will promote valid and reliable data analysis, multistudy and multisite comparison, meta-analysis studies, and advancement of the state of nursing science. The higher education literature advocates the development of student retention databases (3). Although some databases exist on national, state, and local levels, the databases typically aggregate data examining select demographic characteristics of nursing program applicants, enrollees, graduates, licensees, postgraduation employment, and higher educational pursuits. These databases do not compile data about retention strategies implemented and their evaluative results, or about psychometric properties for related questionnaires and assessment tools. In the future, databases on nursing student retention must go beyond documenting categories of learners and their enrollment, progression, graduation, and licensure characteristics to tracking a pathway trajectory and determining strategies that work best with different student groups.

Today, retention studies (and other nursing educational studies) are often disconnected from each other due to lack of definitions, ambiguous definitions, inconsistent definitions, and/or different definitions. Optimally, consistent terminology would encourage the opportunity for multidisciplinary collaboration, comparison, and research. The definitions presented in Table 1.2 and other definitions provided throughout this book seek to provide a beginning point for possible adoption or adaptation in the future.

> What retention-related definitions are used consistently by you, faculty, and administrators in your institution? What recommendations do you propose for the future?

Identify At-Risk Students

Historically, retention (or attrition) research has allocated much attention to the identification of at-risk students using post hoc studies or autopsy studies after the student has already left the academic institution (8). Retention studies in the future must shift the focus from autopsy studies to prospective studies, in which the early identification of at-risk students allows for early intervention, maximizing opportunities for achievement and success. Although at-risk students have been identified on the basis of select student profile characteristics, early identification measures of the future will need to take into account the interaction among many variables, necessitating a different approach. The NURS model may guide a systematic process for identifying at-risk students. Quantitative approaches involving questionnaires (see Toolkit Items 1–5) or qualitative approaches such as focus groups can provide valuable data in identifying at-risk students at the beginning of a semester or nursing program. More approaches are needed that assist students' self-discovery that they are at risk; such approaches may encourage early self-help and/or help-seeking behaviors.

> How have at-risk students been identified within your course(s), by your faculty colleagues, and by your administrators? What else should be done?

Develop Diagnostic and Prescriptive Strategies to Facilitate Success

The profusion of evidence-based nursing practice must expand still further to include nursing education. The increasing diversity of students demands a concerted effort in developing diagnostic and prescriptive strategies to facilitate success. Accurate appraisal of student strengths, weaknesses, perceptions, and concerns is a necessary precursor for any diagnostic and prescriptive intervention. Such an appraisal extends beyond merely identifying students who are at risk for failure and/or attrition.

Diagnostic and prescriptive strategies may be initiated at the individual, subgroup, or larger group level. Proponents of a psychological approach to student retention presume that persistence decisions occur on an individual level (7). Others advocate analysis at the departmental level (3). Past interventions have frequently targeted subgroups of students based on age, ethnicity, nursing program, scholastic aptitude, or other characteristic (9). The NURS model is flexible enough to be used to guide assessment at the individual, subgroup, course, program, institution, or multisite level.

In the future, it will be increasingly essential to develop strategies for success based on individual student assessments. Generally, student assessment has centered on student aptitude measures; yet, current and future research will demonstrate that other forms of student assessment will need to be developed. Practical feasibility and the numerous benefits of student interaction will necessitate clustering and matching students based on strengths and weaknesses in order to create positive and productive cohort strategy intervention groups. The future of diagnostic and prescriptive interventions is contingent upon the future development of reliable and valid student assessment tools that consider the multidimensional phenomena of undergraduate nursing student retention. Nurse educators will need to be adequately prepared in educational measurement and/or be prepared to consult with appropriate experts. Additionally, they will need more expertise to develop innovative strategies that address students holistically, especially as diversity among nursing students and faculty increases.

> What diagnostic and prescriptive strategies have you designed, implemented, and evaluated to facilitate success among diverse students? What will you do in the future?

Connect Retention With Innovations in Teaching and Educational Research

One purpose of the NURS model is to guide innovations in teaching and educational research. What this suggests is that every teaching innovation can potentially impact upon nursing student retention either positively or negatively. Visionary nurse educators of the future will need to consider seriously how various teaching innovations will affect different student groups via academic and psychological outcomes (see Toolkit Item 24). Such considerations necessitate the consistent pairing of teaching innovations and educational research that not only aims to evaluate learning outcomes but also strives to evaluate the direct and/or indirect effects on student retention. The future of nursing and nursing education urgently needs (and will depend upon) the advanced development of the scholarship of teaching (science of nursing education), including theoretically and empirically supported teaching innovations and more educational research (1,2,10–19). However, it will be extremely important to advocate a broad view of the science of nursing education that connects the scholarship of teaching with the other dimensions within the scholarship of nursing education.

> How have teaching innovations been connected empirically to retention results in your course(s), other courses, and total program evaluation? What else should be done?

Evaluate Retention Strategy Effectiveness

Another intended use of the NURS model is to provide a framework for evaluating retention strategy effectiveness. Anecdotal accounts of retention strategy components and their presumed effectiveness are inadequate today and will undermine future efforts to advance the science of nursing education if continued. Additionally, failure to quantitatively demonstrate positive outcomes resulting from retention strategy components will severely limit funding opportunities for future student retention interventions. Although anecdotal accounts and other qualitative data provide important information for nurse educators, current and projected future funding agency criteria will probably continue to emphasize quantitative data. Nurse educators of the future will need to be astute in selecting and gathering valid and meaningful quantitative and qualitative data for future funding and educational, theoretical, practical, and empirical purposes. Furthermore, nurse educators will need to plan carefully formative and summative evaluations that specifically include academic and psychological outcomes if evaluations are to be truly comprehensive and holistic.

Today's limited number of nursing educational instruments and methods for evaluating educational innovations (1,20) will continue to severely limit evaluation capabilities unless the number of nursing faculty specifically prepared for the scholarship of nursing education is substantially increased. Whereas development of new, valid, and reliable instruments may be indicated, the proliferation of instruments to measure the same phenomena will limit comparative studies, meta-analysis studies, and psychometric studies. Retention strategy evaluation studies of the future must include appropriate and ongoing psychometric testing of the instruments used. Partnerships with statisticians who have specialized expertise in educational measurement will offer a wealth of new options and opportunities. As new statistical methods and software become available, more sophisticated analyses beyond those used presently and in the past will decrease error and increase precision with which data can be interpreted. Psychometric study results must be centrally compiled in databases easily accessible to other educators and researchers for future consideration, use, adaptation, and/or testing.

What retention strategies have been consistent and evaluated in your course(s), other courses, and the overall program using? To what extent are the evaluation methods valid and reliable? What types of psychometric analyses have been performed? How have you and your program shared retention program effectiveness evaluation results beyond your institution? What recommendations do you have for the future?

Revitalize Nursing Education

The current shortage of nurse educators is projected to grow well into the future. Half of today's nurse faculty workforce is expected to retire by 2015, yet registered nurse employment is expected to grow approximately 22%, leaving a frightening gap (21). Furthermore, the percentage of nurse educators who have been formally prepared in nursing education will continue to decline, especially as retirement of prepared faculty increases. Advanced practice nurses (clinical nurse specialists and nurse practitioners) are now hired as part-time, adjunct, or full-time faculty, yet may not have received formal preparation in nursing education, the role of the nurse educator, or academia. Without formal preparation, these nurse educators are poorly equipped to meet the needs of diverse student populations and optimize nursing student retention and success. Nursing students' chance for success should not be jeopardized because of inadequacies in poorly prepared nurse educators.

Formal preparation must include opportunities for students to learn both the science and art of teaching; a series of educational courses is insufficient (17). Retention, curriculum, evaluation, and other important educational areas should include didactic learning experiences that incorporate the latest learning technologies and evidence-based best practices for educating diverse learner populations if educators are to be well prepared to engage in and advance the scholarship of nursing education. Nurse educator postmasters certificate programs and nurse educator certifications offer one option for establishing nurse educator expertise; however, they must be partnered with ongoing continuing education to keep updated with new teaching topics, strategies, technology, resources, and student needs. Advanced practice nurses who elect to pursue doctoral education in nursing (or outside of nursing) may also lack formal preparation in nursing education and educational research at the doctoral level, thereby missing the opportunity to develop the necessary skills and expertise to conduct educational research independently. The opportunity to be mentored by expert researchers in nursing education while conducting doctoral research focused on nursing education may also be absent. Consequently, experienced nurse educators and researchers will need to mentor inexperienced faculty and researchers differently than before, especially when novice faculty lack formal courses in nursing education and student teaching experiences.

Presently and in the near future, experienced nurse educators must plan to allocate considerable time in mentoring inexperienced nurse educators and researchers. The literature on nursing faculty recruitment and retention notes the numerous benefits of mentoring within nursing education (22–31). Formalized mentoring programs for new full-time and adjunct faculty coupled with ongoing mentoring through one's career trajectory in academia yields positive outcomes in preparing and retaining highly qualified faculty in forthcoming generations. Mentoring doctoral students interested in pursuing studies in nursing education will extend beyond the doctoral program's faculty. Existing and future technology will make mentoring and collaboration possible beyond geographic constraints of the past. For example, social media tools provide numerous options to engage in formal mentoring (29). Because of the current and future shortage of nurse educators, those experienced in retention and other educational research will be in great demand for consultation, collaboration, leadership, and mentoring. Although initially this demand may require substantial time commitment and energy, nurse educators must invigorate the next generation of nurse educators with excitement about nursing education scholarship.

Visionary nurse educators and leaders must also seize the opportunity to invite diverse undergraduate students, peer mentor-tutors (PMTs), graduate students, and nurses in clinical agencies to consider seriously nursing education (and education research) as a possible career option. Highlighting incentives within the Nurse Reinvestment Act pertinent to nursing faculty development is one strategy. Sharing positive and exciting experiences about nursing education and research is another strategy. Offering a faculty shadowing experience is an innovative strategy to attract undergraduate students early on (30). Reaching out to corporations, institutions, and agencies for support is another strategy that can make a positive difference in recruitment, preparation, and retention of nurse educators who will be equipped to work with forthcoming generations of nursing students. For example, the Johnson & Johnson Campaign for Nursing's Future—AACN Minority Nurse Faculty Scholars program provides financial assistance, mentoring, and leadership development for graduate students from diverse backgrounds who commit to faculty roles post graduation (32). Diversifying the nurse faculty population is an important measure; however, incentives to attract, prepare, mentor, and retain diverse populations into the full-time faculty role must be expanded. "The interdependent nursing and nursing faculty shortages must be resolved collectively" (31, p. 8). Together, nurse educators, other nurses, college administrators, legislators, policy makers, and other stakeholders must take action to revitalize nursing education. Revitalization will improve nursing education overall, and nursing student retention will undoubtedly benefit from this process.

What strategies have you implemented to revitalize nursing education? What else can you do in the near and far future?

CONCLUSION

Today, nurse educators may agree that nursing student retention and success are important, and yet, consensus will not make retention and success instantly happen. However, taking appropriate action will make a difference. Whatever is done (or not done) today will influence what happens tomorrow and beyond. Each nurse educator or future nurse educator is empowered to make a positive difference in the world of nursing education and in the lives of students. As active partners in the complex process of nursing student retention, nurse educators can continually seek to understand the dynamic and multidimensional process of nursing student retention, develop empirically and conceptually supported retention strategies, and make a positive difference.

KEY POINT SUMMARY

- The most persistent trend in nursing student persistence research is that nursing student attrition persists.
- Every nurse educator has the potential to make a positive impact on nursing student retention today and in the future.
- The NURS model can guide future directions in retention research, theory, and practice.
- Future directions include
  1. Stimulating interest and commitment
  2. Valuing retention research
  3. Expanding specialized knowledge base
  4. Testing conceptual and theoretical directions

5. Adopting consistent definitions
6. Identifying at-risk students
7. Developing diagnostic and prescriptive strategies to facilitate success
8. Connecting retention with innovations in teaching and educational research
9. Evaluating retention strategy effectiveness
10. Revitalizing nursing education

APPLICATION STRATEGIES

EASY APPLICATION ACTION STEPS

Planning for the Future: Individual Appraisal

1. List past and present initiatives implemented for each of the 10 future directions, contemplating barriers, advantages, disadvantages, incentives, rewards, and so on for each.
2. Propose future ideas for each of the 10 areas, placing an asterisk (*) next to the ideas you can implement easily by yourself and a double asterisk (**) next to the ideas for which you will require assistance.
3. Highlight the top five priority ideas for self-implementation in one color and a different color to highlight the top three priority ideas for collaborative implementation; list a starting date for initiating each idea.

Planning for the Future: Collective Appraisal

1. After each program faculty member individually completes the three steps above, discuss and prioritize five targeted areas for a departmental (collective) approach.
2. Create subcommittees and a start date for developing each idea.

EDUCATOR-IN-ACTION VIGNETTE

During a faculty meeting, several faculty express current and future concerns. Here are some excerpts:

PROFESSOR NUMBERS: I can't believe we're turning away so many qualified applicants to the undergraduate nursing program because we just don't have enough faculty. Last year four faculty members retired and two more will retire this year. We hired three new instructors but will still be short by three. I hope these instructors won't drop out after 1 year like the last year's new instructors or like a lot of our students. Attrition is expensive.

PROFESSOR CHANGE: First, to address the faculty retention issue, we could develop a formalized mentoring program for new faculty. We can get ideas from the literature and possibly collaborate with another school who implemented a program. Second, we need to look way ahead into the future and realize that we need a proactive plan to recruit nurses and future nurses into the faculty role. We really don't ask students to consider teaching…and I'm not sure they would believe that they could teach. Many of them are struggling with real or perceived factors that interfere with their academic success and ability to complete their education. Third, we need a comprehensive action plan for enhancing our students' academic success and prevent dropout.

PROFESSOR QUEST: About the student retention issue…we should assess what factors restrict or support our students' ability to remain in a nursing course and progress through the curriculum. We need to ask the right questions. By getting a clearer picture or composite of our students' learner characteristics and perceptions, we can design strategies based on students' needs. Perhaps, there are questionnaires and assessment tools or a toolkit already designed and used by others.

PROFESSOR NUMBERS: Yes, there are. We can collect data before and after the strategies we design to see what changes occurred.

PROFESSOR GRANT: We can use the baseline data as a need assessment. This will be valuable in writing up a grant proposal.

PROFESSOR PRONTO: We should do something now before the future creeps up on us. We may want to do a lot later, but we need to do something now. It seems like we can accomplish multiple objectives by developing a peer mentor-tutoring program. The literature mentions that many PMTs become interested in pursuing more advanced nursing education and even the nurse educator role. Students who are mentored often become PMTs later and so the cycle continues. We can become more proactive and advocate and encourage the nurse educator role. Students need to develop self-confidence for this possibility and being a PMT helps. By creating a PMT program that focuses on enrichment rather than remediation, ideally, all students can achieve their academic potential, manage stress, and feel satisfied. So, student retention should improve. We should also check to see if there is a toolkit that can guide us to design or tailor strategies for our students and program.

TOOLKIT RESOURCE BOX

Items 1–30

DISCUSSION QUESTIONS

1. During an initial Doctor of Nursing Practice (DNP) program planning meeting, Professor Light proposes that a required nursing education course titled "Evidence-based teaching and learning practices for

diverse learners" be included as a core course early on in the curriculum. Professor Light further provides rationale, that of these principles "Advanced practice nurses of the future will need this specialized area of evidence-based knowledge to individualize teaching and learning strategies based on learner characteristics and preferences including language, literacy, culture, lifestyle, and so on." Professor Booke says, "Yes, we would not think of eliminating evidenced-based pharmacology, epidemiology, pathophysiology, or other courses in the DNP curriculum. We need to go beyond the comfort zone of the medical model of nurse practitioner programs to recognize the wealth of evidenced-based specialized knowledge concerning teaching and learning in other disciplines, such as education and psychology. We need to emphasize evidenced-based practices. A core course can provide the foundation for integration and application within subsequent theoretical and didactic or clinical learning opportunities within the DNP program." Professor Clock says, "We don't have time to cover everything substantially to prepare a DNP graduate for the nurse educator role. That's not the purpose of a DNP program. We need to prepare expert advanced practice nurses and that requires much time focused on clinical expertise development. DNP graduates who later decide to pursue faculty roles as they get older can just take a post-master's nurse educator certificate course, engage in online CE courses, and/or take the nurse educator certification review class and exam."

As a faculty colleague, how would you respond?

2. A student in a PhD nursing program works as an adjunct clinical instructor at a local college and is bothered by high attrition rates among diverse groups of "passing" students. The PhD student proposes piloting several strategies empirically supported in the literature and evaluating quantitative and qualitative outcomes using transcript data, questionnaire data, and other measures suggested in the higher education literature. A doctoral advisor says, "This is a PhD program in nursing that has traditionally focused on theoretical research. Nursing has moved beyond just studying the same old thing with student populations. Action research is a lower level research that has no place in advancing the scholarship of the nursing discipline. If you wanted to do education research, you should have applied to the adult education program down the hall."

What are your feelings and thoughts about this student–faculty interaction? What potential impact could this have on nursing student retention, nursing education, and nursing scholarship of the future? How would you respond to the student's research interests if expressed to you? What else should be done?

3. A promotion-tenure committee is reviewing two untenured faculty members' recent publications. One committee member says, "Professor Ed only has two publications in a nursing education journal. Although

the well-written articles are based upon grant-supported research, the grant funding is modest and only shows statistically significant changes among two of the student groups serviced through the piloted enrichment/mentoring program. Who reads those educational journals?—A limited audience so the research doesn't reach the broader nursing community. In contrast, Professor Sun has two large grant-supported publications in a clinical research journal comparing the sunscreen practices among different populations in 10 different geographic locations in the United States and Canada. These articles are read by more nurses and even doctors, generated lots of grant money and prestige to the college, and involved international research rather than research conducted at one institution. We should reward Professor Sun with tenure, deny tenure for Professor Ed, and set an example for future faculty." As a committee member, how would you respond to your colleague?

4. Which of the 10 recommended future directions do you think should have the highest priority in your personal agenda? Why? In your work setting? Why? In the nursing profession? Why?

5. How can the snapshot scenarios be used to make positive changes for the future? What did you like best? Why? What did you like least? Why?

REFERENCES

1. Diekelmann, N., & Ironside, P. M. (2002). Developing a science of nursing education: Innovation with research. *Journal of Nursing Education, 41*(9), 379–380.
2. Drevdahl, D. J., Stackman, R. W., Purdy, J. M., & Louie, B. Y. (2002). Merging reflective inquiry and self-study as a framework for enhancing the scholarship of teaching. *Journal of Nursing Education, 41*(9), 413–418.
3. McLaughlin, G. W., Brozovsky, P. V., & McLaughlin, J. S. (1998). Changing perspectives on student retention: A role for institutional research. *Research in Higher Education, 39*(1), 1–17.
4. Tinto, V. (1998). College as communities: Taking research on student persistence seriously. *Review of Higher Education, 21,* 167–177.
5. Diana, T. J. (2011). Becoming a teacher leader through action research. *Kappa Delta Pi Record, 47*(4), 170–173.
6. Bean, J.P., & Metzner, B. (1985). A conceptual model of nontraditional undergraduate student attrition. *Review of Educational Research, 55,* 485–540.
7. Bean, J. P., & Eaton, S. B. (2000). A psychological model of student retention. In J. Braxton (Ed.), *Reworking the student departure puzzle* (pp. 48–61). Nashville, TN: Vanderbilt University.
8. Braxton, J. M., Brier, E. M., & Hossler, D. (1988). The influence of student problems on student withdrawal decisions: An autopsy on "autopsy" studies. *Research in Higher Education, 28*(3), 241–253.
9. Tucker-Allen, S., & Long, E. (1999). *Recruitment and retention of minority students: Stories of success.* Lisle, IL: Tucker Publications.

10. Diekelmann, N. (2002). "She asked this simple question": Reflecting and the scholarship of teaching. *Journal of Nursing Education, 41*(9), 381–382.
11. Riley, J. M., Beal, J., Levi, P., & McCausland, M. P. (2002). Revisioning nursing scholarship. *Journal of Nursing Scholarship, 34*(4), 383–389.
12. National League for Nursing (2007). The need for funding for nursing education research, Available at http://www.nln.org/aboutnln/PositionStatements/nursingedresearch_051807.pdf
13. National League for Nursing (2009). *A commitment to diversity in nursing and nursing education.* [Reflection and Dialogue]. Available at www.nln.org/aboutnln/reflection_dialogue/refl_dial_3.htm
14. National League for Nursing (2005).Transforming nursing education, Available at http://www.nln.org/aboutnln/PositionStatements/transforming052005.pdf
15. National League for Nursing (2003). Priorities for research in nursing education. Available at http://www.nln.org/research/priorities.htm
16. Storch, J., & Gamroth, L. (2002). Scholarship revisited: A collaborative nursing education program's journey. *Journal of Nursing Education, 41*(12), 524–530.
17. Tanner, C. A. (2002). Learning to teach: An introduction to "Teacher talk: New Pedagogies for Nursing." *Journal of Nursing Education, 41*(3), 95–96.
18. Young, P., & Diekelmann, N. (2002). Learning to lecture: Exploring the skills, strategies, and practices of new teachers in nursing education. *Journal of Nursing Education, 41*(9), 405–412.
19. Jeffreys, M. R. (2010). *Teaching cultural competence in nursing and health care: Inquiry, action, and innovation.* (2nd ed.). New York, NY: Springer Publishing.
20. Oermann, M. H., & Gaberson, K. B. (2009). *Evaluation and testing in nursing education.* New York, NY: Springer Publishing.
21. National League for Nursing. (2011). NLN's footsteps heard on the "hill": Board of governors advocates for Title VII and VIII funding. *NLN Nursing Education Policy Newsletter, 8*(5), Available at nln-communications@nln.org.
22. Forbes, M. O., Hickey, M. T., & White, J. (2010). Adjunct faculty development: Reported needs and innovative solutions. *Journal of Professional Nursing, 26,* 116–124.
23. Vance, C. (2011). *Fast facts for career success in nursing: Making the most of mentoring in a nutshell.* New York, NY: Springer Publishing.
24. Vance, C., & Olsen, R. K. (1998). *The mentor connection in nursing.* New York, NY: Springer Publishing.
25. Jacob, S. R., & Sanchez, Z. V. (2011). The challenge of closing the diversity gap: Development of Hispanic nursing faculty through a health resources and services administration minority faculty fellowship program grant. *Journal of Professional Nursing, 27,* 108–113.
26. Cangelosi, P. R. (2004). A lack of qualified faculty: One school's solution. *Nurse Educator, 29*(5), 186–188.
27. Dunham-Taylor, J., Lynn, C. W., Moore, P., McDaniel, S., & Walker, J. K. (2008). What goes around comes around: Improving retention through more effective mentoring. *Journal of Professional Nursing, 24,* 337–346.
28. Sawatzky, J.-A. V., & Enns, C. L. (2009). A mentoring needs assessment: Validating mentorship in nursing education. *Journal of Professional Nursing, 25,* 145–150.

29. Bassell, K. (2010). Social media and the implications for nursing faculty mentoring: A review of the literature. *Teaching and Learning in Nursing, 5*, 143–148.
30. Seldomridge, L. A. (2004). Attracting students to the professorate: A faculty shadowing experience. *Nurse Educator, 29*(6), 256–259.
31. Yoho, M. J., Timpanaro, P., & Fowler, C. (2006). Recruiting and retaining nursing faculty in a Texas community college system: A strategy focused on collaboration and support. *Teaching and Learning in Nursing, 1*, 4–9.
32. American Association of Colleges of Nursing. (2010). *The future of higher education in nursing: 2010 annual report.* Washington, DC: Author.

Index

Note: Page numbers followed by *"f"* and *"t"* denote figures and tables, respectively.